HEALTH ECONOMICS:
Fundamentals and Flow of Funds

Thomas E. Getzen

Temple University

John Wiley & Sons, Inc.

New York   Chichester   Brisbane
Toronto   Singapore

—to my family

Cover Photos:
(*left*) Jonathan Morgan/Tony Stone Images
(*right*) Lois & Bob Schlowsky/Tony Stone Images

ACQUISITIONS EDITOR   Whitney Blake
MARKETING MANAGER   Wendy Goldner
PRODUCTION EDITOR   Melanie Henick
COVER DESIGNER   Madelyn Lesure
ASSISTANT MANUFACTURING MANAGER   Mark Cirillo
SENIOR ILLUSTRATION COORDINATOR   Anna Melhorn

This book was set in 10/12 Palatino by TCSystems and
printed and bound by Hamilton Printing. The cover was printed by Phoenix Color.

Recognizing the importance or preserving what has been written, it is a
policy of John Wiley & Sons, Inc. to have books of enduring value published
in the United States printed on acid-free paper, and we exert our best
efforts to that end.

Figure 7.3, p. 153: By permission of the *New England Journal of Medicine*.
Figure 15.1, p. 315: By permission of Blackwell Publishers.
Figure 19.4, p. 420: By permission of *The World Bank*.

Library of Congress Cataloging in Publication Data:
Getzen, Thomas E.
     Health economics : fundamentals and flow of funds / Thomas E.
Getzen.
        p. cm.
     Includes bibliographical references.
     ISBN 0-471-58648-X
     1. Medical economics. I. Title.
     RA410.G48   1997
     338.4'33621—dc20
                                        96-21162
                                        CIP

Printed in the United States of America
10 9 8 7 6 5 4 3 2 1

Preface

Principles of Health Economics is a primer for the economic analysis of medical markets and the production of health.[1] Its intended audiences are students of medicine, public health, and administration, who wish to engage the central economic issues of their field without prolonged preparatory work; beginning students in economics who wish to study an applied area in detail without recourse to extensive mathematical manipulation; and more advanced students in economics who may be familiar with analytical techniques, but lack knowledge of the many institutional features which make the study of health and health care so unique and rewarding. The first thirteen chapters use a "flow of funds" approach to describe the incentives and organizational structure of the health care system. Transactions between patients and physicians (and others) are examined to see how profits are made, costs covered, contracts written (or implied) and regulations formed. The long-term consequences of exchanging services for money in a particular way are revealed by exploring the historical development of those distinctive features which characterize the industrial organization of health care: licensure, third-party insurance, non-profit hospitals, and government regulation. The continuing evolution of the system in the U.S. is the subject of two

---

[1] This book draws upon the work of many scholars, but in keeping with its design as a primer for introducing students to the principles and concepts of health economics rather than its literature and research methods, the use of attribution, footnotes and references is purposely limited. Some suggestions for additional reading are listed at the end of each chapter. Those students wishing to access the literature should consult the *Journal of Health Economics, Health Economics, Inquiry, Health Services Research* and other journals and books listed in the bibliography, a sourcebook such as Rosko & Broyles *The Economics of Health Care: A Reference Handbook*, a more advanced text such as Foland, Goodman and Stano's *The Economics of Health & Health Care*, and databases such as Econlit, Medlines and GratefulMed. Inquiries to the author are also invited to obtain lists of sources and documentation regarding the numerous pieces of research that are only touched upon in passing or left unmentioned in the text.

chapters on managed care. The last seven chapters take a wider macroeconomic perspective in order to explore the dynamics of change within the health care system, and to explicitly consider determinants of national health spending and the role of governments in public and private health.

The introductory chapter lays out the overall flow of funds and schematically presents the complexity of medical care transactions. Chapter 2 introduces the basic principles of supply and demand, marginalism and equilibrium, using a cost-benefit approach in a clinical context.[2] The more detailed investigation of medical care organization begins in Chapter 3 with insurance, as third-party reimbursement has become the dominant form of payment for medical care. Numerical examples, taxation and competition are addressed in Chapter 4. Physicians, the patient's agent and a central player in all medical care transactions, are the subject of the next three chapters. Chapters 8 and 9 cover the reimbursement, regulation and cost structure of hospitals. HMOs and the other contractual networks used to manage care are discussed in Chapters 10 and 11, with particular attention to payment mechanisms and access to capital. The survey of providers is rounded out with chapters on long-term care and pharmaceuticals.

In order to understand the interactions between the parts, it is necessary to place health care in a macroeconomic context which includes redistribution, taxation, inflation, and growth. The economic history of health is traced in chapter 15, drawing on the cliometric work of Fogel and North, and the contributions of demography. Chapter 16 explores the role of government, and Chapter 17 examines public goods as a particular form of market failure which requires intervention. The dynamics of national health expenditure are presented in Chapter 18 as an application of the permanent income hypothesis. This model is then used to empirically assess the effectiveness of several attempts to control health care costs. Chapter 19 provides international comparisons of health and medical care expenditures, taking Kenya, Mexico, and Japan as illustrative examples. A final chapter addresses the probable trends in health care spending, suggesting that the primary barrier to increased effectiveness and efficiency is poor allocation.

Health economics is fascinating to study, but is not easily summarized or readily captured in neat equations. In part, that is because the study of health economics is relatively new and still in the process of refinement, but primarily it is because the trades organized by doctors and hospitals are not simple, and cut to the heart of what it means to be human. What is the value of life? Who pays the price of pain, and what does it mean to trust a surgeon who profits in crises? Since most medical care is funded through taxes and insurance, there is no direct linkage between the amount paid and the resources used in treatment. As a consequence, "prices" become more ambiguous and are often of less immediate relevance to the transaction than ongoing relationships of trust and professional behavior. It is important to understand how economic forces continue to operate when markets are indirect and inefficient, and how other organizing principles (professionalism, licensure, agency, regulation) act as substitutes for prices. While

---

[2] The special features which make medical care so interesting as a subject for economic analysis also tend to make the application of simple models difficult or implausible. Those students who have the desire and opportunity to do so are well advised to get a firm grasp of basic principles using a text such as Heyne's *The Economic Way of Thinking* or Samuelson's *Economics* before attempting to grapple with the complexities and ambiguities of medical care.

most of the special features of medical markets are there to make people better off, they have also been shaped by those groups who had the power to modify the rules in their own interest, subject to the controls of economic and political competition. Tracing the economic rationale and development of medical care organization, and making those forces more clearly visible and amenable to analysis, is the purpose of this book.

15 May 1996   THOMAS E. GETZEN

ACKNOWLEDGEMENTS _____

The writing of this book incurred intellectual and personal debts sufficient to preclude any complete listing of those who have contributed. The real impetus, to become a professor, and to write, came from my mother and father, Bea and Bob Getzen. My wife, Karen Shirley, and our children, Matthew and Zoa, have generously read and commented on most of the text. Other family members, especially my brother, Bob, my cousins Rufus and Beverly Getzen, Sydney White, Joe Troxell and the many friends of Bill W., have given me the encouragement necessary to endure, to get help when needed, and to accept criticism.

My initial research on these topics began at the University of Washington, with the assistance of Yoram Barzel, Gardner Brown, Steve Shortell, Bill Richardson and Mike Morrisey, and while working under Gordon Bergey, who was an exemplar of the concerned physician and administrator. I am indebted to the texts by Burton Weisbrod and Paul Feldstein which I read at that time, and to the efforts of Joe Newhouse, Mark Pauly, Tony Culyer and others who have done so much to build the field and create a rigorous body of literature in health economics. David Barton Smith, who hired and mentored me at Temple, has inspired me to write as well as to complain. Bill Aaronson, Chuck Hall, Bob Sigmond, Sally Villar, Jackie Zinn and the other members of my department have been an integral part of my team, shouldering a substantial burden down the stretch. Patrick Bernet shaped the health economics course as it was taught, proving that a graduate assistant can be both popular and rigorous. Alan Maynard sheltered and inspired me during my sabbatical at York during which the framework and first chapters were laid down. Michael Kendix lead me through the intricacies of time series analysis. Joel Telles, George Dowdall and Erwin Blackstone and other participants in the Temple health research group have provided the sounding board that refined some of my wilder ideas. Morris Barer took over the iHEA conference and made it possible for me to finish. Francis X. Selgrath and Rosetta Smith taught me the practical application of economics and the challenge of managing health care. Expertise in special areas and useful comments were provided by Michael Drummond, Mark Freeland, Sandra Harmon-Weiss, John Nyman, Rosemary Stevens, and especially Tom Abbott who prepared the chapter on pharmaceutical markets. David Bradford, Jeff Caswell, Connie Koran, Mike Pogodzinski and Bruce Stuart read the book in its entirety and provided numerous useful comments and corrections. Whitney Blake at Wiley first engaged me in writing a textbook, and convinced the rest of the editors to bear with me until the task was done. The usual and heartfelt disclaimer applies, all remaining errors are mine.

ABOUT THE AUTHOR

Thomas E. Getzen is Professor of Health Administration in the School of Business and Management at Temple University, and the founder and director of iHEA, the International Health Economics Association. After receiving an undergraduate degree from Yale University, he worked for the U.S.P.H.S. Centers for Disease Control Venereal Disease program in New York and Los Angeles, and then obtained an MHA degree in Medical Care Organization and Ph.D. in Economics from the University of Washington. Dr. Getzen's main research contributions have been in the areas of contracting, forecasting, and health care price indexes. His consulting work has included employee benefit negotiations, laboratory diagnostics, risk assessment, and capital financing for managed care. He has served as a visiting professor of health macroeconomics at the University of York (U.K.) and of health care finance at the Wharton School of the University of Pennsylvania. Dr. Getzen was a W.K. Kellog Foundation fellow, received the Follmer Award from the Healthcare Financial Management Association, and in 1986 was named "outstanding professor" by the alumni board of the Temple University School of Business and Management. For more than a decade, he has been an active board member of Covenant House, a local community health center in Northwest Philadelphia, and chair of the audit committee for a venture-capital financed managed behavioral health care corporation. He serves on the editorial board of the journal *Health Economics*, and has previously been chair of the Health Economics Committee of the American Public Health Association, and of the Finance Forum of the Association of University Programs in Health Administration.

FOREWORD

Public policy in almost any field depends on specific knowledge of the field, but it usually also depends (or should depend) on general principles of economics. For example, the building of a bridge requires knowledge of engineering, to know what is feasible; it requires knowledge of traffic patterns; and it requires knowledge of economic principles, to see if the traffic that will use the bridge and the value of the time saving to that traffic will justify the costs imposed by the engineering requirements. So, too, is there a need of economic analysis to help in the construction of a system of health care. First of all, indeed, we must know what medical care can do, and how much in the way of skilled professionals, other workers, machinery, and buildings it takes to achieve any given level of medical care. But second, we must analyze how the payment mechanisms to compensate for these supplies affect the delivery of medical care.

Medical care is indeed a more complex economic problem than bridge-building. Like some other professions but unlike many other goods and even services, it is difficult for the consumer (here the patient) to evaluate the quality of the services received. Much depends on the self-control and reliability of the individual practitioner, the supplying group, and the medical profession as a whole, in ways that the patient cannot readily check. Then, too, the service provided is needed only at unpredictable intervals, but it frequently is very important when it is needed.

Further, the costs, a reflection of the resources used, are very uncertain and can be very high. All these reasons lead to the use of some form of insurance, a natural economic institution for improving everyone's welfare. But insurance reduces the incentive of an individual patient or physician to seek the most economical means of treatment. As a result, new institutions and regulations develop to overcome this "moral hazard," as it has been termed—institutions such as health maintenance organizations, managed care by insurance companies, and regulations such as those that govern Medicare expenditures. The standard paradigms of economics have been enriched to discuss problems such as this.

The difficulties of quality evaluation and moral hazard are special cases of a more general phenomenon, differences in information between the two sides of a transaction. These differences, though not confined to medical practice, are especially important there, and have further consequences beyond those already noted, as in the need for licensing physicians or the specially important role of nonprofit institutions.

The economic problems of allocating resources to medical care have long been a major part of government economic policy, more in other countries than in the United States. The steady rise in the expenditures on medical care, outstripping the rise in national income by a considerable margin, has brought these issues to the fore of public attention. Equally important has been the increase of explicit consideration of costs within the medical profession; the historically unwelcome trade-off between costs and treatment has come forcibly to the fore. The need for good education and good texts has become acute, and Professor Getzen's book is a welcome attempt to meet this strongly felt need.

KENNETH J. ARROW

Contents

CHAPTER 1

The Flow of Funds Through the Health Care System

QUESTIONS

1. *Why does health care cost so much?*
2. *Who pays for it?*
3. *What is the average amount spent per person in the United States?*
4. *Does everyone get the same amount of care?*
5. *Why have costs risen so rapidly?*
6. *Do we have too many physicians? Too many hospitals? Too many nurses?*
7. *Is insurance the solution to high costs, or part of the problem?*

Who gets a heart transplant? Why does surgery costs so much? Will insurance pay for AIDS treatment? How many children get immunized? Is Senator Smith's health plan worth voting for? These questions are dealt with every day in hospitals, in doctor's offices, and in peoples' homes. They are the subject of health economics, along with the more mundane decisions that cumulatively have an even larger impact on your personal health: how much exercise to get, the value of reducing cholesterol in your diet, whether to study until 3 A.M. or get a good night's sleep, and so on. Conveying information and using it to make decisions is the stock in trade for both doctors and economists. By the end of this book we will have discussed hospitals, nurses, ambulances, drugs, sex, extortion, kickbacks, government, family ties, love, international trade, sports injuries, and the next generation—all the makings of a box office hit. The perspective will be that of an economist, seeing things in terms of opportunity cost, budget constraints, monopoly, marginal productivity and other analytical concepts. Some people would claim that this takes all of the fun out of drugs, sex, and business intrigues. Not so. Economic principles provide the motivations, and the limits, that shape this story so that it has character development and structure, rather than just one violent scene after another, as in some forgettable action movie. As a sophisticated student of human society, you desire full disclosure: a story revealing the ambitions that lie behind the actions, the deviousness of self-interest cloaked in proclamations of public benefit, the pragmatism of those who use strategy and tactics to make the best of a bad situation, the tragedy of noble aspirations that fail because of human limits, the labyrinthine connections of one of the world's largest businesses, and the growing awareness that behind it all we will find money at the root of much that is evil, and even more that is good, in the search for health. This wealth of behind-the-scenes drama is what makes the economic perspective on health so compelling.

The approach to the economics of health care taken in this textbook is that of a natural scientist or businessperson, looking carefully at how people make deals with physicians, with hospitals, and with each other to improve their health. Tracing the flow of funds through the health care system will make it possible to apply the principles of price theory to situations involving life and death, nonprofit organizations, professional licensure, addiction, and other issues. The powerful generalizations and concepts of microeconomics, macroeconomics, and industrial organization will allow us to see how medical transactions are like, and yet unlike, most of the rest of the economy. As a practical matter, it is helpful if you already have some grasp of economics theory and applications. Reviewing a textbook such as Paul Samuelson's *Economics*, Paul Heyne's *The Economic Way of Thinking*, or Campbell McConnell and Stanley Brue's *Microeconomics* may prove useful before starting out.

1.1 SOURCES AND USES OF HEALTH CARE FUNDS _____

Medical care in the United States is a trillion-dollar business, with an estimated average of $4,226 spent per person in the year 1997.[1] The 278 million citizens of the United States receive services from more than 6,000 hospitals, 30,000 nursing

TABLE 1.1   U.S. Health Care Spending, 1997

$1,175 billion total $4,226 per person

Uses of Funds	Percent of Total	Amount Per Person*	Sources of Funds		
Hospital	36%	$1,509	Medicare	19%	$813
Physician	20%	$852	paycheck deductions		$528
Dental	4%	$175	Medicaid	14%	$593
Drugs & Supplies	8%	$353	VA & DOD	3%	$119
Nursing Home	8%	$340	Workers Comp	2%	$93
Home Health	3%	$123	other government	7%	$297
Eye & Equipment	1%	$55			
Other	9%	$375	Total Government	45%	$1,914
Admin & Ins	5%	$215			
Public Health	3%	$113	Employer Ins.	34%	$1,416
Research	2%	$62	Self Paid	17%	$734
Construction	1%	$54	Charity etc,	4%	$162

*Based on a projected U.S. population of 278 million.

Source: U.S. Office of the Actuary, Health Care Financing Administration 1995 - 2000 (projections).

homes, 550,000 physicians, 1.5 million registered nurses, and 8 million other health care workers. The major sources and uses of health care funding in 1997 are indicated in Table 1.1. Individuals paid $204 billion, or 17 percent of total funding, private (mostly employer-based) health insurance paid 34 percent, and government was the largest payer at 45 percent (19 percent Medicare, 14 percent Medicaid, and 12 percent other government programs). The remaining 4 percent of total health care funding comes from a variety of other private sources (philanthropy, industrial clinics, interest and rental income of providers, etc). The largest use of funds was the $420 billion spent on hospital care, 36 percent of the total.

Figure 1.1 presents this information graphically, highlighting a simple yet important fact: the "sources" and "uses" bars are of equal height because the total amount spent on health care must identically equal the total amount collected by providers. Every dollar spent by a patient, insurance company or government is recorded as a *cost*, but also as *income* to some physician, hospital, agency, administrator, or other employee. The flow of money is circular. Money itself is only a way of keeping track of all the obligations within the economy. Every dollar spent by one person is, of necessity, a dollar of income for someone else. Tracing the flow of funds through this complex system provides some sense of the forces that shape the economy.

1.2   FLOW OF FUNDS_____

Goods and services are provided in a market economy only if the people who want them are willing to pay for them, and if suppliers are willing to accept those payments in return. Exchange is based on voluntary agreement, so that trade between

Flow of Health Care Funds – 1997

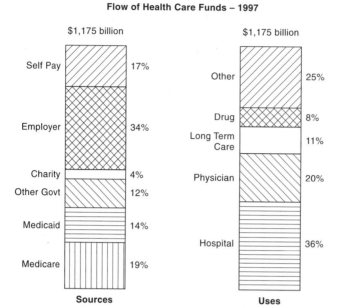

FIGURE 1.1 *Sources and uses of health care funds, 1997, from the National Health Accounts.*

a buyer and seller only occurs when both parties believe that they will be made better off by trading. This central economic insight into the gains from trading is known as the **Fundamental Theorem of Exchange.** In the simplest form of trade, consumers buy from business, exchanging money for services in a **two-party transaction.**

Consumers make up the demand side of this simple service market, while firms make up the supply side. In legal terms, firms are *fictional individuals,* contractual entities that can own property, buy and sell, and pay taxes just like real people. To get the labor, land, and other inputs needed for production, the firm that was a seller in Figure 1.2 must also be a buyer, as shown in Figure 1.3. These secondary two-party transactions are characteristic of **derived demand,** purchases made as an intermediate step in production, rather than for final consumption.

Firms are owned by individuals (or other firms) that provide the capital, labor, and organizational effort necessary to get them started and keep them running. Thus, every dollar that a consumer gives to a firm, whether used for wages, profits, or purchase of inputs from another firm, ultimately ends up in the hands of someone who wants to spend it. When workers or owners spend money, they

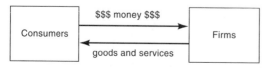

FIGURE 1.2 *Two-party transaction*

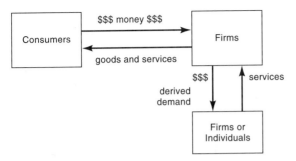

FIGURE 1.3 *Derived demand between firms*

become consumers, and so complete the **circular flow of funds** through the economy as shown in Figure 1.4.

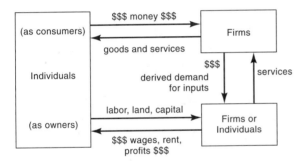

FIGURE 1.4 *Circular flow of funds*

The Role of Government

If individuals buy goods and services from firms, and all of the money is passed on by the firm either to the individuals from which it buys land, labor, or other inputs, individuals who own the business, or other firms that do the same things, what is the role of government? Government can be viewed as a kind of collectively owned "public firm" that is paid to regulate the system, control the money supply, and provide certain kinds of goods such as justice, national defense, and clean air, which are not easily bought and sold in standard two-party transactions (see chapters 16 and 17).[2] In a less complex market economy, perhaps like that of the United States around the year 1900, federal, state, and local governments played a necessary but limited role. As regulators of commerce and arbiters of law, government officials affected almost every transaction, but were few in number. The range of services provided by government has expanded rapidly over the last century; in 1995 federal, state, and local governments accounted for 17 percent of total employment.[3] In addition, there are transfers of funds from taxpayers to beneficiaries through Social Security, AFDC (Aid to Families with Dependent Children), Medicare health insurance for the elderly, and Medicaid health insurance for the poor, so that in total, more than 30 percent of the nation's income passes through the hands of government agencies (see Figure 1.5).

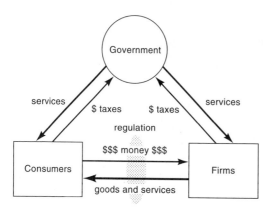

FIGURE 1.5 *Flow of funds with government*

Flow of Health Care Funds

The flow of funds in health care was much simpler in 1900 than it is today. At that time, only about 3 percent of total national income (gross domestic product, or GDP) was devoted to medical services, primarily spent on doctor visits and drugs purchased directly in standard two-party transactions.[4] Hospitals were small and cared for those too poor to be nursed at home, and thus were supported by charity. Nonprofit hospitals and clinics funded by churches or leading philanthropic citizens formed an intermediary that functioned rather like government—funding necessary services that could not be obtained through standard two-party transactions (since the poor did not have the income to pay for the care which they needed). Doctors and pharmacists were also expected to act "charitably," providing care immediately regardless of ability to pay, and then making up the shortfall by charging a little extra to those who could afford it. Figure 1.6 diagrams the flow of funds in medical care in 1900, presenting a picture similar to that of the economy as a whole at that time; a large number of two-party transactions with a small but vital third party acting as intermediary and intervening to close the gaps. In the case of health care, that third party was most likely to be a nonprofit charitable organization funded by donations, rather than a government agency funded by taxes.

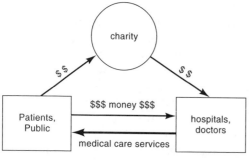

FIGURE 1.6 *Health care flow of funds, circa 1900*

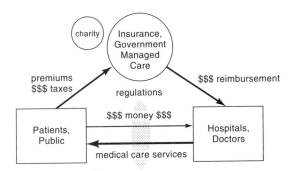

FIGURE 1.7   *Health care flow of funds, circa 1995*

Health care has grown enormously. In 1997, it took 15 percent of GDP and accounted for 1 of every 12 employees in the labor force. That growth has been facilitated by the shift from individual payments to third-party financing. In 1929, 81 percent of all medical expenditures came directly from individual "out-of-pocket" payments and just 19 percent from government and other third-party organizations. By 1997, these fractions had been reversed, with individuals paying only 17 percent directly and the remaining 83 percent of funds flowing through third-party transactions involving government, non-profit charities, and insurance (see Figure 1.7).

All of the elements that characterize health care in 1997 were present in some form in 1900, but their relative importance to the flow of funds has changed so much that the transactions look entirely different today. Payments by individuals directly to doctors, hospitals, pharmacies and retail outlets now make up only 17 percent of the money flowing into medical care; 83 percent of the money comes from third parties (see Table 1.2). Physicians, who in 1900 were tradespeople sometimes making do with partial payment in eggs or flour, have become highly paid and technologically sophisticated professionals who rarely talk to their patients about paying the bills. Hospitals, once a minor support for a few disabled and disadvantaged, are now technological palaces of intensive treatment and the

TABLE 1.2   Sources of Payment, 1929, 1960 and 1997

	1929	1960	1997
Total Health Spending (millions)	$3,656	27,135	1,175,000
Adjusted for inflation (1997 $$)	41,500	146,000	1,175,000
As a % of GDP	3.5%	5.3%	14.8%
Per capita (adjusted)	342	808	4,226
	% Paid by		
out-of-pocket	81%	49%	17%
Third Parties	19%	51%	83%
Government	14%	25%	45%
Private Insurance	<2%	22%	34%

largest user of U.S. health care funds. Whereas in 1900 hospitals were financed by a few donors and some patient fees, they are now financed almost entirely by third parties: either by government insurance such as Medicare and Medicaid or by private insurance provided through employment or purchased directly by consumers. For every hundred dollars spent in the hospital, less than 2 percent comes from charitable donations, and even the 3 percent paid for by patients out-of-pocket does not really flow through a two-party transaction, because it largely consists of copayments, deductibles, and other fees related to third-party insurance payments.

1.3 SOURCES OF HEALTH CARE FUNDS ____

The major changes in health care financing over the last sixty years have been (1) funding had to grow rapidly to provide all the new and technologically sophisticated services people wanted, and (2) the sources of funding have shifted from direct patient payments to third parties (government, in particular) as health care expenditures increased. There are many reasons health care spending has grown rapidly: an increasingly wealthy population desires to spend more on all goods; extra spending on health care has a greater appeal after basic necessities such as food and housing are taken care of; technological advances make modern medicine more and more desirable; insurance now covers more of the cost, an aging population favors health care over other goods.

Third-party private insurance was almost nonexistent in 1929, and then grew rapidly, to control almost a quarter of the funds flow in 1960, and about a third in 1993. However, government is now the primary means of financing health care. It has always been larger than private insurance, and its importance is magnified because government extensively regulates all third-party contracts. For hospital care, the single-largest category of spending, government accounts for 58 percent of the total, and along with other third-party payers controls 98 percent of the funds flowing into hospitals. Shifting the financial burden from individuals to third parties not only changed the way funds flowed, but made more funds available, so that the health care system could grow rapidly and absorb an ever-larger share of total economic output.

Why Shift to Third-Party Payment?

As medical care became more expensive, the potential cost of illness went from burdensome to overwhelming. In 1929, $200 was an unusually large medical bill. In today's high-technology intensive care units (ICUs), hospital costs of $100,000 or more are not uncommon, with extra bills for surgery, anesthesia, laboratory and drugs. Few individuals can afford to pay the high cost of advanced modern treatment for serious illness, but few are willing to forgo treatment if they become seriously ill. Insurance makes it possible for most people to obtain care when they need it without going bankrupt. Regular withholding of premiums and taxes spreads the financial risk across many people, and makes catastrophic expenses bearable.

TABLE 1.3 The Concentration of Personal Health Expenditures

	All	Top 1%	next 9%	Middle 75%	Bottom 15%
Persons (000's)	278,000	2,780	25,020	208,500	41,700
Health $ (millions)	$1,050,000	$367,500	$367,500	$309,750	$5,250
per person	$3,777	$132,194	$14,688	$1,486	$126

Insurance would not be necessary if everyone's medical expenses were near the average of $4,226 per person per year. Instead, there is a great deal of individual variation—much more than for food, housing, clothing, transportation and other major expense categories. Most people are quite healthy during any given year, with 15% having minimal costs (less than $500) for medical care (see Table 1.3 and Figure 1.8).[5] However, the 9 percent of the population that had to go into the hospital during the year each averaged more than $15,000. Only 1 percent of patients cost more than $100,000, but this 1 percent of patients accounted for 30 percent of total health care dollars. Indeed, it took just 10 percent of all the patients to account for 70 percent of the costs.[6]

Although each of us would prefer to pay nothing, most of us can afford to pay for at least some of the cost of the care we expect to receive if we get sick. Even if

Distribution of Individual Medical Care Expenditures

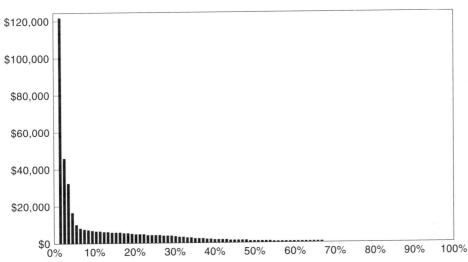

FIGURE 1.8 *Distribution of personal health care expenditures. The 1 percent of individuals with highest cost consume approximately 30 percent of total services, and the top 5 percent consume about 50 percent.*

we are healthy, we can reasonably be asked to contribute something toward the expenses of those who are not. But how much? A $150,000 bill would be staggeringly difficult to pay. We might not even think that we can afford the average annual cost of $4,226 cost a person. But whether we wish to pay that much or not, an average of $4,226 a person must be extracted through taxes, bills paid by individuals, insurance premiums paid by employers (who must therefore reduce wages), or some other means, such as charitable giving, in order to keep the system running. These funds are needed to keep the hospitals open; doctors, nurses, janitors and clerks paid; research laboratories searching, and so forth. Most of us are not aware of the financial burden we bear for health care provided to ourselves and others. For most workers, employers pay about $2 an hour (11 percent of compensation) for health benefits, reducing the amount that can be paid out as wages.[7] Even if an employer does not provide health insurance, something is deducted each week as taxes labeled "H.I." or "MC." This is hospital insurance, not for the employee, but for the elderly and disabled on Medicare. Every time we buy a candy bar or gallon of gasoline, we pay state taxes that fund Medicaid for indigent people. On the other hand, senior citizens might be complaining bitterly about the costs of drugs and hospitals and nursing homes, with little awareness of how much subsidy they are receiving. Even if they pay thousands of dollars out-of-pocket, over 90 percent of the hospital bills, half of the nursing home bills, and almost a third of the costs of their drugs are being borne by other people, mostly younger working people.

Health Care Payments are Complex

Third-party payments are made with taxes paid to government agencies (chapters 16 and 17), employer and employee payments to commercial insurance companies (chapters 3 and 4), for-profit and nonprofit managed care firms (HMOs, PPOs, and other acronyms discussed in chapters 10 and 11), as well as philanthropic contributions to charities (chapters 3 and 17), and each of these major categories exists in endless variations. They are complex, with motivations and internal details that differ widely, but from a flow of funds perspective they all have a similar purpose: pooling funds from many people through a third-party organization to pay the bills of those few patients who are deemed to need care according to the rules of the collective and the opinions of the professionals who run the health care system. In each case, indirect third-party payment weakens the monetary linkage between buyer and seller that characterizes the direct two-party transactions typical in most other sectors of the economy. For most medical transactions, there is no exchange of money between the recipient of services and the provider. The patients (or their families) pay insurance premiums and taxes, and the doctors and hospitals are paid by the government and insurance companies. In the absence of a direct link between the amount paid and the resources used in treatment, "prices" become more ambiguous and less important to the transaction than ongoing relationships of trust and professional behavior. One of the tasks of this textbook is to explain how economic forces continue to operate when prices do not function in a normal way, and how other organizing principles (professionalism, licensure, regulation) serve as replacements.

1.4 INCOME AND ETHNICITY AS DETERMINANTS OF MORTALITY _____

Spending money on medical care is only one of many ways that the economy affects people's health. Economic growth enables people to have a better diet, to avoid hazardous jobs and clean up the environment, as well as to purchase more medical care. A major contribution of higher incomes is to allow people to become more educated, which changes their values and their production possibilities in ways that are favorable to health. Chapter 15 provides a more detailed examination of the complex relationships between economic growth, income distribution, medical care and health, but some basic facts form a useful background for study of the health care system. Table 1.4 presents the results of a study of a group of 320,000 middle-aged men enrolled in a trial of cardiac risk reduction.[8] Income for this study is based not on individual wages, but the community in which the person lived (average per capita income of the zip code of residence). Reading down the columns, it becomes evident that men in poorer communities face a much higher risk of death each year, a finding which holds even as the groups are adjusted for age, unemployment, use of medical care, and other factors. Indeed, the group living in areas with average income below $10,000 per year were twice as likely to die as those in areas with incomes above $30,000 per year. Blacks are more likely to die than whites, largely because of living in lower income areas. Yet even after controlling for differences in income, black mortality is still significantly greater each year. Similar differences in morbidity and mortality rates by socio-economic and ethnic grouping are observed among women, the elderly, and children.

Although the spread of insurance and government assistance has done much to equalize access to medical care, large disparities in actual health and life expectancy have endured. Inequalities in health are found throughout the world. Countries like Sweden and the United Kingdom, which have universal national health systems, also show substantial differences in mortality between groups, as do poorer countries such as Bangladesh and Ghana, where national health infrastructure is almost non-existent. Health economists are still working to understand the persistence of excess mortality among disadvantaged groups despite tremendous increases and redistribution in health care spending.

TABLE 1.4 Annual Mortality Rate Among Middle-Aged Men

	Mortality Rate	
Income Category	White	Black
< $9,999	0.918%	1.234%
$10,000 – $14,999	0.840%	1.123%
$15,000 – $19,999	0.706%	0.899%
$20,000 – $24,999	0.660%	0.867%
$25,000 – $29,999	0.591%	0.603%
$30,000 +	0.542%	****

Source: G. D. Smith et al, American J. Public Health 86:486-504, 1996.

1.5 HEALTH CARE PROVIDERS: THE USE OF FUNDS

Payments by patients, government, and insurance companies have gone up two-hundred fold over the last sixty years; thus, payments received by doctors, hospitals, and other providers of care have increased by the same amount. In general, both the public, as users of the system, and providers, as suppliers of care, have been happy with this large increase in spending. The public has gotten a medical care system that is technologically advanced and responsive to their personal needs. Providers have gained glory in the fight against disease, and substantial gains in income, making them eager to continue the struggle.

Part of the increase from $4 billion in 1929 to $1,175 billion in 1997 is just an accounting fiction due to inflation, because $1 in 1929 is roughly the same as $11 in 1997. Also some of the increase reflects a rise in the number of people who must be cared for. Yet even after adjustment for changes in population and inflation, real per capita spending has increased more than tenfold since 1929. Some of this real increase in spending is due to a real increase in wages. As per capita incomes rise, workers expect more real goods and services per hour of work. Therefore, expenditures on labor intensive services will tend to rise more rapidly than expenditures on goods or capital intensive commodities. Furthermore, the wages of health care workers have risen more rapidly than for other types of labor.[9] This probably reflects both the increased education of health professionals today and the increased demand for their services. Increases in the quantity of services provided (days of hospital care, number of visits to physicians, number of prescriptions) accounts for some of the growth in total expenditures, but growth in quantity has been quite slow since 1960 (see Table 1.5).[10]

After taking all of these factors into account—inflation, higher health care wages, more utilization of services—there is still a tremendous increase in expenditures over the last thirty years, more than 250 percent. How can spending increase so much more rapidly than the increase in the number of services, or in the wages of those that provide them? By increasing the **intensity of services.** More tests are done for a patient in a modern intensive care unit during a single day than would have been done for a patient over the course of a month in their wooden bed in 1929, and many of those tests (MRI scans, blood glucose, heart monitoring) would not have been available back then. The physician who drove to the patient's house and worked alone out of a black bag has been replaced by a team of therapists, technicians, and support staff assisting a group of physicians, many of whom are specialists, with an array of medical equipment. Another factor that explains some of the growth in spending is that as some common acute (short term) diseases have been made subject to cure or prevention, medical care is increasingly applied in cases of chronic disease that would once have been considered hopeless. The shift from simple caring to technologically sophisticated curing is reflected by shifts in the categories of expenditure; more is going to institutional care in hospitals and nursing homes, while the share devoted to personal services by physicians and dentists has declined. The fraction of the health care dollar spent for manufactured goods, such as drugs, has also fallen, while the cost of labor-intensive services has risen.

TABLE 1.5   Changes in the Use of Health Care Funds over Sixty Years

	1929	1960	1997
Spending per person (in 1997 dollars)	$306	$722	$3,777
Percent Usage			
Hospital	18%	34%	36%
Physician	36	20	20
Dental	12	7	4
Drugs	18	16	8
Eye care	1	3	1
Nursing home	na	4	8
Home health	na	na	3
Other	3	3	9
Admin. & insurance	3	4	5
Public health	3	2	3
Research	1	3	2
Construction	5	4	1
Total	*100%*	*100%*	*100%*
Hospital days per 100 people	9.4	10.1	7.3
Hospital Employees per patient	<0.5	1.1	5.3
Physician visits per person	2.6	4.8	6.0

Hospitals

There are about 6,500 hospitals (the subject of chapters 8 and 9) in the United States today, a number that has increased only slightly since 1929, and has actually declined in the last ten years.[11] Today's hospitals are larger, more technologically advanced, and organizationally linked to a broad array of clinics, home health agencies, and purchasing cooperatives. Most (90 percent) are "general acute care hospitals," meaning that they provide a broad range of care with most patients staying from three to ten days. Some special-purpose hospitals address specific areas, such as psychiatry, physical rehabilitation, or eye care, or specific population groups, such as children or veterans.

Research institutions such as the Massachusetts General Hospital or Johns Hopkins are usually quite large (more than 400 beds), closely affiliated with a university, and most of the physicians are "house staff": interns, residents, medical students, and the professors who train them. Much more numerous are the community general hospitals of medium size (100–300 beds) that serve a local area, with most of their physicians being local private practitioners who volunteer to be part of the medical staff (they are not paid by the hospital, but earn income from their own private practices).

Since there is rarely a direct monetary transaction with patients, the flow of funds into hospitals is known not as sales, but *reimbursements*, 98 percent of which comes from third parties. There are some government hospitals and private for-profit hospitals, but the bulk are voluntary organizations with ownership resting in a nonprofit community or religious board. The operations and finances of most acute general hospitals are quite similar, regardless of whether they are owned by government, investors, or voluntary boards, and all three ownership types are represented across the range of specialty and teaching/research categories. There is a small amount of funding from philanthropy and grants for research or outreach. There are usually a number of patients that are treated for free, and uncompensated care is paid for through "cost shifting," raising the price to insured patients to pay for charity care. The average hospital will have about 180 patient beds, 650 employees, a budget of about 44 million dollars, and a "profit" margin of 0 to 6 percent. Around 5,000 cases per year will be handled in the hospital as inpatients, and an additional 64,000 outpatient "ambulatory" visits will be provided in the emergency room, clinics, or medical offices. The average cost per day is about $1,000, and the patient will usually pay less than $20. Although the average case will have a total cost of about $7,000, quite commonly hospital bills exceed $100,000 (see Table 1.6).

TABLE 1.6   Characteristics of Acute Care
Hospitals, 1994

Total number of hospitals	6,539
Average per Hospital	
Beds	180
Employees	650
Inpatient admissions	4,700
Outpatient visits	64,000
Budget	$44 million
Cost per day	$998
Profit margin	4.5%

Nursing Homes

There are about 1,730,000 patients in nursing homes (the subject of chapter 12) on any given day, twice as many as there are in hospitals.[12] Although nursing homes tend to be smaller, averaging only 55 beds, there are many more nursing homes, 33,000, than there are hospitals. About one in four Americans can expect to be admitted to a nursing home for more than thirty days sometime during their life, and those who are admitted will spend an average of three and a half years there.[13] Nursing homes provide long-term care primarily to elderly persons who can no longer take care of themselves, but also serve younger patients who are severely disabled or mentally ill. It is best to consider long-term care as providing a range of support, from ordinary meals and housing in board-and-care homes, to advanced and demanding services such as intravenous medication and monitoring in SNFs (skilled nursing facilities). The cost rises with the level of care, from a minimal $30 a day for room and board, to more than $300 a day for skilled nursing care.

More than half of all nursing home reimbursement comes from Medicaid, the state/federal program for indigent patients. However, many nursing home patients are not "poor," but simply older persons who have outlived their retirement savings, or who were admitted to a nursing home as a private paying patient and then "spent down" their assets until they became qualified for Medicaid. Less than 10 percent comes from Medicare, which covers most medical expenses for the elderly. That is because nursing homes cover custodial rather than curative services. A third is paid for directly by patients or their families, with only 2 percent coming from private insurance.

The flow of funds into the U.S. health care system is determined by reimbursement rules that make a rather sharp distinction between hospitals and nursing homes. This distinction is not so sharp, or is nonexistent, in many other health care systems. In Canada and Japan, for example, many of the "hospital" patients are not receiving intense technological services, they stay for very long periods of time, and they would be placed in nursing homes if they were in the United States. On the other hand, some countries, such as Denmark, provide extensive support and rehabilitation services as part of housing assistance to the elderly and disabled, so that what would be classified as nursing home care in the U.S. is provided outside the health insurance scheme. Table 1.7 presents some characteristics of nursing homes in the United States.

Doctors

There are about 670,000 physicians (the subject of chapters 5, 6, and 7) in the United States, 550,000 of whom are actively caring for patients.[14] That is approximately one physician for every five hundred people. They are among the most respected and highly paid professionals in America, earning an average of $182,400 in 1994. Two-thirds are self-employed in a small business. They work in an office with a number of nurses, clerks, and ancillary workers. About half of the revenues of a physician office practice will go for wages for nonphysician ancillary workers, office rent and equipment, medical supplies, and malpractice insurance. About a third of physicians are "solo" practitioners, but this number is declining as more and more physicians join groups to gain the benefits of closer interaction with colleagues, more professional office management, access to financial services such as billing and payroll, and more regular working hours. Most groups have grown over time as a successful practice acquired more and more partners. The Mayo clinic, one of the oldest and most well known, now has more than 1,230 doctors on staff.

TABLE 1.7   Characteristics of Nursing Homes, 1994

Total number	33,006
Average per Nursing Home	
Beds	55
Employees	30
Budget	$1 million
Cost per day	$48
Profit margin	5%

It is common to divide medical practice into *primary care* (the initial visit by a patient and follow-up for general services) and *specialty care* (for complex illnesses) provided by referral. In reality, the distinction is often hard to make, because many people seek their primary care from specialists, and most generalists or "family practitioners" must have membership on a hospital medical staff and provide some specialized services such as testing or surgery to keep their practices economically viable. The situation is markedly different in some other countries, such as England, where office-based general practitioners working in the community are about half of the total number of physicians. They are entirely separate from the specialists and physicians in training who are based in hospitals, see only referral patients, and work on salary. As shown in Table 1.8, the vast majority of U.S. physicians are "specialists" in that they concentrate their professional practice on a certain set of illnesses. Most have undergone three to five years of specialty training in a hospital-based residency program, and are certified by one of the recognized specialty boards that administer a national examination. Indeed, even family (general) practitioners have, since 1969, been eligible for certification as "specialists" by their own examining board.

Although the title of *doctor* is most commonly applied to those who have received the M.D. (doctor of medicine) degree, those who have completed the D.O. (doctor of osteopathy) degree are also considered physicians and are functionally equivalent in many states (the two professional societies merged in California). There are a number of other types of doctors: podiatrists, chiropractors, ophthalmologists, and clinical psychologists, for example. Each has its own professional association and training program. Physicians have kept incomes high by maintaining high standards—and also by limiting the number allowed into the profession. Such control over entry makes the AMA (American Medical Association) and affiliated organizations into something of a professional monopoly, with economic as well as scientific and humanitarian interests. Conflict between different types of doctors over patients, billing, and standards of care, are recurrent themes in the history of medicine because each group is competing for the same flow of funds. Relations between chiropractors and M.D.s are often quite acrimonious. For other types of doctors, the conflict is more civilized, and many instances of cooperation can be found—not because there is no conflict between, say, psychiatrists (who are M.D.s) and psychologists (who are Ph.D.'s), but because each party has found it more profitable to put up with the other than to try to eliminate it from the field of practice. Fighting for patients and money occurs not just between types of doctors, but between specialties as well. Family practitioners want to do some surgery, cardiologists want to do invasive procedures, and almost every

TABLE 1.8 **Characteristics of Physicians, 1994**

Total number	550,000
Average income	$182,400
Solo independents	33%
Employees	33%
Partners	34%
Specialists	77%

specialty wants to read some X-rays and do laboratory testing, poaching on the fields of radiology and pathology. Over time, professional turf struggles usually disappear below the surface as accommodations are reached. If different specialties attack each other in court, it threatens the flow of funds from patients, who are apt to mistrust both sides. However, the rise of managed care and the pressure to cut costs across the board in recent years has stressed old fault lines and threatened many informal "understandings" that allowed for the peaceable allocation of patient business.

Economic struggles, while important, are secondary in understanding the medical profession. The road to advancement as a doctor comes through the provision of better patient care and research leading to technological innovation, with entrepreneurship playing only a minor role. While accountants, architects, lawyers (and economists) are also "professionals," they are so in a less distinctive way. The archetype of a profession with an ethical creed and special privileges based on service to society and intellectual advancement is still best personified by the physician as healer and scientist, freed from narrow self-interest by the expectation of earning a generous income from a grateful citizenry.

Nurses and Other Health Workers

In tracing the evolution of health care employment, two trends stand out: the fragmentation of medicine into many distinct professions, and the rise in the number of other health workers per physician. In 1880, *medical care* meant physician care. Few patients ever went to the hospital, and most physicians were solo practitioners working from a black bag carried about in a horse-drawn carriage. Per physician, there were only 0.2 ancillary workers (nurses, pharmacists, etc.) of all types to work with. By 1990, there were 16 ancillary workers for each physician, a relative growth rate of 8,000 percent.[15] Thus, in many ways, the story of the growth of medicine is that of organizing and paying for all of the support personnel that make modern medicine possible.

With more than 2 million nurses in practice in the United States today, nursing is the largest medical profession. Yet in many ways, it is the most difficult to define. Originally, nurses were "doctor's helpers" providing patient care at the bedside and usually trained on the job. Later, schools of nursing were opened up in hospitals (with student nurses providing much of the nursing care for free). Such "diploma programs" have increasingly been replaced by formal academic training (bachelor's, master's and doctor's degrees), and the nurses so trained have moved increasingly far from their original role as caring helpers with good hearts but limited training. More and more direct patient care has been taken over by licensed practical nurses (LPNs) who are trained outside of universities, and associate degree RNs trained at community colleges, and a variety of newly emerging professions, such as respiratory therapists, perfusionists, and physical therapists. The number of baccalaureate nurse graduates (B.S.N.s) has declined steadily from a peak of 25,000 in 1979 to under 19,000 in 1995 as other allied health professions have grown (see Table 1.9).[16]

The economic study of nursing has focused on issues of wages and recurrent labor shortages, with 15 percent or more of the nursing jobs within a hospital being vacant at one point in time, and then again several years later. Gender has

TABLE 1.9   **Characteristics of Nurses and Other Health Workers, 1994**

Total number of all health workers	10.5 million	
9 percent of the U.S. labor force		

	Number	Average income
RNs	1,840,000	$34,400
LPNs	700,000	$21,500
Nurse aides	1,400,000	$13,800
Health services managers	302,000	$70,000
Physical therapists	90,000	$35,400
Respiratory therapists	74,000	$32,000
Physician assistants	58,000	$41,000
Radiologic technicians	162,000	$28,300
Medical assistants	181,000	$17,000
Medical records	76,000	$22,000
Clinical lab techs	268,000	$26,300
Paramedics & EMTs	114,000	$28,000
Optometrists	31,000	$75,000
Dispensing opticians	63,000	$26,000
Pharmacists	163,000	$45,000
Chiropractors	46,000	$70,000
Podiatrists	15,000	$100,000
Dentists	183,000	$90,000
Dental hygienists	108,000	$31,000
Dental assistants	183,000	$16,000

Source: Occupational Outlook Handbook, U.S. Bureau of Labor Statistics Bulletin 2450, 1994.

played a tremendous and not always well-understood role in the formation and economics of the nursing profession. Nursing is 97 percent female, perhaps the only sizable profession that is truly woman-dominated, yet it has always had to struggle with issues of physician dominance couched in scientific rather than po-litical terms.

Administration

In 1880 medicine was essentially a private transaction between patients and their physicians. There was no need for organization. Now, with a trillion dollars flow-ing through the computers of insurance companies, 400 billion of those dollars being collected from taxpayers; hundreds of pages of rules covering pharmaceu-ticals, home care, ambulatory surgery, and other therapeutic issues; and more than six hundred employees in the average hospital, organization is essential. Increased efficiency is now apt to come more from improvements in organization than the refinement of production methods. Health care is moving from a "craft" system, with autonomous, skilled individual practitioners making custom thera-peutics based on their own experience, toward a "corporate" system where treat-ment is based more on a body of scientific evidence and carried out by a team of specialists and technicians.[17] Caring will always be a product of immediate human interaction, but reading an X-ray or monitoring antibiotic levels in the blood are tasks that are already well on the way toward being automated. In such a complex system, coordination of all the parts is often more important than how well each part functions on its own, and an increasing amount of resources and people must be devoted to management. The Bureau of Labor Statistics categorizes 208,000 persons, 2 percent of the health labor force, as administrators and managers. The percentage of total effort devoted to management is much higher than that. Consider all the medical records clerks, finance officers, and computer specialists whose sole job is to move information around the system. Next, add to that all the time that doctors and nurses spend meeting in committees, writing in charts, dictating notes, verifying laboratory results, and submitting charge slips for payment. It is easy to see how the tasks of administering the system may take more than half of the total resources used in providing health care.

As medicine has evolved into a health care system financed through a variety of interlocked third-party mechanisms, control over the flow of funds has shifted from doctors and patients to managers and their computer systems. While in some ways inevitable, necessary to support expensive modern technology, and often labor-saving and more efficient, this loss of control has also been frustrating to both patients and physicians. The money is more and more concentrated in the hands of the professional administrators, or simply hidden in a maze of electronic transactions.

Public Health

Many of the most important factors in determining health are public goods: water quality, highway safety, nutritional labeling, and infectious disease control (chapter 17 discusses public goods and public health). Overall longevity and illness rates are less a function of the medical care provided to individuals than the efforts put into educating children, providing safe food, housing and water, and so forth.[18] Since the beginning of civilization, steps have been taken to protect the health of the public, which only government could do well. Public health clinics have been leaders in childhood nutrition, control of epidemics, and service to disadvantaged populations so as to ameliorate social problems. An important task of health economics is to distinguish which tasks are best performed by government, which are best left to unregulated markets, and which need some combination of public and private action.

Research

Technology has been the driving force in the health care system—saving babies, lengthening lives, creating hospitals, linking medical records worldwide, and raising the American public's willingness to spend over a thousand billion dollars a year. One can easily imagine that spending would be doubled again without complaint if the research laboratories could come up with a vaccine for AIDS, a cure for cancer, and a reversal of Alzheimer's. Medical discoveries have most often been fortuitous outgrowths of other activities (Pasteur's discovery of bacteria grew out of an investigation into the causes of spoiled wine and beer) or the refinement of insights from patient care. Historically, what little direct funding there was for research came mostly from philanthropists. Today, taxpayers are the largest source of pure research support, through the National Institutes of Health and other programs. However, a much larger portion of research "funding" is hidden in the cost of patient care, as the work of physicians to develop and refine new technologies is covered through reimbursement. The most prestigious hospitals and clinics are deemed superior because cutting-edge research and innovative therapies are first applied there. Being on the cutting edge is expensive, and charges for patient care at the top academic medical centers are as much as three times higher than those at local community hospitals. This source of indirect funding may be under pressure as the growth of managed care increases price competition in the hospital services market.

Most of the cost of developing new types of surgery and diagnostic tools does not show up as "research" in the national health accounts because it is covered as part of patient care reimbursement. Similarly, most of the research and development (R&D) at pharmaceutical companies is buried as an overhead cost in the production of drugs. Even more hidden is the cost of administrative innovation. Developing new forms of contracting, such as health maintenance organizations, or new methods of delivering care, such as home health companies or life care communities, is very costly, largely because it is a trial-and-error process requiring many expensive failures before a better system can be found. Yet such organizational development is usually not even recognized as being research, and is almost never counted up alongside the laboratories and biomedical scientists.

The cost of continually innovating and changing medical treatments and delivery systems is staggeringly high, yet the forgone *opportunity cost of not innovating* is much greater. What athlete injured today would wish to forgo arthroscopic knee surgery and accept a hot mustard plaster? Senior citizens may say they want to turn back the clock to the good old days, but any politician that threatens to take away Medicare, or even to cut benefits slightly, gets slaughtered at the polls. The American public demands a modern, constantly updated health care system. Research into new therapies and new forms of organization is the force that has made it worth spending 1,175 billion dollars today versus 0.4 billion dollars a hundred years ago. Yet the flow of funds into research is hard to trace, the connection between spending and benefits difficult to make, and the dynamics of technological and organizational change among the most challenging of economic questions.

SUGGESTIONS FOR FURTHER READING _____

Sally T. Burner and Daniel R. Waldo, "National Health Expenditure Projections, 1994-2005" *Health Care Financing Review* 16(4):221-242, Summer 1995.

Victor Fuchs, Economics, Values and Health Care Reform, *American Economic Review,* 86(1):1-24, 1996.

William Kissick, *Medicine's Dilemmas*, New Haven, Conn: Yale University Press, 1994.

Katherine Levit, *et. al.,* "National Health Expenditures, 1993" *Health Care Financing Review* 16(1):247-294, Fall 1994.

U.S. Department of Health and Human Services, *Health United States,* Annual Publication.

SUMMARY _____

1. **Health care costs so much because people are willing to pay for it.** As a wealthy country, the United States is willing to spend a vast amount supporting a dynamic and technologically sophisticated health care system.

2. U.S. national **health spending** in 1997 will exceed 1 trillion dollars, **$4,226 per person.**

3. Health care costs have consistently **risen 3 to 5 percent more rapidly than incomes,** and now account for **15 percent of GDP** (gross domestic product).

4. Due to the uncertain and **uneven distribution of medical care costs,** with 70 percent of total dollars being spent on behalf of that 10 percent of people who become most ill during a year, most health care payments flow through **third-party insurance** intermediaries that pool and transfer funds, rather than the direct exchange of money for services between two parties (consumers and providers) common to most markets.

5. Insurance and government programs have greatly reduced disparities in the use of medical care between income groups, but **socioeconomic differentials in health status have persisted.** People living in poor neighborhoods are twice as likely to die as persons of the same age and sex living in wealthy neighborhoods.

6. **Government** is the largest provider of health care funds (45 percent), and hospitals are the largest user (36 percent).

7. **Physicians** account for about 0.5 percent of the U.S. labor force, about the same fraction as in 1880. However, the number of nurses and other health workers per physician has risen from 0.2 to 16.

8. The use of medical services (visits to physicians and hospital admissions) has grown only modestly, so **most of the 500 percent real growth in health care costs is due to increased service intensity**—more workers per patient providing ever more technologically advanced care.

9. As health care moves from a cottage industry practiced by solo physicians to large-scale **corporate organization of health systems,** improvements in efficiency will depend on managerial innovation (information networks, flexible staffing, risk sharing, managed care).

10. Much of the **improvement in health and longevity** has, and will, come from **social factors** and inexpensive **public health** activities rather than expensive applications of new medical technology.

11. **Research** into new drugs and therapeutic techniques is very expensive, but the forgone opportunity cost of not innovating would be much greater.

PROBLEMS _____

1. {*planning resources per capita*} Using the data in this chapter, calculate the number of physicians, nurses, hospitals, and nursing homes there would be in an average small town with 10,000 people (total U.S. population was approximately 278 million in 1997).

2. {*local estimates*} Use the telephone book for your city and attempt to estimate if the numbers are above or below the expected amount. Why is it harder to estimate the number of physicians than the number of hospitals? Why is it so difficult to estimate the number of nurses?

3. {*distribution of health expenditures*} Thirty percent of total spending is accounted for by the top 1 percent of patients. Take the overall average per capita personal health expenditure ($3,777) and determine how much on average is spent on each of these high cost patients. The top half of the population accounts for 90 percent of total spending. What is the average amount spent on the remaining persons in the bottom half of the distribution? Is the median (i.e., amount spent on the person who is at the middle of distribution, with half of all people spending more, and half of all people spending less) higher or lower than the mean?

4. {*philanthropy, $ versus %*} Has the dollar amount of charitable giving for health increased or decreased since 1900? Has the fraction of health expenditures paid for with charity increased or decreased?

5. {*manpower*} Which has increased more rapidly since 1900, the number of physicians, or the number of ancillary health workers? As medicine becomes more technologically advanced, which will grow faster, the number of more-skilled workers or the number of less-skilled workers?

6. {*utilization*} Did people go to the doctor more or less often in 1995 than 1960? than 1929? Did they spend more or less days in the hospital? Why?

7. {*causality*} Have health expenditures increased because the number of people employed has increased, or has health employment increased because total health expenditures have increased?

8. {*causality*} Would eliminating research reduce or increase the cost of U.S. health care?

9. {*Fieldwork*} Contact six people and find out how much they spent on health care last year. Try to estimate how much they spent out of their own pocket, and how much was spent by their employer, insurance company, or government. Did the people with more serious health problems always end up spending more of their own money on health care? Did they personally end up paying a larger or smaller percentage of their total health bills?

ENDNOTES _____

1. Extrapolated from Sally T. Burner and Daniel R. Waldo, "National Health Expenditure Projections, 1994–2005" *Health Care Financing Review* 16(4):221-242, Summer 1995; Katherine Levit, *et. al.*, "National Health Expenditures, 1993" *Health Care Financing Review* 16(1):247–294, Fall 1994, and additional compilations by the Office of the Actuary, Health Care Financing Administration. The HCFA Office of the Actuary is the source for all expenditure estimates in this and subsequent chapters unless explicitly noted.

2. Joseph E. Stiglitz, *The Economics of the Public Sector*, New York: W.W. Norton, 1986.

3. *Monthly Labor Review*, U.S. Department of Labor, Volume 119, Number 2, Table 20.

4. Committee on the Costs of Medical Care, *Medical Care for the American People*, Chicago: University of Chicago Press, 1932; Odin W. Anderson, *Health Services as a Growth Enterprise in the United States since 1875*, Ann Arbor, Mich.: Health Administration Press, 1990.

5. *Health Care Financing Review, Medicare and Medicaid Statistical Supplement, 1995*, p. 35; Alan Monheit, "The Concentration of Health Expenditures Revisited" *Health Affairs*, 1992.

6. The distribution of costs across individuals can be measured only for personal health care costs which are billed to individuals, not overhead items such as public health, construction, insurance administration, etc. Such overhead items make up about 10 percent of national health expenditures, and hence the "all persons" average in Table 1.3 is only 90 percent as large as the per capita average for all national health expenditures in Table 1.2 and elsewhere. In truth, many costs have overhead components and are difficult to unambiguously assign to a single person, although they are clearly concentrated on the most ill and not evenly distributed. Many economists would argue that costs are even more concentrated than Table 1.3 indicates because hospitals and physicians typically overcharge the least complex patients to subsidize the most difficult and complex cases (see the discussion of "cost shifting" in Section 8.4).

7. Bureau of Labor Statistics, U.S. Department of Labor, *Employment Cost Indexes and Levels, 1975-90*, Bulletin 2372, 1990.

8. G. D. Smith, J. D. Neaton, D. Wentworth, R. Stamler and J. Stamler, "Socioeconomic Differentials in Mortality Risk among Med Screened for the Multiple Risk Factor Intervention Trial, "*American Journal of Public Health*, 86:486-504. 1986.

9. Bureau of Labor Statistics, U.S. Department of Labor, *Employment and Earnings*, Biannual.

10. U.S. Department of Health and Human Services, *Health United States*, Annual Publication.

11. American Hospital Association, *Hospital Statistics: 1994-95 Edition*, 1995.

12. E. Hing, "Use of Nursing Homes by the Elderly," *Advance Data from Vital and Health Statistics*, No. 135, DHHS Publication No. (PHS) 87–1250, National Center for Health Statistics, 1987; *Statistical Abstract of the United States*, 1994, Tables 178, 191, 192, Washington, D.C.: U.S. Government Printing Office, 1994.

13. M. A. Cohen, E. J. Tell, and S. Wallack, "The Lifetime Risks and Costs of Nursing Home Use Among the Elderly," *Medical Care* 24(12):1161–72, 1986; C. E. McConnel, "A Note on the Lifetime Risk of Nursing Home Residency," *The Gerontologist* 24(2): 193–199, 1984.

14. American Medical Association, *Physician Distribution and Licensure in the United States, 1995*, Chicago: American Medical Association, 1995.

15. Michael Kendix and Thomas Getzen, "U.S. Health Services Employment: A Time Series Analysis," *Health Economics* 3(3) 169–181, 1994.

16. Bureau of Labor Statistics, *Outlook 2000*, Bulletin 2352, Washington, D.C.: U.S. Government Printing Office, 1990.

17. Paul Starr, *The Social Transformation of American Medicine*, New York: Basic Books, 1982.

18. Thomas McKeown, *The Modern Rise of Population* (London: Edwin Arnold, 1976); Massimo Livi-Bacci, *A Concise History of World Population* (trans. Carl Ipsen), Cambridge, Mass.: Blackwell, 1992.

CHAPTER 2

Economic Evaluation of Health Services

QUESTIONS

1. *Is there necessarily a trade-off between health and money?*

2. *Is "medical need" the same as "demand?"*

3. *Can the statistical probability of death among teenagers be compared to mortality among the retired elderly?*

4. *Is the effort expended to save one more life a total or a "marginal" cost?*

5. *What is the value of life? Is one life worth less than another?*

6. *Is it more beneficial to screen high risk or low risk people for disease?*

7. *Why will decisions based on average benefits lead to excessive use of medical care?*

8. *Why do economists insist on discussing every choice a person makes as if it could be converted into dollars?*

9. *Which is the better measure of the value of medical care, professional judgement or the choices of patients?*

2.1 COST–BENEFIT ANALYSIS (CBA) IS ABOUT MAKING CHOICES _____

"It is best to think of the cost-benefit approach as a way of organizing thought rather than as a substitute for it."*

CBA and CEA

Economics is about exchange between people and the trade-offs that they make. **Cost-benefit analysis (CBA)** replicates on paper the balancing of pros and cons, of advantages and disadvantages, that occurs implicitly in the marketplace. CBA is also used for public decision making to protect the interests of children, homeless persons, the mentally ill, addicts, and other disenfranchised individuals, as well as those of future generations that are not adequately represented in the marketplace.[1] Moreover, many health care decisions are sufficiently complicated and threatening that the individual, even though otherwise competent, may have to depend on the good judgment of physicians and other professionals to identify alternatives and determine the relative values of medical outcomes, rather than depending on his or her own informed choices. When decisions must be made involving third-party financing or multiparty public issues, an explicit decision-making process such as CBA replaces the independent market decisions of consumers. **Cost-effectiveness analysis (CEA)** is a truncated form of cost–benefit analysis, fully analyzing the cost side but not translating the benefits (lives saved, cases prevented, additional days of activity, extent of sight restored, and so on) into dollars. CEA analysis is used to determine which among several alternatives is cheaper, or as part of an analysis, whereby the reader subjectively evaluates benefits to make a decision. A study of whether cardiac bypass surgery adds a sufficient number of years to life expectancy to justify the cost is a cost–benefit study. A study evaluating whether hypertension screening, nutrition counseling, medication, or bypass surgery would provide the most additional years of life expectancy for each dollar spent, is a cost-effectiveness study.

Opportunity Cost: Looking at Alternatives

"Growing old is a pretty lousy thing to have happen to you, until you consider the alternative."

George Burns

Costs and benefits are not intrinsic or absolute values, but relative. Once a patient is diagnosed with pancreatic cancer or AIDS, all of the alternatives are pretty bad, but four years of life might be a lot better than two years of life, and the ability to play tennis is a lot better than continuous nausea. On the other hand, all of the alternatives facing a student graduating with a master's degree in Medical Information Systems may look good, and yet Baltimore might be much more appealing than Springfield, and the possibility of moving up into corporate systems management within a national health care chain more exciting than staying as

---

*Michael Drummond, *Principles of Economic Appraisal in Health Care* (Cambridge: Oxford Univ. Press: 1981), p.17.

head of records in a small, fifty-four-bed hospital. In order to make a decision, the relevant question is not how good or how bad the situation is, but "What are the options?" The appropriate measure of economic cost is **opportunity cost**, defined by the highest-valued alternative forgone when a decision is made. Thus, in choosing a $45,000 job in Baltimore, the graduating student who gives up a $50,000 job in Springfield is "paying" an opportunity cost of $5,000. The cost of not taking an experimental drug is the forgone chance of living an extra two years, or of feeling better.

Although it might seem excessively obvious and straightforward to state that opportunity cost is the correct measure of costs, many discussions that purport to be logical and objective go off track and distort rather than clarify decision making. A common tactic is for a supporter of a program to compare it with an alternative that is obviously bad, and thus overstate costs and benefits (e.g., "Do you want to go to the dentist today, or would you rather have all of your teeth fall out?" Or, "The proposed health insurance program can save the country from socialized medicine.") Most of us are able to detect such bias in the presentation of arguments, but may miss more subtle distortions. Often a decision is presented as all or nothing, when the real alternatives are between different levels of action. The choice is not between flossing your teeth every day or never, but between flossing occasionally, every other day, or after each meal.

Defining Marginal: What is the Decision?   The term *marginal,* much favored by economists, means *the change in* ___. It is the decision being made that defines the margin. Sometimes, it is how many patients to admit for treatment. For the example in section 2.2, screening for colon cancer, it is assumed that everyone will get screened, so the "margin" is the number of times the test is to be repeated to increase accuracy. Economists use a powerful analytical rule to simplify decision-making; **the decision between alternatives depends only on those factors that change.** Therefore, it is not necessary to examine the full range of possibilities, but only to look at doing a little more or a little less (i.e., to consider changes at the margin) to see whether a decision is optimal. If the marginal benefits of a therapy are greater than the marginal costs, then more should be done. If marginal costs are greater than marginal benefits, do less.

Need versus Demand   Decisions regarding who gets what medical services and when are mostly made by doctors.[2] Physicians tend to consider medical decisions in terms of **need**. This "need-based medical perspective" frames decisions as responses to a technical question regarding the level of service required to adequately treat the illness of a particular patient. A need-based medical perspective focuses on differences in health status and ignores the role of prices and incomes in allocating scarce resources. Medical determinations of patient need are based on physicians' assessments of the presenting illness and the prevailing state of the art in medicine. Physicians try to remove themselves from thinking about who pays (employer, patient, taxpayer) and who gets paid (themselves, hospitals) so as to concentrate on patient needs without the distraction of economic concerns. Their task is to operate within a given system to allocate resources, and to advocate for patients. There is even a certain purposeful forgetting of economic issues, because physicians are supposed to always act in the patient's best interest. Therefore, physicians try to act as if prices were set anonymously by somebody else, as if the bills got paid to some agency unrelated to their personal incomes, and as if insurance payments were really paid by some insurance company rather than taken out of wages.

Economists focus on the choices that must be made. The concept of **demand** adds two fundamental insights: (1) providing more medical treatment means giving up something else (opportunity cost) and (2) as more and more care is provided, the marginal benefits of each additional unit become smaller and smaller (downward-sloping demand). When economists say *demand*, they usually mean the **demand curve**, a graph or schedule *showing how the amount of service that people choose to consume will change as its price changes*. This stands in contrast to the medical concept of *need* as a fixed quantity. Consumers choose to buy less of a good as its price is raised if its price is higher. This common observation is what makes demand curves downward sloping, and is often referred to as the **first law of demand**.

In order to apply principles of maximization and use mathematics to estimate values, economists must abstract from other elements, ignoring some of the complexity of medical conditions and framing the issues in terms of dollars. Prices, costs, taxes, bids, contracts, and so on are the language used by economists to communicate human desires and limitations. The task of CBA is to make that language clear and applicable to the situation at hand, presenting the essential facts and trade-offs in a way that is easily understood by physicians, the public, and political decision makers.

For decisions regarding individual patients, a need-based medical perspective is suitable, and the economic insistence upon prices and trade-offs may seem clumsy and inappropriate. That is because physicians operate within the health care system as it currently stands to do the best for their patients, not to change the system to save money or help people they have never met. We do not ask doctors to determine what is best for taxpayers or employers or insurance companies, yet someone must address those larger questions. Economists are asked to do just that. We are required to think about choices between systems; how choosing one set of insurance regulations means more children will get immunized, but fewer elderly will receive home care, while another plan might protect accident victims, or provide more incentives to work. The trade-offs between medical care and other goods, between different groups of patients, and different types of care, are issues that health economics is designed to address. Although *demand for medical care* is a concept that is awkward when applied to a specific individual, who either is or is not sick, it is a tool that works well when considering groups of people or society as a whole. In these large groups there is always a range of illnesses and a range of treatments available, so that the necessity for choices and balancing at the margin is obvious.* Bringing the structure of economic models together with the

---

*There is often an unnecessary and acrimonious confusion between economists and doctors in addressing medical care because the two are trying to answer different questions. For doctors, the question is "what should I do for this patient acting as if money were no problem?" Economists, even health economists, have no particular skill at answering such a question. They address a different issue, "given that there is not enough for everyone to have all that they need, who should get treated?" It could be said that to some extent, doctors ignore economics, while economists ignore medicine. Health economics, and CBA in particular, have arisen to help these two groups talk and work together.

science of medicine is the interdisciplinary task that has created the field of study now known as health economics.

A Marginal Benefit Curve is a Demand Curve   The **marginal benefit** is the value to the consumer of one more unit of service. Their willingness to pay for additional care declines as more and more is provided, so the curve slopes downward. It looks very much like the demand curve; in fact, the marginal benefit curve and the demand curve are one and the same. To see why, remember that the demand curve is a schedule showing what quantity a consumer will buy at different prices. As long as marginal benefit exceeds the price, consumers will continue to buy. The quantity at which they have had enough and stop buying is the quantity at which the marginal benefit has fallen to the point where it is just equal to price. The quantity bought at price $P is the same as the quantity at which marginal benefit is $P; the marginal benefit (stated in dollars) of one more unit for a consumer who already has quantity Q is the same as the price they are willing to pay for one more unit.

Maximization: Finding the Optimum

More medical care will usually make people healthier. Physicians, rightly, concentrate on benefits, and often try to do as much as possible. However, using more resources to provide medical care means that fewer resources are available for food, entertainment, housing, and other goods that people want. Economics is concerned with trade-offs. What is the appropriate balance between medical care and other goods? How many doctors, nurses, hospitals, and so on should there be? Economists insist that both costs and benefits be considered in making a decision. An economist will also go about the question in a slightly different way than most physicians, asking not what is right or wrong, but whether a little more or a little less would make things better or worse—that is, an economist will use marginal analysis to **optimize,** moving toward a maximum in small steps.

Even though society benefits from having more medical care, the additional increment of benefit from each additional hospital day or doctor visit tends to become smaller and smaller as more services are provided. There are two reasons for declining marginal benefits. As more treatments are provided, they are given to less and less severely ill people, who are less likely to benefit. In emergency rooms or army field hospitals, the process of giving treatment first to those who are most likely to be helped is known as *triage,* and although it does not use all the mathematics or geometry or technical terminology, it operates on the same principles as economic maximization. Second, for any single person, the benefit from having one more medical service tends to decline as more and more are used, just as benefit from consuming additional pizzas or sodas or pretzels per day tends to decline. In Figure 2.1, the fact that more medical care will improve health is shown by the rise in the total benefit curve. The fact that marginal benefits become smaller as more and more services are used shows up as a lower rate of increase, reducing the slope to make it flatter.

Costs are the other side of the decision. Every additional unit of treatment adds to total costs. After start-up, the marginal cost of producing another unit of medical treatment is usually constant or rising as the total number of treatments increases. Each additional hospital bed tends to cost as much or more than the last

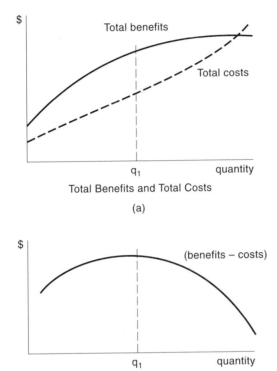

Total Benefits and Total Costs

(a)

Net Benefits

(b)

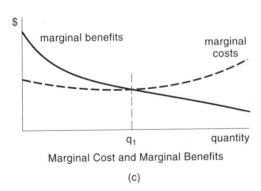

Marginal Cost and Marginal Benefits

(c)

FIGURE 2.1   *Total, Net, and Marginal Benefits and Costs*

one, and each additional nurse who is hired expects to get paid as much or more as the last one. At some point, the additional costs of extra treatments will outweigh the additional benefits. An optimum is where the net gain (benefits − costs) is largest. Diagrammatically, this can be found either by plotting both benefits and costs on the horizontal axis and choosing the point where the distance between them is greatest (Figure 2.1a), or equivalently by plotting net gains on the horizontal axis and then choosing the quantity of care where it peaks (Figure 2.1b), or finally by plotting the marginal benefit and marginal cost curves and choosing the point where they cross (Figure 2.1c).

There is a geometric property of Figure 2.1 that is frequently used by economists to determine the point at which a maximum is reached: at the peak of the net gains curve it is flat (horizontal), so its slope is 0 (Figure 2.1.b). The total benefit and total cost curves (Figure 2.1.a) have a corresponding property: at the point where net gains are maximized, their slopes are equal, so that the difference in the slopes is 0. More generally, since net gains are defined as benefits − costs, $\text{slope}_{\text{net gains}}$ = $\text{slope}_{\text{benefits}}$ − $\text{slope}_{\text{costs}}$, and at a maximum, $\text{slope}_{\text{net gains}}$ = 0. These principles of maximization common to geometry and calculus can be stated in everyday terms. As any curve or function approaches a peak, the incremental increases become smaller and smaller. The maximum occurs at the turning point, where the curve goes from rising (positive) to falling (negative). To the left, marginal gains are positive, and to the right, marginal gains are negative. Here, as the optimum is reached, the marginal gains from adding a bit more or less are 0. To determine the maximum distance between two curves, the focus is on the incremental or marginal change of one curve relative to another. If the additional (marginal) benefit from providing one more treatment is larger than the additional (marginal) cost, then providing more treatments will make society better off (Figure 2.1.c). If the additional benefit from providing one more treatment is smaller than the additional cost, then society will be made worse off. At the optimum, the additional benefit will just offset the marginal cost, and so there is no change in net gains (marginal gain = 0).

maximum net gains at: Marginal Benefit = Marginal Cost, MB − MC = 0

Average, Total, and Marginal Costs

Although it is possible to use geometry or calculus to find the average cost and average benefit as well (they are the slopes of a line from the origin to the total benefit or total cost curve, respectively), these common accounting measures are not especially useful for optimization. The largest average gain usually occurs at a point to the right of where marginal costs have long exceeded marginal benefits. **A society that uses average benefits and costs as a guide to decisions will usually end up providing far too much medical care.** To see why, consider the following illustrative example. Suppose that a new operating suite for cardiac surgery is built. The first operation will be performed on the patient who needs it the most, one who gets a major reduction in mortality (the risk of dying), say 50 percent. The next patient selected will be not quite as needy, and will obtain a significant although smaller reduction in mortality, perhaps only 40 percent. The third and fourth patients may obtain mortality reductions of 30 percent and 20 percent respectively, at which point the operating suite is full. How much benefit would be obtained by increasing capacity so that a fifth patient could be treated? If expansion allowed a fifth patient to be treated, and that patient had a 10 percent reduction in mortality, then the marginal benefit is 10 percent. However, the *average* mortality reduction is much larger, 50% + 40% + 30% + 20% + 10% ÷ 5 = 30%, making the expansion appear much more worthwhile than it really is. Whether that extra patient is scheduled to come in first or last does not make any difference. The relevant issue is that the more limited operating room space would be given to the neediest patients, and so the marginal benefit of adding one more patient (10% gain) is less than the average benefit (30% gain). In other words, the overall average gain per patient treated is a poor indicator of the marginal benefit to be gained by treating one more patient.

2.2 AN EXAMPLE OF MARGINAL ANALYSIS: COSTS AND BENEFITS OF A SIXTH STOOL GUAIAC _____

Colon cancer is a serious illness, with 109,000 new cases being diagnosed in the United States each year, of which 64,000 will be fatal, accounting for about 10 percent of all cancer deaths. One way to reduce such deaths is early detection of asymptomatic cases through screening. A "stool guaiac" is a screening test commonly used. A positive test means that occult blood is present in the feces, and this is taken as possibly indicating cancer (i.e., the cancer is causing minuscule amounts of internal bleeding that shows up in the feces), but a "false positive" may also occur due to bleeding from ulcers, diet, and random errors. Therefore, each positive test is followed up with a more specific test, such as a barium enema, which can look specifically for early and precancerous growths and rule out other causes of a positive test result. Since a single test may fail to pick up these early signs of cancer, it is common to test repeatedly even if the patient is negative the first time. In 1974, the American Cancer Society endorsed a protocol suggesting that all persons receive six stool guaiac tests in a row to screen for colon cancer. If any one of the six tests came back positive, the person screened was to be referred for further cancer evaluation. However, two researchers, Duncan Neuhauser and Ann Lewicki, decided to examine the incremental gains and costs of using five, four, or fewer tests, rather than the recommended six.[3] Their study illustrates the substantial difference between marginal and average costs.

The expected incidence of asymptomatic colon cancer among a group of 100,000 people is about 720 cases (many would die of other causes before colon cancer appeared). It is assumed that the initial stool guaiac, costing about $4, would detect 90 percent of the undiagnosed colon cancer, or 648 cases (.90 × 720, see Table 2.1).[4] However, this test would also give "false positive" results for about 20 percent of the people who did not have cancer, so that the total number of positive tests among the 100,000 persons screened would be 20,648. Each positive, whether true or false, would require a confirmatory barium-enema test costing $100. Following up false positives would account for 80 percent of the $2.5 million total program costs. The cost of cancer detection using a single test on each patient is $2,464,800 ÷ 648 cases = $3,804 per case found. While hardly trivial, this does not seem an outrageous amount to spend for early detection of potentially life-threatening cancer.

The second test would cost $1 and pick up 90 percent of remaining undiagnosed cancers, or 64.8 cases. The incremental cost for the second test, $1.7 million, is less than for the initial test, but the number of additional cases detected is far lower, so that the average cost per case detected with two tests is higher, $5,852. More importantly, the marginal cost of cancer detection with the second test is much higher, $26,335 per additional case found ($1.7 million additional costs ÷ 64.8 additional cases).

TABLE 2.1 Calculating the Costs of Using Stool Guaiac Tests to Detect New Cases of Colon Cancer

Number of Tests	Cases		New Cases Found	# Tests Positive	Costs of Screening Program				Cost Per Case Detected	
	Detected	Not			Testing	Confirmation	Total	Marginal	Average	Marginal
0	0	720	0	0	$0	$0	$0	$0	$0	$0
1	648	72	648	20,648	$400,000	$2,064,800	$2,464,800	$2,464,800	$3,804	$3,804
2	712.8	7.2	64.8	36,713	$500,000	$3,671,300	$4,171,300	$1,706,500	$5,852	$26,335
3	719.28	0.72	6.48	49,519	$600,000	$4,951,900	$5,551,900	$1,380,600	$7,719	$213,056
4	719.928	0.072	0.648	59,760	$700,000	$5,976,000	$6,676,000	$1,124,100	$9,273	$1,734,722
5	719.9928	0.0072	0.0648	67,952	$800,000	$6,795,200	$7,595,200	$919,200	$10,549	$14,185,185
6	719.99928	0.00072	0.00648	74,506	$900,000	$7,450,600	$8,350,600	$755,400	$11,598	$116,574,074

Source: Adapted from "What do we gain from the Sixth Stool Guaiac?" by Duncan Neuhauser and Ann Lewicki, *New England Journal of Medicine*, Volume 293, pp. 226–228 (1975). The table assumes that 100,000 persons are to be screened, and that if perfect, the test would detect 720 cases of colon cancer. Each additional test will find 90% of the undetected cases, so that the first test will find .90 × 720 = 648 cases, the next test will find an additional .90 × 72 = 64.8 cases, and so on. However, the test will also be falsely positive for 20% of the people who do not have cancer. Thus with one test, about 20,000 people with no cancer as well as the 648 with cancer will test positive. With two tests, about 36,000 false positives will occur (i.e., 20,000 from the first test, plus 20% of the 80,000 cancer-free people who were negative on the first test). It is assumed that the cost of stool guaiacs is $4 for the first test, and $1 for each additional test, and that each person who tests positive will be given a barium-enema test to confirm whether or not cancer is really present costing $100.

The third, fourth, fifth, and sixth test would each cost $1 and would each pick up 90 percent of the cancers not yet diagnosed. These additional tests are finding very few new cases of cancer, but are still generating a substantial number of false positives. Since 5 tests will have uncovered almost all (719.9928 out of 720) of the cancer, the additional cases of cancer detected by the sixth test is an almost negligibly small .0065—but the sixth stool guaiac will still account for 100,000 tests and another 6,554 false positives, so that the marginal cost per case detected for the sixth stool guaiac is $755,400 ÷ .0065, an almost astronomical $116,574,074 per additional case found.

In order to complete a cost–benefit analysis, the dollar value of early cancer detection must be estimated. The discussion of valuation methodology is deferred to section 2.9, but in order to illustrate the process, an arbitrary benefit per case of cancer detected of $100,000 is assumed, with comparisons to a range of other values (from $1,000 to $10 million) to see how significantly different measures of benefits would change the results. Total benefits can be determined by multiplying value per case by the number of cases detected. Using one test will detect 648 cases, which, at $100,000 each, implies total benefits of $64,800,000. With two tests, 712.8 cases are detected, for total benefits of $71,280,000. With six tests, 720 cases are detected, for total benefits of $72,000,000. Total benefits and total costs for the range of decisions (0 to 6 tests) are graphed in Figure 2.2a. The total benefit curve is above the total cost curve throughout, indicating that any amount of stool guaiac screening from one to six tests generates positive net gains over the no-screening alternative. The maximum net gains (benefits minus costs) are obtained with a screening program that uses two tests, as can be seen from Figure 2.2b, or using the marginal curves (Figure 2.2c). The marginal cost of the third test is $1,380,600, while it detects only 6.48 additional cases of cancer, for marginal benefits of $648,000. The first test yields very large gains and is clearly worthwhile. The second test has a marginal cost of $1,706,500 and detects 64.8 cases, generating marginal benefits of $6,480,000, and is thus also seen to provide net gains. Marginal analysis shows that the optimal level of screening is obtained by using just two tests. The conclusion that two tests are "better" than three tests depends on the value the analysis places on detecting a case of cancer (here, $100,000). Three tests will find 6.48 more cases, and potentially allow treatment to extend someone's life, but the additional health benefits are deemed to be worth less than the cost—$648,000 versus $1,380,600. The original program with six tests is better than doing nothing, as indicated by the result that the average cost per case of $11,598 is less than the $100,000 average benefit, but the fact that the marginal cost of $116,574,074 is much higher indicates that a screening program using fewer tests will provide greater net gains (see Table 2.2).

The cost per case of cancer detected in this example depends on several factors. If the prevalence of colon cancer in the group being screened were greater than 720 cases per 100,000 population, then more cancer would be detected and the cost per case (both marginal and average) would be lower. Conversely, a population with a lower cancer prevalence would have a higher cost per case, and a larger percentage of those who tested positive would, in fact, turn out to be false positives. A better test would be more specific to colon cancer, with a lower false positivity rate. If the stool guaiac did not so frequently indicate cancer when none was present, then the cost per case detected would be much smaller. The appropriate

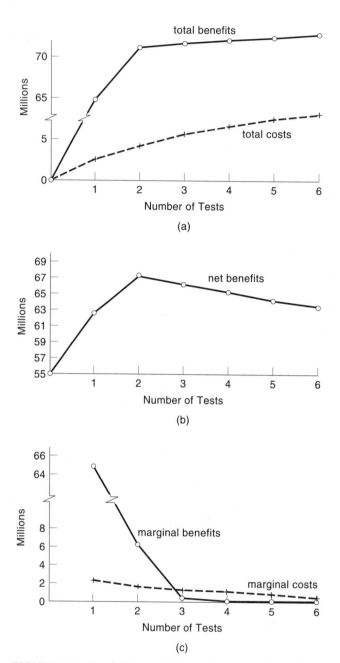

FIGURE 2.2 *Total Net, and Marginal Cost and Benefits—Stool Guaiacs*

level of testing also depends on the estimated benefits of detection. Most of the cases, and most of the benefits, are found with the first test. If the value per case were $10,000, then just one test per person would be optimal. If the value per case were $1 million, then three tests would be optimal. Trying out different assumptions regarding costs, benefits, therapeutic effectiveness and disease prevalence to

TABLE 2.2   Calculating Benefits and Optimal Level of Stool Guaiac Testing
Total, net, and marginal costs and benefits of stool guaiac screening

Number of Tests	Cases Detected	Total Benefits	Total Costs	Net Benefits	Marginal Benefits	Marginal Costs
0	0	$0	$0	$0		
1	648	$64,800,000	$2,464,800	$62,335,200	$64,800,000	$2,464,800
2	712.8	$71,280,000	$4,171,300	$67,108,700	$6,480,000	$1,706,500
3	719.28	$71,928,000	$5,551,900	$66,376,100	$648,000	$1,380,600
4	719.928	$71,992,800	$6,676,000	$65,316,800	$64,800	$1,124,100
5	719.9928	$71,999,280	$7,595,200	$64,404,080	$6,480	$919,200
6	719.99928	$71,999,928	$8,350,600	$63,649,328	$648	$755,400

Source: See Table 2.1. Table 2.2 assumes value of each case detected is $100,000. For alternate assumptions, see text.

see how much they affect the results of CBA is called "sensitivity analysis." Here, a hundred-fold variation in estimated benefit (from $10,000 to $1 million) only changes the recommendations slightly, from one test to three tests. A little algebra and examination of Table 2.2. shows that any level of estimated benefit per case between $27,000 and $210,000 would lead to a recommendation of two tests per person. While the exact value of early cancer detection is hard to estimate precisely, it is unlikely that it falls much outside the range that would support one to three tests, and is certainly less than the $100 million needed to justify doing all six tests, as originally proposed. The Neuhauser and Lewicki article and subsequent cost–benefit studies have been influential in convincing the American Cancer Society to revise their recommendations in 1980, and again in 1992, to take a more conservative stance. Now, routine stool guaiac screening is recommended only for individuals over age 50, or whose family history makes them at high risk for colorectal cancer.[5]

This study illustrates several important elements of cost–benefit analysis. First, the marginal cost is often quite different from the average cost. Second, the direct cost (screening) may be much less than the indirect costs of dealing with unintended side-effects (barium-enema test to rule out cancer among those falsely testing positive). Taken together, these observations suggest the following **rule for making medicine cost-effective: target diagnosis and treatment on those persons at highest risk.** This principle seems so obvious that it hardly needs to be stated, but it is routinely violated. Our desire to do as much as possible for as many as possible means that effective screening programs are extended to everyone—including healthy young people with almost no risk of disease—and so the marginal cost per case becomes very high. At least some of the rapid growth in medical care costs can be attributed to this general failure to distinguish average costs from marginal costs, when it is actually marginal costs that are relevant to the question of "how much" medical care should be provided. Thousands of lives are saved by modern medicine each year—and more than 95 percent of those lives could still be saved even if half of the system were eliminated, so long as we continued to screen and treat those at highest risk.

2.3   AN EVERYDAY EXAMPLE: KNEE INJURY _____

Every decision —whether in the market, the public sector, or the family—involves a form of cost–benefit analysis. Usually the consideration of costs and benefits is informal and internal, so we are not conscious of it. Only the behavior that results from this internal weighing of costs and benefits can be observed. Life, and the medical care system in particular, confronts us with difficult choices every day. Is it worth taking three hours, and maybe having to pay $100, to go to the emergency room so a doctor can look at the throbbing knee you injured playing soccer? Since the pain makes it difficult to think, it can be easier to keep track of your thoughts if you make a list of the pros and cons.

Cost–Benefit Analysis (CBA) of Knee Injury (*first step*)

PROS (go to ER)	*CONS* (don't go)
It might stop the pain.	It will cost $50, $100, or more.
It could prevent long-term injury.	It will take at least two, and maybe four, hours.
I will feel stupid if something was wrong and I did not go.	Even if the injury is serious, surgery could make it worse, not better.
I can't get any work done anyway while I sit here worrying about it.	My buddies on the team will think I am a wimp.

If you think the benefits of going to the doctor outweigh the costs, then you will call a friend to take you to the emergency room. Even if you do not write down the pros and cons, a similar type of mental balancing takes place inside your head. CBA is the explicit and formal presentation of that mental balance sheet. Economics does not provide any answers, or make it easier to take bitter medicine, but it does clarify *how to ask the question* in order to make decisions more rational and more consistent. First, *enumerate* the benefits and costs as was done in the preceding list. Then, *quantify* each of them as well as possible, given what is known about the situation. It is impossible to tell exactly how much time it will take in the emergency room (ER), but you think a range of two to four hours is likely. A *value* must then be placed on each benefit and cost item. A balance sheet can be added up only if every line is expressed in the same terms, usually dollars. It would not make much sense to compare a benefit of $50 with a cost of ¥910 (yen), and there is no rule for determining how many hours of pain are worth avoiding a permanent limp, while it is very clear that a cost of $500 is less than a benefit of $1,000.

This hypothetical knee injury can be used to illustrate cost–benefit analysis. The direct dollar cost of the emergency room visit is expected to be about $80. In addition, you expect to wait for three hours. Since you could have been at a job where you make $7 per hour, we can add $21 for the *opportunity cost* of the waiting time. The possibility that surgery will make you worse instead of better we will take up later. Being made to feel like a wimp seems silly, but it is worth something. How much? Suppose that you were willing to pay $40 for crutches that you really did not need, just to keep your buddies from making fun of you. This **willingness to pay** $40 reveals the dollar value of your revealed preference for avoiding a "wimp" label. Adding all the items together, your estimated comprehensive total cost for going to the ER is $80 (charges) + $21 (time) + $40 (WTP fear) = $141 (see Table 2.3).

It is reasonable to assume that if your knee does not get better, you will eventually seek treatment, even if you don't go to the ER immediately. Let's suppose that before you injured your knee, you had already made an appointment to go to the sports medicine clinic a week from Thursday. Therefore, the relevant costs and benefits are for treatment today versus treatment ten days from now, rather than treatment versus no treatment. *Only count those items that change as a result of your decision—the marginal benefits and costs.* The potential that a visit to the ER will stop the pain is counted on the list of pros and cons as a benefit. The labeling is somewhat arbitrary, and it would have been equally correct to have said that the potential for continued pain was a cost of not going to the ER. A reduction in cost is the same thing as a benefit, since both are expressed in dollar terms. It is this equivalence that makes it possible to create a balance sheet for decision making. If benefits and costs were not expressed in the same terms (dollars) with opposite signs (+ or −), then one could not say which was greater.

What is it worth to stop the pain? Suppose that instead of going to the ER, you could just call the clinic and have them phone a prescription to the pharmacy. How much would you be willing to pay to get the prescription rather than endure the pain? It is hard to study, and may be impossible to work, when you are in pain. It is also hard to sleep, or even to enjoy watching television. You might be willing to pay as much as $150 for relief from pain for the next ten days. This willingness to pay (WTP) is the correct measure of the value of benefit received. WTP is the mirror image of opportunity cost, the "highest valued opportunity forgone." Different people would put different values on what it is worth to endure pain. Furthermore, your estimate of its worth to you will be imprecise, because you don't frequently make deals trading money for pain. However, your refusal to spend $200 for some pills demonstrates that the value of pain relief is less than $200 for you. The value is somewhere between the lower ($0) and upper ($200) bounds. Is it worth $40, $50, $150, or more? There is no way to tell unless we can observe your entire demand curve.

There is an overstatement of benefits here, since the pills are virtually certain to relieve pain, whereas the visit to the ER may or may not. Clearly a chance of reduced pain is worth less than the certainty of reduced pain, but how much less? An approximate **adjustment for risk** can be made by calculating the **expected value.** Assume that we have made enough observations to know that the average person would be willing to pay $150 for relief of this knee pain. If we think there is a 1-in-3 chance that going to the ER now will stop the pain, then the expected benefit of this one third chance of pain reduction is one-third of the $150 I would be willing to pay for certain pain reduction; i.e. $50.

The most important benefit of prompt treatment is probably a reduction in the risk of permanent injury. People are willing to pay thousands of dollars and undergo multiple operations to try to have their knees fixed. Although your personal valuation is the only one that is truly relevant, the values established by other people may provide a useful guide since you have not had hundreds of opportunities

TABLE 2.3   Knee Injury as an Example of Cost–Benefit Analysis

Scenario: I injured my knee playing soccer this afternoon. I called and got an appointment to go to orthopedics/sports medicine clinic in ten days, next Thursday. However, it has now begun to hurt a lot and I wonder if I should go to the emergency room (ER) right away.

CONS (don't go)

Visit to ER will cost $50, $100, or more. *(direct personal cost, ignores cost to insurance)*	average	=	$80
I will have to wait for at least 2, maybe 4 hours. *(opportunity cost)*	3 hours × $7	=	$21
My buddies on the team will think I am a wimp. *(willing to pay $40 for crutches just to look good)*	willingness to pay	=	$40
Even if the injury is serious, surgery could make it worse. *(the issue is treatment today v. thursday, rather than treatment v. no treatment so only incremental costs count)*	sunk cost	=	$0
	Total Costs		**$141**

PROS (go to ER now)

Might stop the pain. *(pills stop pain with certainty, going to ER just a 1-in-3 chance)*	$150 × 1/3	=	$50
Could prevent long-term injury. *(WTP knee surgery $50,000, 1/200 chance, discount 7 years @ 5%)*	$50,000 × 1/200 × .71	=	$178
Will feel stupid if something was wrong and I did not go. *("worried well" WTP for regular office visit)*	willingness to pay	=	$20
I can't get any work done anyway while I sit here worrying about it. *(time has same $ value for benefits and costs)*	6 hours × $7	=	$42
	Total Benefits		**$290**

Observed behavior just gives us a lower bound that benefits exceed costs (>$141). Another observation, that I did not go when the wait was 5 hours and ER charges were $250, could provide an upper bound as well (<$325).

to figure out how much an injury is worth. Let's say that your estimate of the loss imposed by a bad knee is worth $50,000. This is a lot of money, but the chance that going to the doctor this week rather than next week will make a difference is slight, maybe 0.5% (1-in-200). Thus, the expected value of prompt versus delayed treatment is one-two-hundredths of $50,000 or $250. Furthermore, it is likely that if the knee does cause you a problem, it will be some years in the future. While that is still bad, it is not as bad as being harmed today. To take account of the fact that the problem will not occur for a while, we should **time discount** the $250, using the methods provided in section 2.10. This reduces the expected marginal benefit of prompt treatment to $178.

The fear of stupidly failing to seek treatment for a problem that could have been cured if seen promptly is quite common. Indeed, some studies have estimated that over 70 percent of all initial visits to the doctor are made by the "worried well," people who have some vague symptom and just need evaluation and reassurance rather than any treatment.[6] A modest lower bound for the value of worry reduction might be the price of a brief diagnostic office visit, or $20. What about the loss of work time due to pain and worry? These hours should be valued the same as the waiting time in the ER, or $7 an hour. If you think that a prompt visit will help you avoid six hours of wasted time between now and the appointment next Thursday, that is worth 6 × $7 or $42. The sum total of all the benefits is $50 (pain) + $178 (prevention) + $20 (worry) + $42 (time) = $290.

You go to the ER. Although you are doing so because your subjective estimate of total benefits ($290) outweigh your subjective estimate of total costs ($141), no numbers ever get printed inside your brain. You don't find yourself being wheeled into the ER saying "I'm happy because I've got a projected consumer surplus of $149 ($290 − $141) from coming here." You just do it, or you don't. An economist takes that choice as the true indicator of your personal and largely unconscious cost–benefit analysis. Your preferences would be revealed in more detail if we could observe you in another situation where you chose not to go. Suppose you arrived at the ER, found out that the wait would be 5 hours instead of three, the dollar cost to you $250 instead of $80, and you left without waiting to be seen. This would provide the analyst with a second set of costs ($325), which exceeded benefits, and so set an upper bound on estimated total benefits.

2.4 EXPECTED VALUE _____

Expected value is a core concept of risk analysis. If the analysis concerns many people, so that the law of large numbers applies, then the expected value is just the average.* For a single person facing an event that either will or will not happen, the expected value is the value of that event (benefit or cost) multiplied by the fraction of the time that the event will occur.

$$\text{Expected Value of } Z = (\text{Probability } Z \text{ will occur}) \times (\text{Value of } Z)$$

A patient receiving chemotherapy with a 70 percent chance of death may live, while a patient receiving surgery with a 20 percent chance of death may not. Yet

---

*The "law of large numbers" says that the observed average will be close to the "true" mean if the number of observations is large enough.

the decision must be made in advance, and should maximize expected welfare in the face of this uncertainty. Of course after the fact the patient's family may wish that they had done something differently. To say that the optimal choice sometimes turns out worse is just to recognize that life is full of risks. Cost–benefit analysis is based on the best available estimate of probability. It may be a subjective guess, or, preferably, an extrapolation from well-designed studies reported in scientific journals that the analyst references. "I don't know," or "I need more information," are not valid responses, since a decision is going to be made regardless of how much is or is not known. The job of the analyst is to get the best estimate, and to indicate the sources of information and the range of variability—but not to make excuses. A clear discussion of the alternatives in specific terms is required. Under this useful shorthand formula, an option is chosen if:

$$(\text{Probability of Gain}) \times (\text{Benefit}) > (\text{Probability of Loss}) \times (\text{Cost})$$

In this formula, attention is focused separately on the uncertainty and the relative values that interact in the decision process. Judgmental advice, such as "it is better to get the operation and risk dying than not get the operation and remain impaired" jumbles probabilities and values together, hiding information and making communication more difficult. Such commingled statements do not make the patient think about how much it is worth to live impaired relative to dying, nor to consider what the actual probability of partial recovery, or of death, really is. An explicit recognition of benefits, costs, and risks provides a better ground for shared decision making between physician and patient.

For situations involving many people and events with more than one outcome, such as the expected medical costs of a family of six people, each of whom could, over the coming year, be well, slightly sick, or seriously ill, then the expected value is a weighted average of all the possibilities, with the weights being the probability that each outcome could occur (e.g., it may be that family members have a 60 percent chance of remaining well, 30 percent chance of becoming slightly sick, and 10 percent chance of being seriously ill).

$$\text{Expected Value} = \frac{\Sigma[(\text{probability that } Z \text{ will occur for person } i) \times (\text{Value of } Z_i)]}{\text{number of persons}}$$

2.5   MEASURING BENEFITS _____

For most medical programs, the three major types of benefits are:

- Health
- Productivity
- Reductions in future medical costs

Health

Better health is the most direct and important gain from medical care. Yet it is often difficult to determine how much change in health status is actually an effect of the medical program, and how much is just due to waiting for things to heal, random variation, nutrition, and other factors. If a cancer patient lives eight months, is that six months longer than the patient would have without treatment, or six month less, since the chemotherapy is so toxic?[7] Such obstacles to valid measurement of the effects of treatment usually limit CB analysis to studies of large groups of patients where statistics can be used to estimate average effects. After the effect of therapy is measured, the problem of placing a dollar value on the improvement in health must be faced. If faster treatment can save the average heart-attack victim four months of life, is that worth $1,000? $100,000? $1,000,000? or perhaps $19.95? Most people would agree than gaining an extra year of life is worth more than $1,000 and less than $1,000,000, but deciding exactly where, within that range, the appropriation valuation lies is crucial in determining whether it is worth spending $50 million to upgrade the 911 emergency telephone system. Some innovative techniques for measuring the value of life are explored in section 2.9, but it is important to recognize now how difficult and ambiguous the measurement process is. Most health care provides more subtle gains (e.g., physical therapy that improves mobility, medication that lessens the pain from a headache), which are even harder to measure in dollar terms.

A significant fraction of all visits to the doctor, perhaps as much as half, do not make a difference in health status. Either the symptoms that led people to seek care were not serious, or the condition was such that medical care could not change the course of the disease. The remainder provide care, reassurance, and social support, but not cure. The benefits of "caring" are often left uncounted because they are small relative to the gains from a dramatic cure. Also, much the same benefit can often be obtained regardless of the type or scientific validity of the treatment (e.g., a naturopath may provide sympathy as well as or better than a trained neurologist).

Productivity

The earliest economists were not so much interested in the value of health itself, as in how much a healthier work force could contribute to the economy. In 1667, Sir William Petty [8] proposed a plan to improve the treatment of the plague in England, and wrote out an analysis showing that the additional costs would be more than covered by the additional taxes obtained from having more people at work.* When modern economists turned their attention to evaluating health programs in the 1950s and 1960s, the difficulty of directly measuring and valuing health improvements led them to consider increases in earnings due to greater life expectancy and reduced sick days as a proxy measure. Such gains can be measured with precision, are objectively verifiable, and were easy to obtain from existing labor statistics. These advantages made earnings the primary measure of benefits in CBA for the next twenty years, but now they are considered inadequate. Are women's lives to be counted as worth less than men's since female

---

*Petty, arguably the first real economist, was no stranger to self-interest or pride. He asked for 2 percent of the net increase in tax revenues from his plague treatment plan be given to him as a reward from the King for his brilliant idea. He did not fully specify how those gains would be figured. Had he done so, health economists today might be much more effective, competing for millions of dollars in health benefits royalties.

earnings are lower on average? Are old people worthless once they stop working? Contributions to society through the labor market are a clear benefit of health care, but by themselves they form an incomplete and biased measure.

Reductions in Future Medical Costs

Many diseases are less costly to treat if care is given early, and if treatment is done correctly the first time. Vaccination now can prevent hospitalization in the future. Better infection control will allow patients to be discharged sooner. Yet good medical care is not always, or even usually, cheaper. The least expensive way to treat heart attacks is never to attempt resuscitation. A transplant may mean ten more years of life, but it will certainly mean hundreds of thousands of dollars in additional care. Reductions in cost, while not insignificant, can hardly constitute the primary justification for medical care.

2.6 MEASURING COSTS _____

The primary types of costs are:

- Medical care and administration
- Follow-up and treatment damages
- Time and pain of patient and family
- Provider time and inconvenience

Medical Costs and Charges

Three methods are used to obtain the direct costs of medical care: adjusted charges, cost accounting, and extrapolation from comparable services. While the prices charged for transportation, food, and clothing can be taken as reasonable estimates of the costs of providing these services in a market economy, medical prices cannot.[9] Most medical prices are overstated to cover related expenses for education, research, community outreach, and charity care to patients who cannot pay. **Adjusted charges** for U.S. hospital care are usually estimated by multiplying billed charges by the medicare cost-to-charge ratio (see chapter 8, section 2). The actual costs of hospital services are only about 60 percent of the billed charges on average. For some services, such as laboratory and drugs, costs may be as little as 15 percent of charges, while for ER and obstetrical services, costs may be as much as 125 percent of charges. Per-unit costs are always estimates, and are somewhat ambiguous and subject to interpretation, since they depend on numerous assumptions regarding overhead allocation, counting, and averaging of quality and quantity. **Cost accounting** for CBA uses the same principles as job costing in other industries. Resources (nursing hours, technician time, space, supplies, etc.) are estimated from direct observation and costed using prevailing wages, prices, and so on, and then an overhead charge is applied for administration, utilities, and other central services. Specialized job costing studies for the most expensive elements of care are often combined with the more readily available adjusted charges for other types. **Extrapolation from comparable services** is used when charges are not available and cost accounting is too time-consuming. For example, the costs of keeping patients in the hospital when they need only custodial care could be extrapolated from the cost of a day in a nursing home. Likewise, the cost of services provided by salaried physicians in a public health clinic may be extrapolated from adjusted charges for similar services in nearby communities.

Follow-Up and Treatment

While the direct costs are almost always counted, most medical care also creates **secondary treatment costs.** In the colon cancer example earlier, the largest cost is not the screening test itself, but all of the additional laboratory work done on those who never had the disease but whose initial test results were falsely positive. Also extended recovery in a nursing home may be far more costly to a seventy-year-old than the charges for the knee operation that put him there. It is also necessary to include as a cost the risks of serious complications and death that attend any surgery. The general point is that most medical care (and other human attempts to do good) involve many secondary or unintended effects that must be included for a comprehensive accounting.

Time and Pain of Patient and Family

The time that patients lose and the pain they suffer often outweighs any direct medical costs. It is common to value patient time at the average wage rate for all employed workers.[10] Using different rates for men and women, children, elderly, or minorities usually contributes little to the analysis, and may incorporate institutionalized discrimination. However, such differentials may do quite a lot to explain individual differences in behavior because they are very real to the person choosing whether to obtain care. Pain, suffering, anxiety, and death are most appropriately valued according to that person's willingness to pay. A reason many "obviously" beneficial treatments are not sought is that the analyst has not considered the patient's point of view, and neglected the costs of time and pain.

Provider Time and Inconvenience

The supply-side reason for not undertaking many medical activities is that the time and inconvenience to providers is not compensated. For example, while there is a tremendous need for organ donations, the physicians who must obtain the families' consent are not the transplant surgeons who benefit from doing additional transplants, but the ER physicians, neurosurgeons, and internists who are present at death and who find the effort of explaining to families and harvesting organs a burden. Managed care plans (chapters 10 and 11), by requiring documentation for every hospital admission or specialist referral, are able to reduce utilization. The provider "hassle cost" of such administrative requirements, rather than denials of medically inappropriate care, is responsible for as much as half of the reduction in medical costs obtained by managed care firms. While some people have considered this reduction in services a sign that managed care plans ration care to reduce costs and make profits, it is important to remember that the services forgone were those for which the patient's physician was unwilling to write a letter or make a phone call to support, and therefore are unlikely to have been considered critically important.

2.7 COMPETITION AND INCREASING EFFICIENCY

In order to raise productivity, meet the challenge of competition, and improve the health of citizens, a health care system must address five issues:

What processes should be used?	*technical efficiency*
Which combination of inputs is best?	*cost efficiency*
How much should be produced?	*allocative efficiency*
How should contracts be formed with customers and suppliers?	*transactions costs*
How should production change over time?	*dynamic efficiency*

Carrying out production so as to obtain the maximum amount of output for any given set of inputs yields *technical efficiency* and defines the production function. Choosing inputs so as to minimize cost of production yields *cost efficiency.* Yet the production of output is not an end in itself. The task of organizations is to provide benefits to customers, and also to satisfy the vendors who supply inputs, salaried workers, unions, government, and other interested parties. Both demand and supply-side considerations must enter into deciding how much to produce, the distribution of goods to consumers, and of incomes to producers. Jointly maximizing the total value of output is necessary to achieve *allocative efficiency.*

It is not easy, or cheap, to coordinate the complex exchanges necessary for a modern economy. Salespeople, insurance agents, lawyers, clerks, computer programmers, and accountants are all components of *transactions costs.* In health care, insurance, finance, and other complex systems, the costs of transacting and exchange are especially high, and far exceed the direct costs of production. Structuring organizations to economize on transactions costs and promote efficiency through property rights, professional associations, and regulations is the underlying theme of most of the chapters in this book. Understanding *dynamic efficiency,* how to create technological and organizational change so as to improve economic efficiency in the future, is even more challenging. In his justly famed *History of Economic Analysis,* Joseph Schumpeter[11] attributed growth in a mature market economy to a process of "creative destruction," yet little is really known about how entrepreneurial renewal occurs, except that some current efficiency must be sacrificed. Scientists must spend time tinkering to make new discoveries, managers must have some slack to come up with ideas for new products and service delivery systems, and a purely cost-minimizing organization is not likely to be the most creative one.

How can an organization lower the costs of production? Why would it want to? Do not assume that more competition and greater efficiency is always good and desired by everyone. Competition is beneficial for the system as a whole, but for any given individual, more competition means more anxiety, working harder, and more chances of failure. Greater efficiency comes at a cost to the individuals involved. First of all, change itself is difficult and often painful. Some workers will not be able to make the transition. Those that do are usually those that try harder, that go and spend some time learning new techniques, and that are willing to make mistake after mistake in order to perfect the production process. All of the effort required to increase productivity is clearly beneficial to the firm, and to the economy, but is worthwhile to the worker only to the extent that he or she shares in the benefits from increased production through higher wages, more time off, and so on. If workers are paid by the hour regardless of the organization's output, why should they innovate or exert themselves? Capturing the benefits of increased productivity requires managers that know what gains are possible, an awareness of the costs to all of the people in the organization, and a willingness to share some of the gains with them.

2.8 PERSPECTIVES: PATIENT, PAYER, GOVERNMENT, PROVIDER, SOCIETY _____

How much has to be paid, and how much it is worth, depends on whose perspective the cost–benefit analyst is taking. From the point of view of the individual, treatment that makes an infectious disease less communicable is of no direct benefit, and medical costs may be relatively unimportant because of insurance. From a group perspective, reducing communicability to neighbors is a major benefit of treatment, and hospital charges are important because total insurance premiums for the group as a whole will rise. The broadest perspective is that of society as a whole, including future generations.

Many of the conflicts over health policy arise from the difference in perspectives of different groups. For gay men in San Francisco, a quarter or more of whom have the HIV virus, AIDS research and prevention is the most important health issue of our time, while finding drugs to assist in stroke rehabilitation is not.[12] For residents of the Christian Acres Retirement Community in a small midwestern town, those priorities are reversed. An economist hired by Medicare to do a CBA on whether or not a new type of surgery should be covered must ask, "Am I to consider primarily the effects on the Medicare budget, or should also I include benefits to hospitals, doctors, and state legislatures?" The treatment of taxes and transfers is crucial in this regard. If new Medicare regulations cost Medicare $100, but reduce state Medicaid expenditures by $40, is that reduction to be counted? From the perspective of the state, it is a windfall gain of $40. From the perspective of the U.S. budget, and the Medicare administrator, it is a cost of $100. From a social perspective, the shifting of costs from state to federal budgets is irrelevant, and the cost is the net amount, $60. Consider, also, the effect of taxes. If a 10 percent tax on health care makes the effective price of a $20 visit to the doctor $22, the extra $2 is a relevant cost to the patient or the insurance plan, but not to society. If there were no "health tax" then that $2 would have to be obtained elsewhere by raising other taxes, or by reducing government spending on roads or defense, for example.

Distribution: Whose Costs and Whose Benefits?

In the real world, people may feel that they should consider benefits to society as a whole, but they act according to a more immediate calculus of benefits and costs to them as individuals, and to the groups (teenagers, steelworkers, residents of Lancaster, hispanics, senior citizens, etc.) to which they belong. A major barrier to actually implementing a project is raised by the following question: what about the losers? Laser surgery for cancer may help thousands of people who would not have survived with the chemotherapy previously used, but it will also kill some people who would have lived. Development of a new home health system means that the hospital down the street will find even more of its beds empty, and have to lay off some employees. It is almost impossible to make a major change that hurts no one. Unfortunately, it is also almost impossible for a politician to vote for a project that clearly hurts some identifiable person. Programs are more likely to pass when the costs are diffused over a large number of people, and thus difficult to identify. For example, a requirement for more extensive testing of drugs or better disposal of toxic wastes leads to a general rise in the cost of medicine. Even though in total it amounts to millions of dollars, it takes only a few pennies per prescription and thus is ignored. Conversely, imposing a loss of just a few thousand dollars on a single individual or firm is sufficient to get them to file a lawsuit to stop the program. The relative power of the group that must bear most of the costs often determines political feasibility of any change.

CBA is a Limited Perspective

While CBA is a powerful tool for policy analysis, it can also be quite limited. It is impossible to do an economic analysis unless the medical facts are well known. How many people have the disease, what is the cure rate from therapy, and what levels of disability are likely to result? These are all clinical questions that must be answered before any assessment of costs and benefits is attempted. The strength of CBA as a tool lies in its ability to interpret medical issues as choices in a market. Yet to do so it must force health and human caring into such a rigid economic model that it tends to overemphasize efficiency, and may entirely fail to recognize the most important ethical and social values that underlie medical practice. Medicine as a profession rests on the dignity and sanctity of life, a philosophy and practice that resists overt commercialization.

CBA and Public Policy Decision Making

Cost–benefit analysis is a way of looking at past behavior, at decisions actually made, so that future decisions can become more clear, rational, and consistent. A decision being made by a single person was used in the illustrative knee injury example. In practice, CB analyses are almost never done for a single case since it takes too long, costs too much, and depends on statistical assumptions that are more valid for large groups. When a single person is involved, that person knows their personal costs and willingness to pay better than any analyst can. Formal analyses are apt to be most useful when:

1. Large amounts of resources ($millions or $billions) are involved.
2. Responsibility for decisions is fragmented (government agencies, large corporations).
3. The goals and objectives of different groups are at odds or unclear.
4. Alternative courses of action are radically different.
5. The technology and risks underlying each alternative are well understood.
6. A long time frame is involved (e.g., strategy versus management).

Econometrics, balance sheets, surveys, decision trees, and other tools of the economics trade are usually applied to large projects or problems of long standing: is screening blood donors for AIDS and hepatitis worthwhile? How often should they be screened, and with what tests? Is inpatient alcohol treatment better than outpatient, and if so, is it enough to justify the increase in costs? The treatment of millions of people costing billions of dollars over many years is involved in each of these issues that have been given full formal cost–benefit analysis. The test of what is important ultimately lies in the judgment of those who are most affected by the decision. Health CBA almost always counts two things, death and money, because they are routinely recorded. A good analysis is able to capture those other factors that are significant, and yet keep the presentation simple enough that the costs and benefits of alternative courses of action are clearly seen.

2.9 THE VALUE OF LIFE _____

"A man who knows the price of everything and the value of nothing."
Oscar Wilde's definition of a cynic.

Isn't health priceless? Some patients and physicians protest that it is impossible to measure the priceless benefits of medical care with the crude yardstick of money. Whether or not you think you can do so, whether it is right or proper, your actions place a dollar value on human life and injury whenever a decision is made to provide treatment. If an 87-year-old in heart failure transferred from a nursing home is placed in a Cardiac Care Unit for ten days, then the physician has stated through his or her actions that living another six months in a nursing home is worth more than $15,000. Immediately discharging that patient back with a prescription to take four aspirin every six hours says it is not. It is not a matter of whether or not we want to value life and health in money terms. Our acts place a dollar value on life even if we do not choose to recognize it. We live in a world of scarce resources, and have to make decisions within those limitations. Perhaps the most important role of economists in the cost–benefit analysis of health care is that forced reality check—if you don't want to have to deal with the problem of who to save, who to fire, who to charge, who is to be *responsible*, then you should accept that such irresponsibility makes you irrelevant. We place a value on health whether we want to or not, and money is the most generalized form of expressing those values.*

Valuing human life places special, but unavoidable, demands on economists. For activities that are traded in the market such as medical care, work time, drugs, and transportation, valuation may be complicated by risk and discounting, or blurred by overhead allocation and wage differentials. However, the process of connecting resources used and program effects to specific dollar amounts is understandable and even familiar. Considerations of life and death, or pain and suffering, are not so clear. Since there is no explicit market for post-operative pain and mortality, some way must be found to reflect the value that people place on these events. By choosing to buy a car that is cheaper but less safe, a person is making an implicit trade between money and the risk of dying. That trade is also made in buying smoke alarms, choosing to accept a more dangerous job assignment for higher pay, refusing to fill a prescription because it costs too much, and flying to the Mayo clinic to get the best possible treatment for a rare disease. People buy and sell health all the time, but they do not do so in some organized market like the New York Stock Exchange. *Economists do not put a value on life or illness; they measure the value that consumer's put on life and illness as shown by their behavior.*

One attempt to provide an explicit dollar value for life is described by Michael Jones-Lee.[10] It was observed that people would run across a highway (at some small but noticeable risk of dying) rather than spend the time going around to a pedestrian overpass.[13] Through observations and questionnaires, it could be established that people were willing to accept a risk of .000002 of death in order to save seven minutes (0.117 hours) of walking. Valuing their time by an average wage rate of $20, the value of life as can be extrapolated:

Value of Life: Jones-Lee Approach

$$\text{Value of life} = \frac{(\text{Value of Time}) \times (\text{Hours Used})}{(\text{Risk of Death per hour saved})} = \frac{\$20 \times .117}{.000002} = \$1,170,000$$

A somewhat more sophisticated approach is to take as the value of life the amount of additional earning required to get someone to take a more dangerous job. A statistical regression[14] of the association between wages and risk showed that for each .0001 increase in risk of death, there was an additional $240 in annual salary, so that the estimated value of life in this method for this study was

---

*A decision maker's preferences are said to be "lexicographic" when everything depends on one factor, with other factors allowed to affect choice only when they are all equal on that primary factor. For example, a parent might order a physician "Do whatever you can to maximize my child's chance of living. Given that, if one treatment will be less painful, or cost less, you can do that one." This decision is lexicographic since one factor, the probability of the child's survival, dominates all others. In such a case there are no trade-offs, and hence no necessity to make an economic analysis such as CBA. Computers sort alphabetic lists lexicographically: rank by the first letter, then by the second, and so on. People often claim that there is one thing which is important above all others (survival, honor, religious purity) even though most behavior indicates that in fact trade-offs are made. Even saints respond to pain, and a parent is not acting nobly if they do everything trying to save one child and in the process ruin their own lives and that of their other children. Arguing that medicine should only consider costs when there is no chance that it will affect quality or risk lives is the same as saying that money does not matter in the real world.

$240/.0001 = $2.4 million. Other studies using similar methods have estimated values of life from $800,000 to $6 million.[15] One problem with occupational risk estimates is what is called "selection bias"; the people who are less risk-averse or mistakenly underestimate the true risk are the ones most likely to apply for the more dangerous jobs. A study that captures the behavior of the more safety-conscious individuals was carried out by Rachel Dardis.[16] She measured the number of people purchasing smoke detectors as a function of price to construct a demand curve (Figure 2.3). In 1974 the price of smoke detectors was $52 each, and only 1.8 million were sold (adjusted for inflation, $52 in 1974 is worth $150 in 1995, and Dardis estimated an annualized operating cost per household of $20 in 1995 dollars). By 1979, the price had declined to $12, and 10 million were sold (which is $24, inflation-adjusted, and yields annualized cost of $3 a year). Each smoke detector was estimated to result in a .000036 reduction in the risk of death, and a .000023 reduction in the risk of injury. Using these probabilities, Dardis estimated that those who purchased smoke detectors when they first came on the market at $150 made decisions consistent with a value of life of $2 million; waiting until prices dropped to below $25 implies a lower value of life, less than $350,000. The Dardis smoke detector study brings home the relevance of the first law of demand: even for life itself, people will buy less as the price increases.

We must all die sometime, and therefore no medicine or miracle can truly "save" a life. A problem with efforts to estimate "the value of life" is that the rhetoric itself reinforces denial, making it seem as if the purpose of medical care is to "save lives" rather than the real task of trying to reduce suffering and anxiety while extending the expected length of life by a few years. Such glorified language can frustrate clear thought and practical action. It may provide a convenient way to avoid admitting in public that the life of an eight-year-old child is valued more than an eighty-year-old grandparent. Such avoidance does not make the difference in valuation any less true. Economists use the decisions made by the state legislature, families, and patients, to show that they value the length and quality

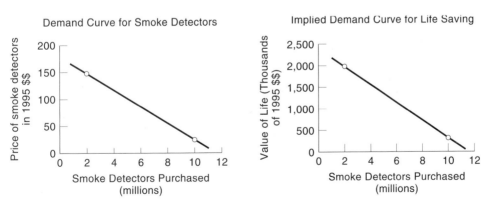

FIGURE 2.3 *Changes in the number of smoke detectors purchased as prices fell from $150 in 1974 to $24 in 1979 are interpreted as a derived demand for life saving, implying a "value of life" demand that exceeds $2,000,000 for early purchasers, and $305,000 for late purchasers. Source: Dardis, Am. Econ Review, 70:1077–1082, Dec. 1980.*

of life, which can be changed by medical care, rather than the fact of mortality, which cannot.

2.10   QUALITY-ADJUSTED LIFE YEARS, "QALYS"

The average dollar cost of providing one additional year of life expectancy has become a standard method for evaluating many health programs. Yet a year spent sick and in pain is worth less than a year lived in perfect health, free of symptoms. A significant risk of surgical mortality may be worth accepting in order to treat the disease and alleviate pain. How much? Researchers use econometrics, surveys, and professional judgments to estimate the value of a year spent in different states of disability. Such **Quality-Adjusted Life Years** (QALYs) rate quality of life between 0.0 (death) and good health (1.00). In the survey results presented in Table 2.4, respondents indicated that living for three months confined to a hospital for tuberculosis treatment was worth only 1.8 months (.60 × 3 months) of regular time.[17] The value of living in the hospital declines further when it is not temporary, but permanent. Living ten more years, all of it confined in a hospital being treated for contagious disease, was considered to be worth only 1.6 years of normal

TABLE 2.4   Quality of Life Adjustment Factors

Duration	Health State	Adjustment
	Reference State: Perfect Health	**1.00**
3 months	home confinement, tuberculosis	0.68
3 months	home confinement, contagious disease	0.65
3 months	hospital dialysis	0.62
3 months	hospital confinement, tuberculosis	0.60
3 months	hospital confinement, contagious disease	0.56
3 months	depression	0.44
3 months	home dialysis	0.65
8 years	mastectomy for injury	0.63
8 years	kidney transplant	0.58
8 years	hospital dialysis	0.56
8 years	mastectomy for breast cancer	0.48
8 years	hospital confinement, contagious disease	0.33
life	home dialysis	0.40
life	hospital dialysis	0.32
life	hospital confinement, contagious disease	0.16
	Reference State: Dead	**0.00**

Source: Sackett, D. L., and G. W. Torrance, (1978). "The Utility of Different Health States as perceived by the General Public." *Journal of Chronic Diseases* 31(11):697–704.

life. Although such conditions were not included in this survey, people consider some illnesses to be worse than death, so that each additional year lived in such misery actually has a negative value.

Discounting Over Time

The value of an additional year of life fifteen years from now is worth less than increasing the probability of living today. The *present value* of an additional year of life obtained fifteen years from now is calculated by discounting over time, the same as the present value of an additional dollar obtained fifteen years from now. If the rate of discount (interest rate) is 5 percent, then the present value of receiving a dollar next year is $\$1 \div (1.05) = \$0.952$, and the present value of receiving a dollar in fifteen years is $\$1 \div (1.05)^{15} = \$0.479$. Analogously, the discounted value of an additional year of life fifteen years from now is about half the current value.

QALY League Tables

The costs of medical care can be compared to benefits by calculating the cost per adjusted life year gained. On the benefit side, each additional life year is discounted for risk (expected value), time, and quality of life. On the cost side, adjustments are made for any differences between charges and actual costs, expected reductions in days lost from work, and reductions in cost of medical care for related conditions. Consider the illustrative hypothetical example in Table 2.5. The

TABLE 2.5 Hypothetical QALY Calculation Example

	year 1	year 2	year 3	year 4	year 5	total
Time discounting factor	1.00	0.95	0.91	0.86	0.82	
Baseline						
Quality of life	.60	.50	.40 (death)			
Discounted value	.60	.48	.36	.00	.00	1.44
Quality adjusted life expectancy without surgery, 1.44 years						
Successful surgery						
Quality of life	.90	.80	.70	.60	.50 (death)	
Discounted value	.90	.76	.63	.52	.41	3.23
Quality adjusted life expectancy if surgery is successful, 3.23 years						

Net gain in QAYLs	1.79	(3.23 - 1.44 discounted years)
Probability	40%	
Expected value	.72	
Less surgical mortality	−.04	(3% of baseline 1.44 years)
Expected net QALY gain	.68	
Cost of surgery	$30,000	
Cost per QALY gained	$44,000	($30,000 ÷ .68)

TABLE 2.6   QALY "League Table"

Treatment	present value of extra cost per QALY
Physician advice for smoking cessation	$450
Pacemaker implantation for heart block	$1,900
Hip replacement	$2,000
CABG for severe angina LMD	$2,800
Control of total serum cholesterol	$4,600
CABG for severe angina 2VD	$6,200
Kidney transplant	$8,200
Breast cancer screening	$9,500
Heart transplant	$14,000
CABG for mild angina 2VD	$35,000
Hospital hemodialysis	$38,000

CABG: "coronary artery bypass graft" LMD" "left main disease"
2VD: "two vessel disease"

Source: A. Williams, "Economics of Coronary Artery Bypass Grafting,"
British Medical Journal, 291:326–329 (1995).

patient can expect to live three years with medications alone, but will live five years if the surgery is successful, and have a better quality of life. However, the surgery is effective only 40 percent of the time, there is a chance (3%) of surgical mortality causing immediate death, and the surgery costs $30,000. The estimated cost per QALY gained is $44,000. Similar sorts of estimates have been made for a number of medical interventions so that relative costs can be calculated and presented in QALY league tables, such as Table 2.6.[18] From these results, it can be seen that it costs 7 times as much ($15,000 v. $2,000) to increase quality adjusted life expectancy by one year with a heart transplant as it does with a pacemaker implant. Trying to extend and improve life by using coronary artery bypass grafting to treat minor two vessel disease with mild angina is still more expensive, $42,000 per QALY gained. QALY rankings can be used to assess which medical treatments should be more expanded and which should be cut back so as to optimize system efficiency. When the state of Oregon decided in 1993 to enroll more poor residents in their Medicaid program, funding those extra persons by eliminating coverage of medical services deemed to be of lowest benefit, legislators used a decision-making process analogous to the construction of a QALY league table.

SUGGESTIONS FOR FURTHER READING _____

Michael F. Drummond, Greg L. Stoddart, and George W. Torrance. *Methods for the Economic Evaluation of Health Programmes.* Oxford: Oxford University Press, 1987.

Willard Manning, Emmet Keeler, Joseph Newhouse, Elizabeth Sloss, and Jeffrey Wasserman. *The Costs of Poor Health Habits.* Boston: Harvard University Press, 1991.

Mark S. Thompson, "Willingness to Pay and Accept Risks to Cure Chronic Disease." *American Journal of Public Health,* 76(4):392-396, 1988.

W. Kip Viscusi, *Fatal Tradeoffs: Public and Private Responsibilities for Risk.* New York: Oxford University, 1992.

Kenneth E. Warner and Bryan R. Luce, *Cost-benefit and Cost-effectiveness Evaluation in Health Care: principles, practice and potential.* Ann Arbor, Mich: Health Administration Press, 1982.

SUMMARY _____

1. **Every act is a judgment about value.** When a person does something, they show by that act that they think the gains are worth more than the costs. Economists look at decisions patients and physicians have made in the past to estimate the value they place on health outcomes.

2. **Cost–Benefit Analysis (CBA)** does not make decisions. It is a **framework** that can be used to make the process more rational, more consistent, and more clearly communicated. The CB analyst organizes the facts provided by clinicians and the values of the public to present data in a way that is useful for making policy decisions. Although some form of cost–benefit trade-off occurs in virtually all decisions by consumers, a formal CB analysis is used only for large-scale government or corporate projects with a long time frame and many parties involved in the decision-making process.

3. **Need** is used to refer to services medically indicated given the current state of the art and the patient's condition technically required without regard for prices, costs, incomes, taxes and other constraints on resources. **Demand** emphasizes the economist's concerns that benefits from treatment decline as more and more services are provided, and that each additional service is costly, implying fewer resources available for other purposes. **Demand, even the demand for life itself, is downward sloping.** As the price of good health or risk prevention rises, people buy less of it.

4. The appropriate measure of costs is the **opportunity cost**, what is given up. The appropriate measure of benefits is **willingness to pay** (WTP), what the patient or society would be willing to give up to attain this improvement in health.

5. In choosing between alternatives, it is the change in benefits (**marginal benefits**) and the change in costs (**marginal costs**) that matter, not the average or per person value.

6. The primary **benefits** to be accounted for in health care projects are:
   1. Health (extend life or reduce morbidity and pain)
   2. Productivity (less time lost from work)
   3. Reductions in future medical costs

7. The major categories of **costs** to be accounted for are:
   1. Medical care and administration
   2. Follow-up and treatment damages
   3. Time and pain of patient and family
   4. Provider time and effort

8. Since marginal benefits are usually declining and below average benefits as health programs increase in size, it is important to **target treatment toward**

those most in need. Many useful medical technologies become wasteful when their use is expanded to low-risk individuals.

9. Benefits are rarely certain. The **expected value** of a medical treatment is the product of the likelihood of success times the magnitude of the health gain that will occur if treatment is successful. A useful shorthand for dealing with risk is to examine whether:

(Probability of Gain) × (Benefit) > (Probability of Loss) × (Cost)?

10. Years of life must be discounted if the quality of life is reduced. Questionnaires are used to estimate how many years of life with a disability a person would be willing to give up in order to gain one additional year in good health, or to reduce the risk of death. In this way, **comparisons can be made between treatment alternatives in terms of "quality-adjusted life years" or QALYs.** Since an additional year of life expectancy in the distant future is worth less than an increase in health now, it is also necessary to use an interest rate to discount benefits over time.

11. Comparing medical therapies in standardized units, such as cost per quality adjusted life year gained, can help to make decisions regarding which programs should be expanded and which should be cut back, and thus lead to better public policy.

PROBLEMS _____

1. {*expected value*} (A) Successful rehabilitation of a shoulder injury obviates the need for reconstructive surgery costing $6,000. However, rehabilitation is successful only 70 percent of the time. What is the expected value of rehabilitation?

   (B) Treatment for endocarditis is risky. The patient will either (a) die in the hospital, (b) partially recover or (c) fully recover. With full recovery, the patient can expect to live for another 20 years, but only 25 percent of patients fully recover. With partial recovery, the patient can expect to live 10 more years. However, 20 percent of patients have no recovery and die in the hospital. Assuming patients would usually live just one year without treatment, what is the expected value of the treatment expressed as additional years of life?

2. {*marginal cost*} (A) A course of chemotherapy costs $8,000. If given to patient A, it will increase life expectancy by 2 months; for patient B by 6 months; for patient C by 1 month; patient D by 5 months; and patient E by 4 months. If all five patients are treated, what is the average cost per year of life gained? If only one patient can be treated, which one should it be? Only 2 patients? What is the marginal cost per additional year of life for the patient most likely to benefit? What is the marginal cost per additional year of life for the patient among these five who is least likely to benefit? Draw the total and marginal benefit curves (label the Y-axis "Years of life gained" and the X-axis "Number

of patients treated"). If all five patients are treated, what is the average cost per year of life gained? The marginal cost? If patients are treated in alphabetical order, which one determines the marginal cost per year of life gained, patient A, patient E or some other patient?

(B) {*demand curve*} Assume that each additional year of life is worth $60,000 and draw the demand curve for chemotherapy. Draw in the supply curve. What is the relationship between the demand curve and the benefit curves drawn in part A?

3. {*downward-sloping demand*} Government programs sending doctors in to reduce infant mortality direct most of the doctors to poorer neighborhoods. Pediatricians setting up new practices are more likely to locate in wealthier neighborhoods. Explain how it is that both can be said to be obeying the "law of downward-sloping demand," even though they move toward opposite ends of the income distribution.

4. {*direct v. indirect costs*} A school district determines that less than 70 percent of first-grade children have completed all recommended immunizations. A task force suggests that there are two ways to reach their goal of 95 percent immunization: hire 20 visiting nurses to do outreach in the community or pass a law mandating that children will not be allowed to attend school unless they bring documentation showing evidence of complete immunization. Which plan is more cost-effective? How is the distribution of costs and benefits different under the two plans?

5. {*need v. demand, opportunity cost*} Many experts recommend that people get at least 30 minutes of vigorous exercise three to five times a week; the actual participation in exercise less than the amount (a) needed or (b) demanded. Why do most college students get more exercise in the summer than the winter? Does need, demand, or differences in opportunity cost of time account for the fact that most actors get more exercise than most accountants?

6. The World Health Organization (WHO) is considering sending a team of experts in to deal with an outbreak of schistosomiasis in a distant country. Sending a larger team will allow them to prevent more fatalities, and they estimate the following effectiveness:

# of team members	# of deaths
0 (i.e., no action)	1,200
5	500
10	200
15	100
20	60
25	40
30	30
35	25
40	22
45	20
50	20

(A) It costs $5,000 for each team member sent. Calculate the *total, average,* and *marginal* cost of life saving through this effort and display it on a graph. If saving a life is valued at $100,000, what is the optimal number of people for WHO to send to combat the epidemic? If saving a life is valued at $10,000, what is the optimal number? What size of team gives the most "bang for the buck," i.e., the largest number of lives saved per dollar spent?

(B) Each person sent must be taken away from a disease-fighting team at work elsewhere in the world. What is the appropriate opportunity cost measure of sending people to fight the new epidemic; the transportation cost of $5,000 or the reduction of life-saving efforts from the job they are pulled away from?

7. {*willingness to pay*} What determines the value of a cure for Acne? of ALS (amyloid lateral sclerosis, or "Lou Gehrig's disease")? of Alzheimer's Disease? Which discovery is worth more to a pharmaceutical firm that is able to patent a cure?

8. {*QALYs*} Patient BN is a 36-year-old female with a type of organ failure that reduces her quality of life to just half of what it would be in good health, and without treatment she can expect to live for only two years. With a successful transplant, BN can expect to live four years, and to have a quality of life that is near (80%) of what she would enjoy in good health. However, the transplant costs $100,000 initially, plus $10,000 each year for drugs and follow-up care, and carries a 15 percent risk of rejection with immediate death. What is the cost per additional year of life gained (without discounting for time or quality of life)? What is the cost per discounted QALY gained (assume a 5% time discount rate)?

**9. {*interest rates and future value*} As a health economist for the Health Care Financing Administration, you have been asked to analyze a number of programs targeting different diseases and recommend which should receive priority, given that budgets are limited. As part of your analysis, you will have to determine what interest rate is appropriate for discounting future costs and benefits. You are going to be visited by an economist from the American Association of Retired Persons, and another economist from the Children's Defense Fund. Which group will lobby harder for a lower discount rate? Why?

ENDNOTES _____

1. Several sources and texts are listed at the end of this chapter as "Suggestions for further reading." Good current examples of cost–benefit analyses and reviews of the literature can be found in journals such as *Health Economics, American Journal of Public Health, Medical Decision Making, New England Journal of Medicine* and *Journal of the American Medical Association.*

2. John Eisenberg, *Doctor's Decisions and the Cost of Medical Care,"* Ann Arbor, Mich.: Health Administration Press, 1986.

3. Duncan Neuhauser and Ann Lewicki, "What do we gain from the sixth stool guaiac?" *New England Journal of Medicine,* Vol. 293, pp. 226–228, 1975.

4. Some of the assumptions used by Neuhauser and Lewicki have been modified slightly

to facilitate exposition. For a more current assessment of the sensitivity and specificity of stool guaiac screening tests, see J. E. Allison et. al., "A Comparison of Fecal Occult-Blood Tests for Colorectal-Cancer Screening," *New England Journal of Medicine* 334:155–159, 1996, and for a critical assessment of the assumptions presented there, the editorial by D. F. Ransohoff and C. A. Lang in the same issue, pp: 189–190.

5. American Cancer Society, "Guidelines for the Cancer-Related Checkup: Recommendations and Rationale," *CA - A Cancer Journal for Clinicians,* 30:230, 1980; Bernard Levin and Gerald Murphy, "Revision in American Cancer Society Recommendations for the Early Detection of Colorectal Cancer," *CA -A Cancer Journal for Clinicians,* 42(5):296–299, 1992.

6. S. R. Garfield, et al. "Evaluation of an Ambulatory Medical Care Delivery System," *New England Journal of Medicine,* 294(8):426–431, 1976; P. J. Wagner and J. E. Hendrich, "Physician Views on Frequent Medical Use: Patient Beliefs and Demographic and Diagnostic Correlates," *Journal of Family Practice* 36(4):417–422, 1993.

7. Michael Ibrahim, "Rules of Evidence," in *Epidemiology and Health Policy,* Rockville, Md.: Aspen Press, 1985, pp. 39–49.

8. Sir William Petty, *The Economic Writings of Sir William Petty* (includes *A Treatise of Taxes and Contributions,* 1662, *Political Arithmetik,* 1676, and other writings), edited by Charles Henry Hull, New York: AM Kelley, reprinted 1963, pp. 108. Petty's plan primarily involved the forced closure of houses where the plague appeared, with resettlement of the families at government expense at farms forty miles ouside of London for three months.

9. Thomas E. Getzen, "Medical Care Price Indexes: Theory, Construction and Empirical Analysis of the U.S. Series 1927–1990" *Advances in Health Economics* 13:83–128, Greenwich, Conn: JAI Press, 1992.

10. See the discussion in the "Suggested Readings" by Drummond et.al. and Warner & Luce.

11. Joseph Schumpeter, *History of Economic Analysis,* New York: Oxford University Press, 1954.

12. T. R. Fanning et al. "The Epidemiology of AIDS in the New York and California Medicaid Programs," *Journal of Acquired Immune Deficiency Syndromes* 4:1025–35, 1991.

13. Michael W. Jones-Lee, *The Economics of Safety and Physical Risk,* Oxford: Blackwell, 1989, page 67, based on data and extrapolations from S. J. Melinek, "A Method of Evaluating Life for Economic Puroposes," *Accident Analysis and Prevention,* 6:103–114, 1974.

14. *Regression Analysis* is covered in virtually all standard statistics textbooks. There is also a short description provided on pages 77–94 of *The Economics of Health and Health Care* by S. Folland, A. Goodman, and M. Stano, New York: Macmillan, 1993.

15. M. Moore and W. Kip Viscusi, "Quality Adjusted Value of Life," *Economic Inquiry* 26:369–388, 1988.

16. Rachel Dardis, "The Value of a Life: New Evidence from the Marketplace," *American Economic Review* 70:1077–1082, December 1980.

17. D. L. Sackett and D. W. Torrance, "The Utility of Different Health States as Perceived by the General Public," *Journal of Chronic Diseases* 31(11):697–704, 1978.

18. Alan Williams, "Economics of Coronary Artery Bypass Grafting," *British Medical Journal,* 291:326–329, 1985.

CHAPTER 3

Insurance

QUESTIONS

1. *Who takes care of people when they need medical care they cannot afford?*
2. *Who pays for losses—the insurance company, or the people who buy insurance?*
3. *How does pooling of funds reduce exposure to risks?*
4. *Is a favor from a friend like a loan from a bank?*
5. *Do insurance companies take risks, or price risks? What is an "actuarially fair" premium?*
6. *Are people who think they will be sick more likely to sign up for insurance?*
7. *Are people with insurance more likely to have a loss?*
8. *Does insurance increase or decrease the demand for medical care?*

Breaking an arm, catching pneumonia, having a heart attack—there are a dizzying array of risks that could disrupt your life. You hope none of these bad things will happen, but if they do, most of us can rely on insurance to cover some of the financial losses. From an individual perspective, insurance generates net benefits by allowing for trade between two possible states of the world: a little money in the usual state (not sick) is given up in order to get a lot of money in the unusual and more difficult state (sick). From the point of view of society, insurance is a method of pooling risk so that one person's loss is shared across many people rather than being borne by that person alone. If all contribute, then the pool of collected funds will be sufficient to compensate the unlucky few. All participants gain peace of mind, knowing that they can obtain necessary medical care with limited financial risk. The next two chapters examine the operations, history, and theory of health insurance. To grasp how it works in the real world, it is necessary to understand that insurance is both a means for individual maximization of utility, and social promotion of group values such as respect for life, care of the disabled, equality of opportunity, and political cohesion.

3.1 METHODS FOR COVERING RISKS _____

What would you do if you broke your arm? Who would take care of you? How would you eat and pay your rent while you were out of work? Who would pay for the doctor and hospital care? There are several ways this loss could be covered.

Savings

The first economic consequence of a loss is apt to be that some savings will be withdrawn to pay for current expenses. *Savings* can be thought of as a trade between time periods. No person saves just to have money pile up. They save so that they can consume more in the future, either because they plan to do so (e.g., retirement, summer vacation) or to protect themselves against the unexpected (e.g., accident, illness). Savings provides a buffer against random losses, smoothing out consumption over time so that you can still eat if you are not working, still pay the rent if you get hit with a $600 doctor bill just after your vacation, and still pay tuition bills if you need expensive prescription drugs to get through finals. The ability to smooth out the amount of consumption over time improves utility. The difference between a plan (spring vacation) and a risk (broken leg) is the element of uncertainty. Saving is limited as a risk management tool because it only allows the individual to trade with his or her self at different time periods; it does not spread a rare and catastrophic loss over a large group of people where it could be more easily borne. Although a person can plan a vacation or retirement within their budget, they may face an extraordinary loss (e.g., spinal injury or cranial fracture) that is far too expensive to be handled within their own resources.

Family and Friends

Young people who have not had a chance to accumulate their own savings must depend on their families' financial resources to carry them during an illness.

Although family assistance may be freely and generously given, it creates an obligation to "pay back" when you are well, to be grateful, and to help other family members in the future when they need it. Thus, the family engages in a form of exchange between persons as well as between time periods.[1] Your current loss is covered by someone else's current savings, which gives you an obligation to cover someone else's loss in the future. Whereas individual savings allowed the one person to trade among their own time periods to optimize consumption, families trade over both time and people, and so can absorb the shock of a loss without a disastrous decline in living standards more effectively than any individual alone.

The favors that friends do for each other occur so frequently and unconsciously that it seems strange to look at them as *trades*. When I carry books for someone whose leg is in a cast, or take notes for a classmate who has the flu, I am just being nice, and not usually looking to gain anything by my helpful actions. Yet ultimately, families and friendship are based on a sense of mutual obligation and reciprocity.[2] If someone consistently fails to help me, then eventually I will stop being helpful to them. Furthermore, I might let others know how inconsiderate and selfish that person is so they won't waste their time showing sympathy and giving assistance. It is through such means that the informal rules of exchange that constitute circles of friends and families are enforced. Helping out might not be legally binding, but it is socially binding.

Charity

The obligation to help extends beyond friends and family to people we have never, and will never meet, and who can do nothing for us in return. We still *care* about people even if we don't know them. It is mutual caring that makes people into a society rather than just a random collection of individuals.[3] The first hospitals were caring institutions, substitute "homes" for people who did not have a home, or for the sick and disabled whose own families were too poor to take care of them.[4] Charity as a means of social exchange predates formal insurance contracts by thousands of years, and has been far more important as a means of paying for medical bills for most of that time. Yet charity is quite limited in scope. People only care so much for strangers, and the extent to which most people feel responsible for someone else's misfortune has declined as formal market institutions have arisen for risk coverage.

Private Market Insurance Contracts

Bad things happen. We cannot always do anything about them, and when we can do something, it often costs a great deal of money. Suppose that I am one of a hundred middle-aged executives being sent by XXumma Corp to Eastern Europe. We can be pretty sure that several of us might get sick over the coming year. Suppose we knew that exactly one of us was going to have a heart attack. There is an operation that can help, a coronary artery bypass graft (usually known by its initials CABG and pronounced like "cabbage"), but this operation, with all of the attendant after-care, costs about $50,000. The one who has the heart attack will suffer financially as well as physically. A way of making a bad situation a little better is for us to form a club. Each person puts in $500, and then the unlucky one who has a heart attack gets the operation paid for. This is known as "risk pooling," and it is the essential feature of all insurance.

Although no one can predict who will be the unlucky one, for large numbers the **risk**—the expected value of all losses averaged over all people—is quite predictable. From the individual perspective, insurance is a trade between two possible states of the universe—one in which that person has a heart attack, and one where he or she does not. Money is shifted from the state in which individuals have more (not sick) to the state in which they have less (sick), much the same as saving shifts money from good periods to bad. From a societal point of view, insurance is a collection of trades between people. Money is shifted from those who still have plenty (not sick) to those who do suffer losses (sick). Note that insurance pools losses; it does not get rid of the losses or even reduce them. The group members must pay for all losses (plus some administrative fees) with the **premiums** they pay. Insurance companies do not like to take on risks. They like to sell insurance to large groups of people with predictable (average) losses. The insurer's revenues and expenses, and therefore its profits, are very stable and predictable from year to year. Insurance companies specialize in *pricing* risks, not in *taking* risks. They try to figure out in advance exactly how large premiums will have to be to cover all the predicted losses. This specialty, known as actuarial science, uses historical information on what losses have been in the past to make accurate predictions of the amount of money required to pay for future benefits. In this example, it is assumed that the probability (1-in-100) and size ($50,000) of the loss is well known, making it simple to determine the **actuarially fair premium**, $1/100 \times \$50,000 = \$500$. An actuarially fair premium is the same as the *expected value of a loss* discussed in Chapter 2 with regard to cost–benefit analysis.

Variability, the chance that the insured group will have extraordinarily high or low losses, *declines sharply as the number of people in the group increases.* Figure 3.1 shows how the risk declines with the size of the risk-bearing pool. It assumes that each person in the group has a 1 : 100 chance of having a $50,000 loss. The expected loss ($500 per person) is the same regardless of the number of people insured. With just 10 people insured, it is virtually impossible for the loss to be equal to the expected loss of $500. With 100 people in the risk pool, it is quite possible (37% of the time) that one of that hundred will get sick so that the loss equals the expected value of $500. Just as often (37% of the time) however, no one will get sick and losses will be 0. About 18 percent of the time two people will get sick, making the average loss $1,000, and 8 percent of the time three or more persons in the group of one hundred will become ill. With 1,000 people in the group, it is very unlikely (0.005%) that no one will have an illness. Most of the time (99%) the average loss will be between $1,000 and $900 per person. These are known as 99% confidence intervals, and are shown in Figure 3.1 by the dotted lines that start off far from the mean and gradually move closer as the number of people in the group increases. With 10,000 people in the risk pooling group, the chances of no one getting sick are vanishingly small, as are the chances that the average loss will be in excess of $1,000. The group will experience losses between $370 and $630 per person 99% of the time. An insurance company is quite confident doing business with a group this large. On the other hand, a company with less than twenty five insureds has a sizable chance of losses that are more than double the expected value (about 22% of the time).

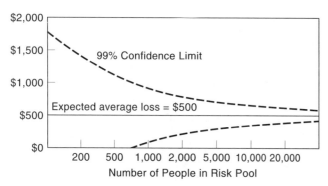

FIGURE 3.1 *Variability Declines as the Size of the Risk-Sharing Pool Increases*

- If the risk pool is one person, then they either get sick (1% of the time) and expenses are $50,000, or they do not (99%) and expenses are $0. Expected losses are $.01 \times \$50,000 = \$500$.
- With ten people in the risk pool, most of time (90.4%) losses are $0. One person will get sick 9.1% of the time, so losses average $5,000 per person, and 0.4% of the time two or more people get sick, so losses average $10,000 per person or more. Expected losses are $500.
- With 10,000 people in the risk pool, the average loss is within $150 of the expected loss ($500) more than 99% of the time.

All real insurance must be priced above the actuarially fair premium to cover the expenses of administering the insurance plan, and to provide some profits to the owners who put up their expertise and capital. The difference between the actual premium and the actuarially fair premium is known as the *load.* Most commonly, it is presented as a percentage of the total benefits paid and is referred to as the *loading factor.* The loading factor may be as small as 5 percent or 10 percent for routine large group business, and may exceed 100 percent for some individual policies.

Social Insurance

Market contracts are mutually beneficial to all those who purchase insurance, and to the companies that act as financial intermediaries as well. However, they do nothing for the poor who cannot afford to buy insurance, or for the disabled and other excluded groups of people. They do not pay for medical research or education programs to promote healthier lifestyles, nor do they provide outreach to teenage mothers or the mentally ill. In short, they do nothing to strengthen the social contract that binds the people of a nation together in support of each other. The informal obligations of citizens to society expressed in charitable giving are extended and formalized in social insurance programs such as Medicare and Social Security in the United States, the National Health Service in the United Kingdom and Canada, and indeed the health care systems of most countries in the world.[5] Contributions to social insurance are not voluntary, but mandatory through the tax system. Who shall pay and who shall receive are a function of concerns common to all; and are determined through the political process rather than through individual choices made in the marketplace.

As was pointed out in Chapter 1, the U.S. health care system is a blend of private and public financing. Medicare, a social insurance program that covers medical bills for 99 percent of all the elderly persons in the United States, is larger than all of the private for-profit companies combined. Furthermore, even when insurance is paid for privately and managed by profit-making firms, government regulations mandate who is to be covered, what services are to be offered, and how prices are to be set, so that even private insurance is forced into some conformity with social insurance principles.

Strengths and Weaknesses of Different Forms of Risk Spreading

Individual savings are quite limited as a form of risk management since the resources of only one person are used. There is no way that a person born with a genetic defect can "save" to cover that risk. Most young people cannot save the $15,000 or so required to treat a broken leg, and a serious illness would exceed the financial capabilities of all but the wealthiest individuals. Trade with more than one person is needed for coverage. Taking money from family and friends spreads the risk more widely, but this larger group may have difficulty telling if you really "need" assistance, and, if they do contribute toward your medical bills, they may also want to give you lots of unwelcome advice and intrude in your personal affairs. Charity brings in an even broader group, but the sick individual has less incentive to minimize waste, since that person is now spending other people's money. Charity also tends to be unreliable and even more meddlesome. The extent of resources available is limited by how much people care, and charity alone could never fund a modern medical system.

WHY DO POLICE OFFICERS AND FIREFIGHTERS HAVE
SUCH COMPREHENSIVE INSURANCE?

Medical coverage for those who put their life on the line for the good of the community remains comprehensive even when many firms and government agencies are cutting back on benefits. There is a symbolic importance to this insurance that goes beyond financial consideration. If the community is not willing to do everything possible to protect the health of these public servants, why should they continue to risk it all in order to save lives? Similar considerations lie behind the willingness of an army troop to go to great lengths to recover a wounded (or dead) comrade when such effort seems not to be worthwhile from a cost–benefit perspective, and has led to the creation of a $16 billion system to care for disabled veterans.

Markets create impersonal contracts to pay for services. They can draw upon financial resources from around the world. Your insurance may be handled by a company in the Netherlands that neither knows nor cares about you as a person, but fully meets your needs as long as all the doctor bills get paid on time. Yet markets are driven by profits, not love, and each participant must pay his or her own way. Nothing will be done for a child with a genetic defect unless a parent has a policy that includes dependents. A lawyer's interpretation of a contract replaces family concerns as the factor determining what kind of medical care is to be provided. The movement from individual to group to market financing reveals a trade-off: the individual is most sensitive to his or her own needs, but has the smallest span for risk pooling (savings, or trade over time periods). The market is global in reach, but impersonal and willing to help only when there is a profit to be made (see Table 3.1).

Social insurance combines the humanitarian thrust of charity and financial strengths of the market, but it provides only a compromise, not a reconciliation. Social insurance can be comprehensive only if contributions are made compulsory through taxes. As the funding base grows broader, it grows ever more divorced from personal empathy and becomes just one more government service provided through the political process. The doctor's self-interested desire to please a paying customer may be lost when medical care is provided by a bureaucracy. Forcing all taxpayers to contribute more so that the poor, the disabled, and the mentally ill can get medical care is generally approved of; it is determining exactly who should pay and how much they should pay that becomes contentious. Even when motivated by the highest ideals, social insurance, like the market, requires full payment by the participants, and is thus bound to the same actuarial projections. As taxpayers, we are willing to provide some medical care for everyone, but not necessarily the best quality in the best rooms of the most modern hospitals, and some taxpayers may be downright hostile about spending millions of dollars on patients who spent their own money on entertainment rather than medical care, for example, or who have worsened their own illnesses through substance abuse or unhealthy lifestyles. Social insurance requires that society reach a broad consensus on who deserves what and how medical care is to be delivered. Such a consensus currently exists in the United States only for the elderly under Medicare, and even that can fall apart, as it did in 1989 when revisions to cover pharmaceuticals and catastrophic expenses were passed, implemented, and then repealed by Congress after a revolt by older taxpayers.[6]

TABLE 3.1 Types of Risk Protection

Method	Reduces effects of loss by:	Depends on:
Savings	Shifting consumption between periods	How much I personally have now
Family, Friends, Charity	Sharing between people	How much people care about me
Insurance Contract	Trading between possible states of the world through financial markets	Ability to price risk

3.2 RISK AVERSION _____

Why would someone be willing to pay even a 10 percent load (mark-up) just to get the premium money back as benefit payments? To the extent that the person can easily fund losses through personal savings, they won't be willing. That is why most routine losses are not insured. Only large and potentially catastrophic losses are worth paying extra to insure. Suppose the premiums required in the earlier heart attack example were not the actuarially fair $500, but $750, or $1,000, or even $1,500? That is still better than having to sell your house, or being in debt for twenty years, or—perhaps worse—not being able to have an operation that could save your life. The fact that people are willing to pay more than the expected value of the loss for insurance is evidence to an economist that they think they are better off with it than without it. The desire to replace an uncertain loss with a steady and certain premium payment is known as **risk aversion.** Some people feel very strongly about risk, and will go to great lengths to avoid it. Most people choose not to take financial chances unless they have to, or are well paid for it (for example, risky investments give a higher rate of interest than safe government bonds). Others are willing to take some chances. To some extent this is a matter of taste, like how spicy you like your food. It also depends to some extent on how much income you have—going from $2 million a year to $50,000 is not nearly as scary as going from $200,000 to $5,000 — that is less than $100 a week for food, rent (forget it—you're at your parents' place again, or homeless), and travel (mostly by bus).

Given that most people are risk-averse, why aren't all risks insured? Life is full of chances. I buy an airplane ticket for spring vacation even though I might die before I ever get to use it. My bicycle might get stolen. Some people study for a profession, such as accounting, or computer science, only to find that job market conditions have changed by the time they graduate. As you take the exam for this class, at least some of the result (hopefully not all) will be random—what questions are asked, when the commercial breaks occurred during your study time. Only a few of the risks in life are insured. Why? For one reason, it is costly to write up and specify insurance contracts, pay claims, and so on. Most small losses will, on average, balance out over time, and thus can be handled by savings. There are also several structural incentive problems with insurance (e.g., moral hazard, adverse selection) that reduce its value which are discussed later in this chapter. In most property and casualty insurance, the losses that are insured are those that are large, infrequent, and random (unpredictable). Many medical expenses meet these criteria, but not all do. For example, most visits for colds and flu are small, frequent, and fairly predictable. Although the magnitude of the financial losses incurred might explain why some medical expenses are insured, it does not

---

ARE YOU RISK-AVERSE?

Here's an easy test. Imagine your boss offering to flip a coin over your monthly paycheck—double or nothing. If the prospect of losing your paycheck is much more unpleasant than the chance of doubling it, then, like most people, you are risk averse and a good candidate for insurance.

explain why insurance is so extensive in health care, covering many minor and routine services as well as catastrophic events. Two special factors must be recognized in considering the market for health insurance. One is the belief that everyone has a right to medical care. The other is the effectiveness of medical providers in promoting insurance because it provides benefits to them, not the least of which is removing the doctor–patient relationship from the grubby world of commercial trade and haggling over price.

The fact that not all risks are insured raises an interesting question: If people are so risk-averse, why do they gamble? It is clear why people may "gamble" with an investment in stock or land. They are compensated by getting (on average) higher returns than can be obtained with less risky investments. But in gambling you don't get paid for taking risks, you have to pay for the privilege of taking on risk. The truth is, people mostly gamble for fun. It is something exciting to do, like going to the movies. Sometimes people gamble because they do not understand that the odds are against them, that if they keep playing long enough they are bound to lose. And then there are a few people who gamble because it is their job, and like casinos, they almost always win when you and I put our money on the table. Don't envy the professional gambler too much, though. For that person it is work rather than a fling, and the hardest thing is finding willing customers—just as it is for an insurance salesman.

3.3 ADVERSE SELECTION _____

Risk pooling works well because everyone in the group is at risk, and therefore has an interest in making sure that solid insurance benefits are provided. Consider the heart attack example again, and suppose that instead of the risk being purely random, you knew that you were the one who would end up in the hospital. Then you would make sure that you got insurance, and might even be willing to pay an astronomical premium to get it. However, if you were certain that you were not going to be the one, then you would not try very hard to be part of the insurance group, and might not be willing to pay $500, or even $50. Differences between the people who choose to buy insurance (the high risks) and those who choose to avoid it (the low risks) is known as "adverse selection."

If higher risks are due to something objective that the insurance company can observe in advance, and that both parties can agree on, then varying premiums by risk category causes no problems (i.e., pricing by age is common, such as $30 up to 35, $50 for ages 35 to 50, $65 for ages 51 to 60, and $85 for ages 61 and over). Adverse selection creates difficulties when some risk factors are known to the purchaser, but not to the insurance company (my chest hurts every time I go walking, I enjoy fried foods and/or lots of drugs, my brother and sister recently died of heart attacks), or because even if the risks are well known, it is considered "unfair" to charge for them (female employees paying less than males; doubling the premiums for age 61 and over; charging more to unmarried men because of risk of AIDS, etc.). If an employer subsidizes an optional health plan for its workers, then those at high risk are more likely to buy insurance. This adverse selection means that the average losses in the insured group will be larger than the expected value for the employees as a whole. If the young, healthy workers choose not to participate, premiums will have to rise. At the extreme, the plan may be left with only those who were ill to begin with and who knew that they would collect benefits—which is not insurance at all, since there is no risk pooling. It is for this reason that most insurance companies require that all (or at least a majority) of the employees in a firm be insured.

A more subtle form of adverse selection occurs when a company offers two kinds of plans, a basic plan and a more comprehensive option for which the employee pays extra for the additional coverage. Who will choose the comprehensive plan? Some people will choose it because they are very risk-averse, and so they will be willing to pay extra for the more comprehensive benefits. This causes no problem for the insurance company. The difficulty arises because there will also be a disproportionate number of the high-risk individuals (older, overweight, etc.) who take the comprehensive plan. As more and more high-risk people sign up for the plan with more coverage, their medical expenses will exceed the expected value, and even the "high" premium will not be sufficient to pay the bills. Thus, the extra premium for comprehensive insurance must be raised still higher. As the premium goes up, fewer and fewer low-risk people are willing to pay for the better coverage. Eventually, only the chronically ill who are certain to have a big loss will sign up for the comprehensive plan. As the difference in premiums between the basic and high option plan becomes larger, fewer and fewer good risks are left in the high option pool. The principle of risk sharing is defeated by the progressive separation of risks between the classes. The more differences there are in expected costs of illnesses, and the more inside information people have about their own health, the greater is the potential for adverse selection. The elderly are particularly problematic because many of their medical expenses are for chronic illnesses that are well known to them, and not random. Insurers' major method for reducing adverse selection, insisting that all employees within a company be included in the group plan, is not available for the elderly, since most of them are retired. The ultimate solution for adverse selection is just to include everyone in a social insurance system, and this is what the United States did for the elderly by creating the Medicare system.

DO PEOPLE CHOOSE TO DIE?

Actuaries have found that the people who buy life insurance are more likely than average to die prematurely.[7] The reasons have less to do with the drama depicted in *Death of a Salesman* (since suicide invalidates most policies), but mundane adverse selection—people who know that their parents died young, or that their heart palpates sometimes, or worry about their lack of exercise since their fiftieth birthday party, are more apt to buy insurance when it is offered. Conversely, those who buy annuities (policies that pay $X per year as long as you go on living) show positive selection, and are less likely to die than average. Questionnaire respondents who reply "yes" when asked, "Do you expect to live a long time?" do, in fact, enjoy longer lives than those who respond "no," even after adjusting for the effects of age, blood pressure, cigarette smoking, and all other measurable health risks, indicating that individuals do have private knowledge that can be used to select coverage that is most favorable to them, but costly to the insurer.

3.4   MORAL HAZARD _____

A different insurance problem, *moral hazard,* arises when people's behavior changes because they are insured so that their losses become larger. For example, a person with medical insurance is more likely to go to the doctor to have a sore throat checked than someone who is not insured. If sent to the hospital, the insured person is more likely to pick a nicer and more expensive facility. These changes in behavior cause the expenditures of people with insurance to be greater than what an actuary would have predicted from observing the records of people without insurance, and this increase in loss is known as *moral hazard.* One form of this behavioral change can be illustrated using ordinary demand curve analysis. Consider the Figure 3.2. The demand for physician visits without insurance is the line D. With insurance picking up 80 percent of the costs, the net "price" that (P_i) the patient personally has to pay is just 20 percent of the actual price, so consumption will increase to Q_i. The increase in visits due to the insurance are attributable to moral hazard.

Is it likely that people will consume care with little medical benefit just because it is free? For heart surgery, no. Pain and the loss of time is sufficient to keep most people from undertaking surgery "just for the fun of it." But what about routine office visits? Many of them are for minor symptoms that will fade away without treatment. Insurance makes people much more likely to seek treatment for minor symptoms, and thus to increase the overall cost of insurance. Even some surgical procedures are of limited value and are likely to be undertaken only if the insurance pays. Suppose seventy-six-year-old uncle Al has a liver infection. It is probable that he will die whatever we do, but there is a chance that he could live several more months or even years longer with a liver transplant—at a cost of $100,000 for the surgery and $5,000 per month after that for drugs and after care. If he, or the family, had to pay directly out of their own pockets, it would probably be decided that it was not worth paying so much for such an expensive operation that is not likely to be successful. However, if insurance is picking up the tab,

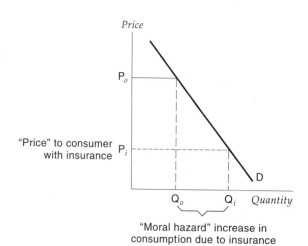

FIGURE 3.2   *Moral Hazard*

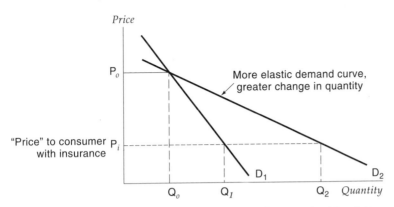

FIGURE 3.3 *Amount of Moral Hazard Depends On Price Elasticity of Demand*

or if Medicare is passing the cost on to all the other taxpayers, then the family might go ahead and try for an improbable cure.

Looking at Figure 3.3, it can be seen that the extent of expenditure increase due to moral hazard increases with the price elasticity of the demand curve. For services that are not very price sensitive, (D_1) being insured will not cause many more to be purchased, and so there will not be much of a distortion in consumer behavior due to insurance. On the other hand, for services that are very price elastic, (D_2) insurance can cause a very large increase in the quantity consumed and paid for, and moral hazard is a large problem. This theoretical result provides us with a hypothesis about what kinds of care will be insured. Since moral hazard reduces the gains from risk pooling, types of medical care that are subject to lots of moral hazard (have high price elasticity) should be less likely to be insured than services for which there is very little moral hazard (low price elasticity). A number of studies have shown that this is, indeed, the case.[8] Services such as hospital care and surgery with lower price elasticity of demand are more likely to be insured than services such as nursing home care, physical therapy, mental health, dentistry, and drugs, which have a higher price elasticity of demand. Exchange must make all parties better off, and whenever problems such as moral hazard reduce the value of transacting, there will be less pooling of risks through the insurance market.

3.5 WELFARE LOSSES FROM HEALTH INSURANCE ————————————————

The extra services that people consume just because they are covered by insurance are, to some extent, an economic waste. When it costs $20 to produce an X-ray, but that X-ray is only worth $5 to the patient, then there is a net loss of value of $15. This loss of value is often called the **welfare triangle** because the area of the triangle between the price that the insurance company must pay and the demand curve yields a good measure of the size of the loss. Consider the example in Figure

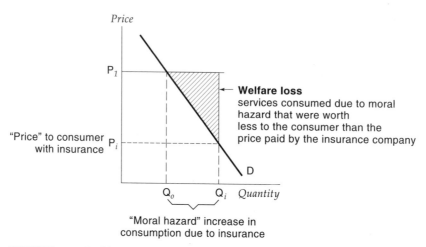

FIGURE 3.4   *Welfare Loss Due to Moral Hazard*

3.4. With insurance that pays 80 percent of the bill, the number of X-rays con-sumed rises from five to nine. The cost for each X-ray stays the same, $20. The sixth X-ray is worth only $16, for a loss of $4, the seventh is worth $12, for a loss of $8, the 8th is worth $8, for a loss of $12, the ninth X-ray is worth $4, for a loss of $16. The total amount paid for the four extra X-rays is $80, and the welfare loss is about half of that, $40.*

Who loses? All members of the insured group lose because their premiums must be higher to cover this excess use. In fact, even the person getting the extra service would prefer a tighter contract that provided only worthwhile services at a lower premium. That is why so much work is done using contract exclusions, fee limits, second opinions, and so on, to make sure that only necessary services get reimbursed. There is a demand for the "hassle" of making patients and physi-cians justify their use of services because it reduces premiums. Evidence for this demand is that consumers choose policies that include restrictive contractual lan-guage rather than policies that pay for everything without question but cost more. That does not mean that it is pleasant when you are sick to go through all sorts of bureaucratic hoops to get a claim paid; it does mean that the effort is justified in terms of reduced premiums—or else you would choose a different plan. Insurance companies will give customers whatever they want, including aggravation, in order to make a profit.

Welfare losses due to moral hazard are to some extent unavoidable. They are just a part of the cost of insurance, the way that an unwanted orange peel is just a part of the cost of an orange. On net, people are better off with the insurance (in-

---

*The size of the welfare triangle is $(P_{original} - P_{insured}) \times (Q_{insured} - Q_{original}) \div 2$, which for this ex-ample would be $(\$20 - \$4) \times (9 - 5) \div 2 = \$32$. This is slightly less than in the numerical example be-cause with discrete units (i.e., one, two, . . . eight, nine X-rays, with no fractions) the demand curve is not a continuous straight line, but a step function, and so the area between the original $20 line and the demand curve is somewhat larger. In most cases, economists use the continuous formula, since with many consumers buying many units of service, the individual bumps are less important and the demand curve approximates a continuous line.

cluding moral hazard) than without it. If people are buying insurance, then the gains from trade due to risk pooling must be exceeding the welfare losses from moral hazard. If the losses were larger than the gains, people would not buy. However, when the purchase of insurance is subsidized by the government, this may no longer be the case. The extra insurance bought due to tax subsidization creates additional excess utilization of services that are not highly valued by consumers.[9]

There is a system-wide welfare loss caused by insurance that is more difficult to see. Insurance tends to increase demand and make patients less price-sensitive, and so increases prices overall. Whether or not one person becomes insured will have little effect on the price of X-rays. Yet if everyone who now has insurance had it taken away, then demand would fall and the price of X-rays would surely decline. People who are uninsured are made worse off because other people are insured, because it raises the price that uninsured people have to pay.* It is even possible that we would all be better off if we were all uninsured, even though each one of us taken singly is better off with insurance. This paradoxical (and quite unlikely) result will occur if the gains from risk pooling are smaller than the increase in prices due to universal insurance. If one person gave up insurance, that person alone would give up the benefits of risk pooling, but if all people (or, at least a large percentage of all people) gave up insurance, lower prices would benefit everyone. The systematic distortion of prices due to insurance raising overall demand probably creates a larger welfare loss than moral hazard welfare triangle attributable to tax subsidy. Such system-wide effects are difficult to gauge because looking at individual behavior may not tell us what is really happening to the system as a whole. One way to measure system-wide effects is to compare different health care systems in different countries that use different types of insurance to see how well each one works and what they cost, but this ambitious effort is left for later (see Chapter 19 "International Comparisons").

SUGGESTIONS FOR FURTHER READING————

Institute of Medicine, *Employment and Health Benefits: A connection at risk.* Washington, DC: National Academy Press, 1993.
Mark V. Pauly, "Taxation, Health Insurance, and Market Failure in the Medical Economy," *Journal of Economic Literature* 24(2):629–675, June 1986.

SUMMARY————————————————————————————

1. From an individual perspective, **insurance is a form of trade** between time periods, or between different possible states (sick or not sick) of the future. From a societal perspective, insurance is a method of **pooling risks** so that the burden of financial loss is distributed over many people. **Savings** can spread

---

*However, it is *sometimes* the case that the profits that hospitals make from insured patients are used to provide charity services to the uninsured (see the discussion of cost-shifting in chapter 8, section 4). Whether or not an uninsured person is made better or worse off depends upon whether or not they receive services for free (or with sufficient subsidy that the price to them is less than the market price would be without insurance).

the cost of illness over time. **Family, friends, and charity** allow for voluntary risk spreading across people. **Private insurance contracts** spread risks through organized markets. **Social insurance** uses taxation to spread the risk over all citizens.

2. The **actuarially fair premium** is equal to the **expected value** of a loss, the dollar amount multiplied by the probability of occurrence. The "law of large numbers" means that higher losses for some will be offset by lower losses for others, so that for a large group the overall loss will usually be close to the expected value. If each person contributes an average amount, the pooled funds will be enough to pay for all the individual losses.

3. **Insurance companies do not pay for losses**, people do. The entire cost of medical care, plus some extra for administrative expense and profits, is paid through premiums, taxes, or patient coinsurance (deductibles, copayments, etc.) collected for each service rendered. Therefore only large, random, infrequent losses are worth insuring. Insurance for small, regular losses raises costs while providing few benefits from risk reduction.

4. People would rather have an income that is certain rather than the same average income subject to random fluctuations. Consumers are willing to pay more than the expected value of a loss to obtain insurance coverage due to **risk aversion**. From the supply side, the excess of premiums over benefits paid out is called the *load* or **underwriting gains** of the insurance company.

5. People who know in advance that they are more likely to have a loss are more likely to purchase insurance, resulting in **adverse selection**, a change in the composition of the group being insured. This difficulty in the grouping of people for insurance is to be distinguished from a change in individual behavior due to behavior. Moral hazard occurs when insurance leads an individual to increase the risk of loss or spend more.

6. The **welfare loss due to insurance** occurs because people who do not have to pay the bills will consume some care that is worth less to them than what it costs to provide. The gains from risk reduction must be worth more than these welfare losses or people would choose to go without insurance. However, the subsidy provided by exempting employer-provided health insurance benefits from taxes encourages extra insurance coverage. There may also be a general rise in the price of medical care because insurance increases the demand for services. This clearly causes a loss of welfare to those who are uninsured, and, by increasing overall costs, creates a system-wide distortion which reduces economic efficiency.

PROBLEMS _____

1. {*cost sharing*} Find four people who have been treated for illness in the last three years. Ask:
    a. How much did they pay for insurance?
    b. How much did the insurance really cost (i.e., what they paid plus what employer or government paid)?

c. How much did they pay in medical bills?

d. How much did the medical care really cost (including payments by insurance company or government)?

2. {*actuarially fair premium*} A firm with 617 employees had the following experience in 1990:

	Cost (each)
14 hospitalizations	$5,600
37 physical therapy	$340
9 births	$1,800
4.1 physician visits per employee	$55
2.4 prescriptions filled per employee	$21

Assuming that the cost of medical care rose 7 percent over the next year, what would the actuarially fair premium per employee be for 1991?

3. {*size of risk pool*} Use the information in Figure 3.1, pertaining to a loss of $50,000 that occurs randomly with a probability of 1:100. If the insurance company charges $750, what is the load above the actuarially fair premium? If there are 100 people in the group, will they usually show an underwriting profit? Will it ever break even? How likely is it that the plan will show a loss next year? With 50 people in the group, is it more or less likely that the plan will show a loss? With 500 people? How large does the group have to be before the insurance company can be 99 percent sure that it will show an underwriting gain for the year?

4. {*savings, social insurance*} Explain which mechanism (savings, charity & contributions from friends, private insurance, or social insurance) you think would be covering losses due to each of the following conditions:

seasonal hayfever
birth defects
schizophrenia
Alzheimer's disease
preventive dental cleaning
post-traumatic jaw reconstruction
cigarette-induced chronic pulmonary obstruction

5. {*adverse selection*} In each of the following pairs, which situation would pose the largest problems with regard to adverse selection?

a) A policy covering accidents for all children attending YMCA camps or b) A policy covering accidents for college students traveling abroad.

c) Inclusion of AIDS treatment in the standard benefit package offered to teachers or d) An optional rider providing AIDS coverage for an additional premium.

e) Basic medical services insurance package offered to entering college students or f) Basic medical services package offered to professors seeking early retirement.

g) Optional mental health coverage offered to employees of ABC Inc. or h) Optional mental health coverage offered to children of ABC Inc. employees.

6. {*moral hazard*} Explain which of the following types of insurance coverage would be most likely to cause the most problems due to moral hazard.
   a) Indemnity payments of $10,000 for each eye or limb lost or b) Indemnity payments of $50 for each day spent in a nursing home.
   c) Treatment in an emergency room or d) Treatment in intensive care.
   e) Arthroscopic surgery for knee injuries or f) Amputation for foot injuries.
   g) Family counseling or h) Electroshock therapy.
   i) Decongestants or j) Antibiotics.

7. {*moral hazard*} The table below gives Ralph's demand curve for doctor visits without insurance. Assume Ralph responds only to the amount he must pay out of pocket when deciding how much care to use. Calculate what Ralph's new demand curve with insurance would be if he had insurance paying 80 percent of the bill by filling in the blank lines. If the charges are $100 (i.e., Ralph pays $20 out of pocket), how many of the additional services Ralph uses are worth (to him) less than their cost? less than what he pays?

Price per visit	Number of visits	Out-of-pocket cost with insurance	Number of visits with insurance
$0	20	____	____
$20	18	____	____
$50	15	____	____
$100	10	____	____
$150	5	____	____

8. {*welfare loss*} Bill's new insurance has a prescription plan that provides all drugs through a local pharmacy with a $2 copayment. Under the old insurance, Bill had to pay for his own medication and purchased 9 inhalers at $17 apiece to help control his asthma. With the new plan, he keeps some spares in his glove compartment and desk and purchased 15 inhalers, since he only had to pay the $2 copayment for each one. How much are the 6 additional inhalers worth to Bill? How much do they cost him? How much do they cost the insurance company? Is Bill better or worse off under the new plan?

9. {*incidence*} When medical care is reimbursed through employer-provided insurance, whose welfare is ultimately affected when the cost of medical care rises: the owners of the firm that pays the premiums, the people in government whose revenues are reduced because insurance benefits are not taxable like wages, or the public at large in their roles of workers, consumers, and taxpayers? Is there any difference between short-run and long-run effects?

ENDNOTES _____

1. Gary Becker, *A Treatise on the Family*, Cambridge, Mass: Harvard University Press, 1981.
2. Robert H. Frank, *Passions Within Reason: The Strategic Role of the Emotions*, New York: Norton, 1988.
3. Edward O. Wilson, *On Human Nature*, Cambridge, Mass: Harvard University Press, 1976; Jerome H. Barkow, Leda Cosmides, John Tooby, eds., *The Adapted Mind:*

Evolutionary Psychology and the Generation of Culture, New York: Oxford University Press, 1992.

4. Rosemary Stevens, *In Sickness and In Wealth: American Hospitals in the Twentieth Century,* New York: Basic Books, 1989; John D. Thompson, *The Hospital: A Social and Architectural History,* New Haven: Yale University Press, 1975.

5. William A. Glaser, *Health Insurance in Practice: International Variations in Financing, Benefits, and Problems,* San Francisco: Jossey-Bass, 1991.

6. William Aaronson, Jacqueline Zinn, and Michael Rosko, "Medicare Catastrophic Health Insurance," *Journal of Health Politics, Policy and Law,* 1993.

7. Lewis C. Workman, "Life Annuities," pp. 155–195 in *Mathematical Foundations of Life Insurance,* Atlanta, GA: Life Office Management Association, 1982.

8. Kevin F. O'Grady, Willard G. Manning, Joseph P. Newhouse and Robert H. Brook, "The Impact of Cost Sharing on Emergency Department Use," *New England Journal of Medicine* 313:484–490, 1985; Mark V. Pauly, "Taxation, Health Insurance and Market Failure in the Medical Economy," *Journal of Economic Literature* 24(2):629–675, June 1986.

9. Martin S. Feldstein, "The Welfare Loss of Excess Health Insurance," *Journal of Political Economy,* 81(2):251–280, 1973.

CHAPTER **4**

Health Insurance Contracting and Flow of Funds

QUESTIONS

1. *Who benefits from insurance: patients, physicians, or insurance companies?*
2. *Who is the third party? Who controls the flow of funds?*
3. *Who is the biggest insurer of medical care?*
4. *Do taxes cause employees to prefer insurance benefits to a wage increase?*
5. *How is a state mandate to cover alcoholism treatment like a tax?*
6. *Why are so many Americans uninsured?*
7. *Which is more competitive, the market for health insurance or the market for medical care?*
8. *Is money the dominant force regulating health care?*

Insurance modifies the nature of economic exchange by redirecting the flow of money. It changes who negotiates prices, who bears responsibility for mistakes, and who has the right to profit from directing business to one hospital rather than another. The standard market model with one group (consumers) determining demand and a different group (firms) determining supply is left behind when we enter a medical world with patients (who receive care but do not directly pay for it), insurance companies (who neither supply nor consume, but pool risk and profit from handling funds) and providers, who are reimbursed by this *third party* (insurance) for a group of patients rather than being paid directly.

4.1   THIRD-PARTY TRANSACTIONS _____

What do each of the three parties in an insurance contracting network gain? *Patients* gain by pooling risks to eliminate financial uncertainty, as discussed in Chapter 3. *Insurance companies* benefit from profits. Even when the **underwriting gains** (the difference between premiums paid in and benefits plus administrative costs paid out) are negative, an apparent loss, the company may still make money because they will hold the premiums for six to twenty-four months before paying out benefits. At 8 percent, the interest on a million dollars in premiums for two years is $(1.08)(1.08) \times (\$1,000,000) - (\$1,000,000) = \$166,400$, which is not a bad profit for a firm that some reports might claim made no money (because benefit payouts exceeded premium revenues). In addition, insurance companies usually get higher returns on investments than individuals because they are so large, with better opportunities and specialized investment staffs. Insurance companies are regulated and taxed as large financial investment institutions, with underwriting gains and losses treated as secondary.[1] This does not mean that underwriting and risk selection are not important, only that expected investment returns are already built in to the price of the premium.

Providers gain from an increase in demand and regularity of payment. When patients are covered by insurance, they are more apt to come in for care and are less likely to argue about price. Traditionally, patients have expected doctors and hospitals to be more lenient than landlords and bankers about late payment, and many medical bills went unpaid or were paid only in part. Falling demand and irregular payment during the Great Depression in the 1930s forced many hospitals to close due to bankruptcy, and led to the start-up of the largest private insurance plan (Blue Cross) in the world as a method of insuring patients so that provider revenues could continue.[2] Like all great ideas, insurance had to benefit all parties so that they would enthusiastically cooperate.

Benefits from Exchange

patients	insurers	providers
risk pooling	*profits*	*increased demand*

Tax Benefits

There is a less visible and more diffuse "fourth party" to most insurance transactions—the government. Many governments take on the social obligation to provide medical care directly, as is done by the British National Health Service or the Swedish Health System. Some countries have chosen to build on employee health insurance plans to create universal coverage for all citizens, such as the German Krankenkassen or the Japanese employment societies. The United States is somewhat unique in that insurance is encouraged but not universally required. The U.S. government directly provides insurance for all those who are over 65 through Medicare, and for many people who are classified as being indigent or disabled through Medicaid. It also provides tax incentives for many others to be insured through the private sector. The primary tax incentive is that health benefits are nontaxable compensation for the employee, and still allowed as deductible expenses for the employer. The example below shows how this tax incentive works.

Employee Pays for Medical Care		*Employer Pays for Insurance*
$1000	company labor cost	$1000
none	insurance premium	−200
$1000	gross paycheck	$800
−350	taxes (@ 35%)	−280
$650	net paycheck	$520
−200	medical bills	*none*
$450	**available for spending**	**$520**

The company is spending the same for labor either way, and does not care whether insurance premiums are taken out of the paycheck or paid later from the employee's bank account. With insurance taken out, the employee's gross is smaller, and therefore the taxes paid are smaller. The employee with the larger paycheck has, after paying for medical care with after-tax dollars, less money left for spending than the employee whose health insurance premiums paid for the same amount of medical care on a pre-tax basis. So long as the administrative load is less than the tax rate, it is cheaper to buy medical care pre-tax using employer-paid insurance than for the employee to pay the bills directly. This tax break for employer-paid health insurance is a substantial and important part of the voluntary system of health care that Americans have come to depend on. Without the tax incentive, most working people would not have health insurance as an employee benefit.

4.2 FLOW OF FUNDS IN HEALTH INSURANCE _____

Three factors explain why more than half (57%) of the U.S. population is covered by employer group health insurance; (1) covering a large group under a single contract reduces transactions costs, (2) group coverage mitigates adverse selection, and (3) employer payment yields a tax benefit.[3] Seven percent of the population, mostly people who are self-employed or who work for small companies that do not provide employee benefits, purchase private health insurance individually. Since the elderly do not belong to employer groups and would be subject to severe adverse selection when purchasing insurance individually, government has created the Medicare programs for the 12 percent of the population over age 65, and some disabled persons. The poor cannot pay for insurance, and many of them (10% of the population) are covered under the government Medicaid program, which also provides supplemental coverage for a substantial number of elderly, including a majority of those in nursing homes. Unfortunately, despite the wide variety of health insurance plans, about 14 percent of the U.S. population has no health insurance. If these individuals need care, they must try to pay out of their own limited resources, find some special government program, depend on charity, or simply present themselves at a hospital or clinic and ask to be treated for free.

Private Insurance

Most private insurance is provided as a benefit of employment. The employee participates by choosing one of the offered options, deciding whether to include children and other dependents, and contributing a small amount toward the total premium. Almost all large employers provide health insurance benefits, but less than a third of small employers (fewer than 10 employees) do so, and often make the employee pay a large part of the premium, so that a smaller number choose to participate. Self-insured (i.e., the employer bears the risk although they may use an insurance company to administer benefits) employee groups covered about 64 million people in 1992, as did commercial insurance group coverage. Individual insurance covered 9 million. Blue Cross/Blue Shield plans enrolled 68 million (individual and group), and for-profit and not-for-profit HMOs 46 million.[4]

Medicare and Medicaid

Most of the money for Medicare comes from a tax of 2.9 percent on all wages and earnings, paid half by the employer and half by the employee, with the remainder coming from general tax revenues and premiums. **Medicare** is split into two parts, part A (hospital) and part B (physician & outpatient services), which are described in more detail in Table 4.1. Part A coverage is provided automatically to persons over 65, and to those entitled to specified disability programs such as Social Security and End Stage Renal Disease. For part B coverage, beneficiaries must pay a premium ($46.10 a month in 1995), which is supposed to cover a quarter of the actuarial cost but usually falls short because of the reluctance of politicians to offend elderly lobbying groups. Since part B coverage is so heavily subsidized, and since part A beneficiaries are automatically enrolled unless they explicitly choose to opt out, almost all (98%) Medicare insureds have both parts A and B. In addition, more than 75 percent of those with Medicare purchase supplemental "Medigap" insurance that covers copayments, deductibles, drugs, and some other expenses (see Table 4.2).

Medicaid is jointly funded by the states and the federal government. The federal government may pay as much as 80 percent of the total program cost for low-income states, but only half for wealthier states. Program design (which differs from state to state), beneficiary enrollment, and other factors, as well as per capita income, can affect both the total cost and the financing split. Although Medicaid

TABLE 4.1 Breakdown of Medicare Coverage
Medicare (part A): Hospital Insurance Covered Services for 1995

Services	Benefit	Medicare Pays	You Pay
HOSPITALIZATION Semiprivate room and board, general nursing and other hospital services and supplies.	First 60 days 61st to 90th day 91st to 150th day* Beyond 150 days	All but $716 All but $179 a day All but $358 a day Nothing	$716 $179 a day $358 a day All costs
SKILLED NURSING FACILITY CARE Semiprivate room and board, skilled nursing and rehabilitative services and other services and supplies.*	First 20 days Additional 80 days Beyond 100 days	100% of approved amount All but $89.50 a day Nothing	Nothing Up to $89.50 a day All costs
HOME HEALTH CARE Part-time or intermittent skilled care, home health aide services, durable medical equipment and supplies, and other services.	Unlimited as long as you meet Medicare requirements for home health care benefits.	100% of approved amount; 80% of approved amount for durable medical equipment.	Nothing for services; 20% of approved amount for durable medical equipment.
HOSPICE CARE Pain relief, symptom management, and support services for the terminally ill.	For as long as doctor certifies need.	All but limited costs for outpatient drugs and inpatient respite care.	Limited cost sharing for outpatient drugs and inpatient respite care.
BLOOD When furnished by a hospital or skilled nursing facility during a covered stay.	Unlimited during a benefit period if medically necessary.	All but first 3 pints per calendar year.	For first 3 pints.***

* 60 reserve days may be used only once.

** Neither Medicare nor Medigap insurance will pay for most nursing home care.

*** To the extent the three pints of blood are paid for or replaced under one part of Medicare during the calendar year, they do not have to be paid for or replaced under the other part.

Source: U.S. Health Care Financing Administration, *Your Medicare Handbook 1995*, page 3.

TABLE 4.1
Medicare (part B): Medical Insurance Covered Services for 1995

Services	Benefit	Medicare Pays	You Pay
MEDICAL EXPENSES Physician's services, inpatient and outpatient medical and surgical services and supplies, physical and speech therapy, diagnostic tests, durable medical equipment and other services.	Unlimited if medically necessary.	80% of approved amount (after $100 deductible). 50% of approved amount for most outpatient mental health services.	$100 deductible,* plus 20% of approved amount and limited charges above approved amount.** 50% for most mental health services.
CLINICAL LABORATORY SERVICES Blood tests, urinalysis, and more.	Unlimited if medically necessary.	Generally 100% of approved amount.	Nothing for services.
HOME HEALTH CARE Part-time or intermittent skilled care, home health aide services, durable medical equipment, and supplies and other services.	Unlimited as long as you meet Medicare requirements.	100% of approved amount; 80% of approved amount for durable medical equipment.	Nothing for services; 20% of approved amount for durable medical equipment.
OUTPATIENT HOSPITAL TREATMENT Services for the diagnosis or treatment of an illness or injury.	Unlimited if medically necessary.	Medicare payment to hospital based on hospital costs.	20% of billed amount (after $100 deductible).*
BLOOD	Unlimited if medically necessary.	80% of approved amount (after $100 deductible and starting with 4th pint).	First 3 pints plus 20% of approved amount for additional pints (after $100 deductible).***

* Once you have had $100 of expense for covered services, the Part B deductible does not apply to any other covered services you receive for the rest of the year.

** Federal law limits charges for physician services.

*** To the extent any of the three pints of blood are paid for or replaced under one part of Medicare during the calendar year they do not have to be paid for or replaced under the other part.

Source: U.S. Health Care Financing Administration, *Your Medicare Handbook 1995*, page 13.

TABLE 4.2 Chart of the Ten Standard Medicare Supplement Plans

Medicare supplement insurance can be sold in only 10 standard plans. This chart shows the benefits included in each plan. Every company must make available Plan "A". Some plans may not be available in your state.

Basic Benefits: Included in All Plans.

Hospitalization: Part A coinsurance plus coverage for 365 additional days after Medicare benefits end.

Medical Expenses: Part B coinsurance (generally 20% of Medicare-approved expenses).

Blood: First 3 pints of blood each year.

A	B	C	D	E	F	G	H	I	J
Basic Benefit	Basic Benefit	Basic Benefit	Basic Benefit	Basic Benefit	Basic Benefit	Basic Benefit	Basic Benefit	Basic Benefit	Basic Benefit
		Skilled Nursing Coinsurance	Skilled Nursing Coinsurance	Skilled Nursing Coinsurance	Skilled Nursing Coinsurance	Skilled Nursing Coinsurance	Skilled Nursing Coinsurance	Skilled Nursing Coinsurance	Skilled Nursing Coinsurance
	Part A Deductible	Part A Deductible	Part A Deductible	Part A Deductible	Part A Deductible	Part A Deductible	Part A Deductible	Part A Deductible	Part A Deductible
		Part B Deductible			Part B Deductible				Part B Deductible
					Part B Excess (100%)	Part B Excess (80%)		Part B Excess (100%)	Part B Excess (100%)
		Foreign Travel Emergency	Foreign Travel Emergency	Foreign Travel Emergency	Foreign Travel Emergency	Foreign Travel Emergency	Foreign Travel Emergency	Foreign Travel Emergency	Foreign Travel Emergency
			At-Home Recovery			At-Home Recovery		At-Home Recovery	At-Home Recovery
							Basic Drug Benefit ($1,250 Limit)	Basic Drug Benefit ($1,250 Limit)	Extended Drug Benefit ($3,000 Limit)
				Preventive Care					Preventive Care

Source: 1995 Guide to Health Insurance for People with Medicare, National Association of Insurance Commissioners and U.S. Health Care Financing Administration, page 14.

was designed to cover poor mothers and children, it has become the dominant funding mechanism for nursing homes. This has occurred primarily because Medicare has very limited nursing home coverage, so that as the elderly pile up expenditures during long nursing home stays, they become poor enough to qualify for Medicaid, and switch to government financing.

Other Government Programs and Charity

Charity paid for about $15 billion in health care in 1995. Workers' compensation, automobile accident insurance, and similar programs paid more than $20 billion. The Veterans Administration took $17 billion in funding, with a somewhat smaller amount being paid for dependents through the Department of Defense. Maternal and Child Health, Drug Abuse, Mental Illness and Mental Retardation, Bureau of Indian Affairs, Vocational Rehabilitation and a variety of other programs accounted for about another $40 billion.[5]

The Uninsured

Thirty to 40 million Americans, almost 15 percent of the population, have no health insurance during any given year.[6] While some of them will pay out of pocket when they get sick, a much larger number simply stay healthy and pocket the cash, or will become charity cases when they get sick. That is why the problem is so intractable—for many of the uninsured, not having insurance is a rational economic decision. Three-fourths of the uninsured are under age 35, and people this young tend to be healthy, and to be in school or earning low wages. For them, paying $300 a month or even $100 a month does not make sense. Those who are working and over age 35 and are in low-paying jobs usually need the money to eat and pay rent more than to provide protection against uncertain medical bills. There is also a small number of people who are chronically ill and would not pass even a cursory medical exam, and hence can be insured only if they take a job in a large firm that provides group coverage. It would be easy to insure everyone by mandating universal coverage, yet this is unlikely to happen in the United States. Most of the suggested reforms intended to bring about a voluntarily increase in coverage would affect only a few people at the margin, and will not have a major impact, since those currently without insurance are often uninsured because of rational economic choices made by themselves or by insurance companies.

Who Pays?

There is a popular misconception that when insurance pays for something, it is free. Unfortunately, while we may not realize who pays because third-party transactions are indirect, every dollar spent on medical care is paid by you, or by me, or by someone just like us. Insurance companies and the government never really "pay" for anything. For the most part, individuals pay for medical care by paying higher taxes and/or taking home lower wages. Even the tax advantage for employee benefits does not mean that we are able to get something for nothing. (This is an economics textbook—there are no free lunches!) The government still has to pay its bills. If fewer dollars are collected through wage taxes, then more dollars must be collected through gasoline taxes or property taxes or income taxes or Social Security taxes or some other tax to make up for the difference. When a hospital provides "free" care to someone as charity, it must raise charges to those who are insured (and the few who cover their bills from their own pocket) to pay for it. Insurance does not reduce the cost of medical care, rather, it redistributes costs so that different people end up paying.

4.3 HOW ARE BENEFITS DETERMINED? A SAMPLE INSURANCE POLICY _____

Insurance is a legal contract, and must be quite specific regarding how much will be paid, under what conditions, the evidence of loss required, and who will arbitrate disputes. "Health" insurance isn't based on sickness at all, but rather, on incurring an expense for medical treatment. Most people will never see the complete contract drawn up by their employer and the insurance company, but only informational pamphlets, descriptions during new employee orientation, and so on. All such benefit descriptions, even in an advertisement or in a simplified brochure printed in Spanish, are legally binding contracts. If a policy says it covers eye examinations, then it covers eye examinations. If it says it will pay $16 for filling a tooth cavity, then it will pay $16. In some sense, every set of documents constitutes a slightly different insurance plan. Whatever a court decides a reasonable person reading such descriptions would expect them to pay for, the insurance plan must pay for. Furthermore, any benefits routinely paid in previous years, and not explicitly revoked, become a precedent, even if those benefits are not mentioned in the contract. The use of "fine print" to leave the insured burdened with thousands of dollars of unexpected bills is simply not allowed—and, in fact, would be self-defeating for an insurance company. In the long run, insurance companies make their money by holding on to premium dollars, not by overcharging. Over time, premiums will be adjusted upward to cover whatever medical costs are incurred.

While the complexity of insurance contracts can easily become overwhelming, certain basic forms are common. Many large employers will provide a comprehensive set of medical benefits that includes Blue Cross and/or Blue Shield with a "wrap around" major medical to cover most other expenses, plus special policies for dental and optical, and an employee assistance plan for counseling and substance abuse (although recently many employers have moved from regular indemnity insurance to managed care plans—see Chapters 10 and 11). The easiest way to understand how benefits are determined is to go through a sample plan and analyze what would be paid for in a hypothetical illness. Note that here we are talking about how the expenses billed to the patient are covered, not how much the doctor or hospital actually receives, which is usually quite different, and is discussed at length in chapters 5–9.

Suppose "George," our hypothetical patient/insurance beneficiary, gets sick, and ultimately is hospitalized for surgery to remove his gallbladder. The total charges of $3,750 (listed in Table 4.3) began with two visits to his family practitioner ($24 each), an X-ray ($38), and some laboratory work ($53). After this, he was sent to a surgeon, who charged a total of $780 for the gallbladder removal, in-

TABLE 4.3 Insurance Benefit Calculation Example

George's Expenses:

2 visits @$24	$48	surgeon	$780	3 days @650	$1,950
X-ray	$38	anesthesia	$140	4 X-rays @40	$160
laboratory	$53	X-ray	$42	op room	$230
drugs	$94	out-pt lab	$80	in pt lab	$135

Total Expenses: $3,750

#1 *Major Medical* with $200 deductible and 10% coinsurance.

    Insurance pays 90% of (3750 − 200)   = 3,195

    George pays $200 + 10% of 3550   = <u>555</u>

                                              $3,750

#2 *Blue Cross* inpatient in full with $20 per day copay.

    BC pays $1,950 hospital daily room charges, $230 O.R.,

      160 X-ray, 135 lab, less $20 × 3 copayment   = 2,415

    George pays copay, all outpatient charges   = <u>1,335</u>

                                              $3,750

#3 *Blue Shield* up to $25 per visit with $8 deductible; Surgeons up to $400

    for appendectomy, $650 gallbladder, $1,200 femur; Anesthesia up to

    1/3 of surgeon; outpatient x-rays @$40 each; outpatient laboratory in full.

    BS pays $650 for surgery, $140 for anesthesia, $320 for 2 office visits,

      $116 for X-rays, and $80 for lab   = 1,018

    George pays for hospital, drugs, surgeon above $650 = <u>2,732</u>

                                              $3,750

#4 *BC/BS with Major Medical wrap-around*

    BC pays same as #2   = 2,415

    BS pays same as #3   = 1,018

    Major med pays 90% of remainder, less copays

      3,750 − 2,415 − 1,018 − 60 − 200 = $57 coverage @90% = 51^{30}

    George pays copays, deductible, 10%   = 265^{70}

                                              $3,750

cluding all pre- and post-operative visits, plus $42 for another X-ray and $80 for additional outpatient (not in the hospital) diagnostic laboratory charges. The anesthesiologist charged $140. George spent three days as an inpatient in the hospital at $650 per day, and also received four inpatient X-rays ($40 each) and $135 of inpatient lab services. The hospital also charged $230 for the operating room and supplies. Over the course of his illness, the charges for George's medication totaled $94. Whichever insurance plan is used, the total of insurance payments plus George's direct payments out of pocket must be $3,750.

First, consider #1, a major medical policy with a $200 deductible and 10% coinsurance. The first $200 is paid out of pocket, leaving $3,550 covered, of which the insurance company pays 90%, or $3,195. George pays the remaining $355 plus the $200 deductible, for a total of $555 in out of pocket expenses. *Second*, George has only Blue Cross policy #2 with inpatient service benefits, subject to a $20 per day copayment. In this case, Blue Cross pays all of the hospital bills, $1,950 in daily room charges, $230 for the operating room, $160 for X-rays, and $135 for lab less $60 in copayments, for a total of $2,415. George pays everything else—a total of $1,335. Even though the anesthesiologist only works in the hospital, those charges are considered a physician bill, and thus not covered as inpatient charges by Blue Cross (or most other insurance). *Third,* consider a Blue Shield physician services policy, #3, that pays up to $20 per visit for outpatient services, with an $8 per visit deductible. Surgeon's fees are paid according to the following schedule: up to $400 for an appendectomy, up to $650 for gallbladder removal, and up to $1,200 for reduction of a fractured femur, with coverage of anesthesia up to a third of the surgical coverage. Outpatient laboratory services are covered in full, X-rays up to $40 each, but there is no pharmaceutical coverage. This Blue Shield policy will pay the following amounts for George's illness; $650 for the surgery, $140 for anesthesia, $32 for the two visits to the family practitioner, $116 for X-rays (two at $38 and one at $40, for which George must pay the remaining $2), and $80 laboratory, for a total of $1,018. George will pay the remaining $2,732.

Finally, consider a comprehensive Blue Cross/Blue Shield with major medical wrap-around (each having the contractual terms as in #2 and #3), policy #4. The Blue Cross payment will be as above, hospital daily room charges (less copayment), OR, inpatient lab, and X-ray, for a Blue Cross total of $2,415. Blue Shield will pay outpatient visits, x-ray and lab, surgeon and anesthesia (as per fee schedule), paying $1,018. Of the $317 not covered by Blue Cross or Blue Shield, $60 is copayments that are excluded from major medical, leaving $257. The first $200 is deductible, so major medical covers $57, paying 90% of that or $51.30. George must pay out of pocket for the copayments ($60), deductible ($200), and the co-insurance ($5.70), for a total of $265.70.

4.4 INCENTIVES TO PATIENTS _____

Which kind of insurance plan encourages patients to use a more expensive, higher-quality hospital? Which plan encourages longer stays? The Blue Cross plan (#2 in Table 4.3) does not make the patient pay anything for hospital care, no matter how high the charges. This provides an incentive to use the best-quality care available for as many days as you want, and also causes the most moral hazard. With major medical (#1 in Table 4.3), the 10 percent patient coinsurance provides some disincentive to using a more expensive hospital, or to staying longer; thus moral hazard is reduced. This Blue Shield plan alone (#3 in Table 4.3), with no hospital coverage, makes it likely that a patient will choose a cheaper hospital and try to get discharged as soon as possible.

What are the incentives with regard to the patient's choice of the quality and quantity of surgery? This Blue Cross plan (#2) alone does not cover surgery, and hence eliminates any moral hazard, but may force the patient faced with the prospect of a large bill to forgo a needed operation or to compromise on quality. However, since hospitalization is a complement to surgery, patients with Blue Cross will use more surgery than patients without any insurance. For the Major Medical plan described (#1), the 10 percent coinsurance factor will again create some disincentive on both the quality and quantity of care dimensions. The incentives under our Blue Shield only plan (#3) are more complicated. For anything above the fee schedule amount ($650 for a gallbladder removal), the patient bears the full marginal cost. Thus, the patient is unlikely to choose a more expensive surgeon unless the difference really seems worth it. There is no moral hazard with respect to quality. This is an example of how the insurance contract can be customized to eliminate inefficiencies due to insurance paying a high rate for services of little value to the patient. However, there is moral hazard with respect to quantity of surgery under Blue Shield, since as long as the patient finds a surgeon charging less than the fee schedule, the patient bears no out-of-pocket cost for having the appendix removed, a bent toe straightened, and so on. It is not surprising that Blue Cross plans provide the greatest incentive for patients to use more hospital services, since Blue Cross was created by the hospital association (see "The History of Insurance," section 4.7). Similarly, Blue Shield was created by physician associations and provides the greatest incentives to use more physician services. The contract specifications reflect not only patient's interests in efficient insurance, but also the self-interest of the provider groups that sponsored the insurance programs.[7]

Adverse selection is inevitable with any insurance plan that covers only part of the population. A Blue Cross service benefit plan would be more attractive to someone who thought he or she had cancer and expected to spend many days in the hospital. On the other hand, a Blue Shield plan with extensive outpatient coverage might attract a patient with arthritis who expected to make many visits to a physician but have few inpatient admissions. It is even possible for an insurance company to design benefits in such a way that they attract "healthy" people. For example, if an employer offers a choice among several plans, and one has much better pediatric coverage (immunizations, well-baby care, etc.) it is likely to attract young families, who are, on average, much healthier than other groups. Similarly, coverage for sports medicine or abortions attracts people who expect to have expenses of this type, but are relatively young and healthy and do not have high expenses overall. On the other hand, chronically ill people run up large out-of-pocket expenses for medications, so good pharmaceutical coverage is apt to draw a disproportionate share of this group that also is at high risk for hospital, outpatient, and ancillary (laboratory and X-ray) utilization.

4.5 FIXED PREMIUMS, ASO, AND SELF-INSURANCE: A RANGE OF RISK-BEARING CONTRACTS _____

An employer can purchase insurance at a fixed price and bear no risk, or it can pool its own funds, handle all claims, and self-insure while bearing all risks. In between are a range of contracts that split the risk and claims-processing burden: experience rated, retention ratio, minimum premium, and administered services only (ASO) plans (Table 4.4). Negotiating price is a major problem in contracting for insurance. **Experience rating,** by allowing the price to rise or fall to match the dollar amount of claims submitted by the employees during the previous year ("experience"), avoids costly and contentious haggling. A **retention ratio** agreement makes a similar adjustment, but in the current year. The employer and insurer estimate losses, and if claims turn out to be less than expected, then the insurer will return most of the difference, retaining only a percentage (the retention ratio) for administrative expense and profit.

TABLE 4.4   Range of Insurance Contracts

Insurer bears risk, processes claims				*Employer bears risk, processes own claims*
Fixed Premiums	Experience Rated	Retention Ratio	ASO	Self-Insurance
pay pre-set amount for coverage	premiums changed each year to reflect last year's actual claims	if losses are less than expected, insurer gives back part of premium	administrative services only, insurance company pays claims using the firm's own funds	firm pays claims, acts as their own insurance company

Two things make it difficult for an employer to act as its own insurance company: catastrophic losses and claims processing. To some extent these difficulties can be ameliorated through contractual arrangements. Economies of scale in risk-bearing can be obtained contractually through **reinsurance,** which is a kind of major medical for employers, a policy for the group as a whole that covers 90 percent of the cost of any individual above some specified high amount (perhaps $50,000) or for some aggregate loss of the group as a whole that is above the expected value (perhaps anything above $5 million). Of course, reinsurance is quite costly, and so coverage is usually purchased only for extraordinary losses. Claims processing is also apt to create difficulties, because the firm is usually better at its own line of business than at the business of managing and paying insurance benefits. Economies of scale in claims processing can be obtained contractually through **ASO** or **administered services only** contracts in which an insurance company processes the bills, pays the claims, and settles disputes, for a set fee per year or per claim, but all of the funds for paying the benefits come directly from the employer.

Under "normal" circumstances, the costs of experience rated and retention ratio, ASO and self-insurance contracts should converge toward the same amount, but things are rarely normal. When a firm accepts bids for an experience rated plan, it is not uncommon for an insurance company to try to "buy the business" by setting the premiums very low in the first year. Then it will use the bad experience in that year to force a high premium in the following year. The employer who got such a good deal is now stuck, and must accept a substantial premium increase or incur the costs of going out to bid again, often finding that with such a record of underwriting losses, few insurers want to bid. Also, a group with higher-than-expected losses may find that their insurer starts to give poor service and gets very nasty about paying claims (and thus is able to hold onto premium dollars longer). On the other hand, employee groups often try to take advantage of insurance companies by dropping them after a bad year (thus allowing no time to make up the extraordinary losses through experience rating), or repeatedly going into the market search for low bids. The more flexible retention ratio agreement is more like a partnership. The insurance company and the employee group get together in a long-run arrangement where initial pricing is not so important. The year-to-year conflicts are avoided. However, the downside of this more integrated contract is that if things do go sour, it is much worse for both parties.

4.6   ERISA, TAXES, AND MANDATED BENEFITS _____

The employee benefits offered by a company are determined largely by competitive conditions in the labor market, as it tries to hire new workers, or directly through negotiations with the unions that represent the workers. Firms see benefits as a way to retain workers, and workers see benefits as a way to protect themselves against losses. The interest of both firms and workers will be represented in the final outcome. Sometimes a broader public interest is imposed in the form of **mandated benefits**—regulations promulgated by the government stating that specific benefits (e.g., substance abuse, AZT for AIDS) must be provided. If such benefits are a good thing, why don't they arise naturally in the course of competitive contracting? Consider the case of substance abuse benefits. Without such benefits, insurance will pay for treatment of liver damage, but not for the excessive drinking that caused it. From a social perspective, it is much more efficient to treat the underlying cause (alcoholism) that to treat just the symptom (liver damage). However, a firm is not interested in the productivity of society as a whole, but in the productivity of its work force. A quite reasonable profit-maximizing response to alcoholism is to fire the employee and push him out on to the streets, where the burden is borne by the rest of society. Adverse selection can also play a role. A firm with especially generous benefits for AIDS will find its premiums going higher and higher as more chronically ill people try to get jobs there. Eventually, if adverse selection were severe enough, only people with a very high risk of AIDS would be willing to accept the low wages paid by this firm in order to get the benefits. Mental illness poses similar problems of adverse selection because the benefits are highly concentrated, with most of the dollars being spent on just a few people, and those people or their families are much more aware of the risks than the insurance company. In a competitive market, insurance contracts reflect the interests of firm and (most) employees, but not society as a whole. If such benefits are not made mandatory, then only a few firms will offer them.

Insurance is regulated largely by the states. Some states, such as Arizona, impose very few mandates, while Massachusetts has over thirty. Employers operating in multiple states need uniform national laws because it would be difficult to maintain many different sets of benefit plans and give more or less to an employee depending on place of residence. Under the "Employee Retirement and Income Security Act of 1974" (ERISA) and later amendments, self-insured firms are regulated under national **ERISA** rules and thus exempt from state mandates. Since only large firms are able to self-insure, the attempt to increase coverage through mandates may have the paradoxical effect of reducing the number of people insured, as small firms opt to provide no health insurance at all.

State taxes provide another incentive to self-insure. Most states impose a premium tax of 1 to 2 percent that can be avoided through self-insurance or ASO contracts. Minimum premium plans where the employer pays the first $X million (usually about 90% of estimated losses) and the insurer the rest exist primarily to avoid state taxes, since they are no different from fixed-premium full insurance with regard to risk or claims processing. Several innovative state health care financing plans have been challenged under ERISA. For example, New Jersey funded a special program for the uninsured through a 30 percent surcharge on all hospital bills. After large firms won ERISA exemption, only small employers and individuals were left paying the surcharge, so the state was forced to dismantle its program.[8]

If mandated benefits are a good idea, why don't the states just pay for them? The answer is that they would have to raise taxes to do so. A mandated benefit, although it operates like a tax on firms, is counted as a regular cost of business to the firm. It does not appear on the government's budget, and thus is not recognized by many voters. Although the public ultimately will lose more in forgone wages than in taxes avoided, that is not obvious to voters when they go to the polls. It is for this reason that any national insurance plan enacted in the United States is almost certain to be based on employer contributions. People who would never vote to increase taxes to fund national health insurance will calmly vote to have government insist that every employer provide benefits—and so our government will rationally follow the path of least resistance.

Insurance, by channeling funds through different organizations and contractual arrangements, has a tendency to obscure the actual costs of medical care. Pretending that a mandated insurance benefit will somehow make these services cost less than if they were funded through a tax increase has misled some people, while firms have misled the public by claiming to have paid a "fair share" for their own workers, but never dealing with the issue of how health care for the homeless, the mentally ill, and people with AIDS will be paid for. A health care system that helps only the healthy is cost-effective in one sense, and worthless in another. Perhaps the worst aspect of the complex system of health insurance that has arisen in the United States is this obfuscation of reality that allows interested parties to avoid responsibility and never face up to the hard decisions of how to pay for health care. It is, therefore, worthwhile to examine how this complex system came to be, and why some organizations and contracts have dominated in the U.S. while different forms of insurance developed in other countries.

4.7 THE HISTORY OF HEALTH INSURANCE _____

In some sense, risk pooling has always existed—people have always taken care of each other during times of need. Financial contracts for pooling risk did not become important until the Industrial Revolution, when economies moved from the medieval manor system, where most people worked the land, to a wage-based economy centered in cities and towns. Freemen who left the medieval estates and gathered in town to practice skilled trades, such as printers or goldsmiths, often became quite wealthy, but potentially subject to catastrophic losses should they become ill. While gaining freedom, they had given up the protection and security that went with being part of an estate. If sick, they might become destitute. The guilds were organized to further their interests collectively, and became natural vehicles for sharing risks. Initially this took the form of soliciting donations from all of the other guild members—"passing the hat"—when someone became ill or died. Then more formal institutions evolved that accumulated funds over time. A "subscription" would be regularly collected that could be used to pay benefits. In this early form of insurance, there was no distinction made between the loss of wages due to illness and the costs of medical care (or burial). Insurance was simply a way to provide money in time of need. The guild members knew each other well, and so the definition of loss was made by a consensus of the leadership, not the existence of a doctor's bill.[9]

Early industrialists also recognized the need to provide wages and medical care for workers when they were sick. It is unlikely that funds were set aside for this purpose. Rather, sickness funds were drawn out of daily business receipts. Also, most such benefits were informal, provided at the discretion of the owner, and not as part of the employment contract. In this sense, early industrial benefits were quite similar to the set of paternalistic obligations that the lord of the manor owed the serfs who worked his land, except that as factories and wages replaced farms and tenant shares, the benefits were money payments rather than direct care. By the nineteenth century, some industries that were particularly dangerous and in remote locations had developed contracts with a "company doctor" so that there was always regular medical care available. In other industries, it was the workers who organized to provide sickness benefits. As unions became an important means for furthering the interests of workers, they found that they needed some way to keep the membership involved (and paying dues) throughout the year and not just when a strike was threatened. Medical coverage became the preferred union benefit. It was always needed, made the workers and their families grateful. In those days it could be provided at relatively low cost through clinics or "dispensaries" staffed by young doctors hired by the union to practice several nights a week. Company and union clinics, mutual benefit societies, and other forms of prepayment had become common by 1850, but still provided medical care financing to only a small fraction of the population, probably less than a twentieth. As wages rose above the subsistence level and workers became more assertive, it became evident that insurance would have to be extended to cover more of the population.

The first national health insurance program was implemented in Germany in 1893. Bismarck, the chancellor who had unified the German *Lander* (provinces) into a nation, saw that his political successes were threatened by the popularity of socialist causes among the workers. By putting together a social security system with medical insurance and retirement benefits for industrial workers, he accomplished one of the main goals of the socialist movement, and was able to maintain popular support. National health plans were established in England in 1911, Sweden in 1914, and France in 1930. At first, only salaried workers in the major manufacturing plants were covered, with usually a lesser degree of coverage for dependents. Other workers—such as agricultural and retail workers, day laborer, shopkeepers, and the self-employed—had to take care of themselves. Over the next fifty years, coverage was successively broadened. By 1980, almost every developed country had health insurance coverage for all citizens, either through a national health service (U.K.), a universal insurance plan (Canada), or by coordinating all of the employer-based plans and providing government insurance for the rest of the population (Germany, Japan).[10] Evolution of health insurance in the United States was much different, and a large segment of the population still lacks health insurance today.

The United States depended mostly on voluntary private initiatives to develop health insurance, with much less reliance on government. There was a recognition that the population needed protection against losses due to illness, and in 1929 the independent Commission of the Costs of Medical Care began a fact-finding study, eventually producing a twenty-eight-volume report that has been very influential in shaping the growth of voluntary insurance in the United States.[11] In this same year, Baylor hospital proposed to the local teachers' association that it would pro-vide all the care needed to anyone who would pay a premium of $0.50 a month. The plan proved to be very popular, and similar plans were started by other nearby hospitals. One problem with this "hospital prepayment" plan was that a patient whose doctor worked in a different hospital, or who needed a special type of care elsewhere, got no benefits. The solution was to combine all of the separate plans under the sponsorship of the state hospital association so that one plan cov-ered all hospitals, and thus Blue Cross was born. It grew rapidly, from 3,000 mem-bers in 1930, to more than 10,000 in 1932, and more than 1,000,000 by 1936. In 1994, 64 million people were insured through Blue Cross/Blue Shield plans.

The rapid spread of Blue Cross can be attributed not only to the gains from risk pooling for patients, but also to the particular economic conditions faced by hos-pitals during the Great Depression. At the beginning of the century, hospitals were still mostly charitable institutions for the poor that were funded by philanthropy. But by the 1930s, they were becoming curative institutions that depended on pa-tient fees to support modern technological advances. Yet the history of charity meant that hospital bills were always among the last to be paid, since no hospital could turn you away if you were sick. The Depression reduced philanthropy and patient fee income just as the drive to build many new hospitals and more mod-ern hospitals began. Blue Cross hospital insurance promised a source of steady in-come to support the building of operating rooms, radiology suites, and all of the other technology that doctors needed to practice the new medical advances. It was much easier to get patients to pay $0.50 each month than to get them to come up with $100 or $500 when they got sick.

During the same time period, medical associations in the Pacific Northwest started the first Blue Shield plans to pay for physician services.[12] Here, competi-tion from alternative organizational forms was an important factor leading to the development of private voluntary insurance. Railroad and timber were dominant industries, and as dangerous occupations carried on in remote locations, had de-veloped a tradition of providing on-site medical services through company doc-tors who were paid on salary. Hungry young doctors with few patients were will-ing to bid aggressively for such "contract practice," driving the remuneration down far below what an established doctor would have expected to receive in fees for treating the same number of cases. Local doctors saw a steady decline in stan-dard fee-for-service practice as more and more clinics were set up. Their response was to establish a medical service plan that provided, in return for monthly pre-miums, services from any physician who was a member of the local medical soci-ety. At the same time, they prohibited member physicians from accepting any con-tract practice or salaried patient care. By splitting the market so that contract practice became unattractive to most junior doctors, the medical association acted as a cartel to promote the interests of its members and keep prices high.

The establishment of Blue Cross plans for hospital coverage and Blue Shield plans for physician services set the stage for a system of comprehensive voluntary insurance against losses due to medical expenses. Insurance companies eager for profits tried to grab a share of the rapidly growing market. However, "The Blues" had several advantages. First, as the official programs of the hospital and physician associations respectively, they had professional and popular support that the commercial insurance companies did not have. As nonprofit organizations, they escaped many business taxes, particularly the premium taxes levied on commercial health insurance. Blue Cross had contracts with all of the local hospitals, often provided a substantial fraction of total revenues, and could therefore negotiate complete "service benefits" at a discount. A commercial insurer, in contrast, might account for only a small amount of business in each hospital, did not have the access to administrators and detailed financial data that the hospital association (and therefore Blue Cross) had, and thus often had to pay full charges, substantially above the Blue Cross reimbursement rates. For physician services, Blue Shield could use its extensive information on fees and utilization to pay a contractually defined UCR ("usual, customary and reasonable" see Chapter 5) amount that also was less than commercial insurers were charged.

In order to offset these considerable cost advantages, commercial insurers developed "major medical" plans. The use of deductibles and coinsurance meant that protection against catastrophic losses could be offered at lower cost. Also, commercial insurers were willing to target companies that had healthier employees and experience rate the premiums, further allowing them to cut prices below those offered by community rated Blue Cross and Blue Shield plans. Although eventually both Blue Cross and Blue Shield accepted experience rating and patient cost-sharing, they fought as long as they could to retain community rating and first-dollar coverage. Why? The answer lies in the nature of third-party contracting. Insurance companies were actively involved in only one side: the financial contract with patients for risk pooling. Insurers were essentially passive with regard to hospitals, paying charges at the going rate. Blue Cross, on the other hand, was (until 1969) managed by the hospital associations. It was far less interested in generating profitable insurance than in increasing and stabilizing revenues for hospitals. Community rating made sense because the hospital had to treat the whole community. There was little benefit to them if only a select group was insured. Nor did they care how the prices were set for different groups of employees. They wanted to increase total hospital revenues to provide more services to the community as a whole. While the deterrent effect of deductibles and coinsurance might help reduce premiums and/or increase profits for insurance companies, it would tend to hurt the hospitals, since they would have a smaller and more price-sensitive market. Thus Blue Cross, acting on behalf of the hospitals, supported both community rating and first-dollar coverage, because such contracts tended to maximize hospital's revenues.

In World War II, wage and price control regulations exempted employee benefits, giving a powerful push toward increased insurance coverage.[13] Companies that wanted to attract workers (and they all did, with wartime production booming and many laborers drafted into the military) used health insurance to replace prohibited wage increases. In a short period of time, health insurance went from being an occasional perk that covered just 5 percent of the population, to a routine benefit that was expected to be part of any good job, and covered more than 50 percent of the population. Even with favorable tax treatments and active encouragement, however, voluntary insurance could not be extended to cover two of the groups who needed it most, the elderly and the poor. The poor were simply not able to afford health insurance. Furthermore, while policy makers and hospital administrators might think that paying premiums to prepare for future medical expenses was one of the most important things a family could do with its money, many of the poor did not. Since there was always some form of care available, usually in city clinics and hospitals, the poor often chose to spend what little discretionary money they had on better housing, better food, or some entertainment, rather than insurance premiums.

The difficulties of the elderly in obtaining insurance were largely attributable to adverse selection and the discounting of consumption over time.[14] While younger people were formed into risk pooling groups on the basis of employment, older people were not attached to an employer. There was no natural grouping by which risks could be shared, and there were no tax advantages to insurance premiums paid out of savings or retirement benefits rather than wages. Furthermore, the differences in the expected costs of medical care between individuals are much greater for older people, making it more difficult to constitute risk-sharing pools. Whereas many of the illnesses that strike younger persons are essentially random events of low probability, many medical expenses of the elderly are for chronic conditions. There is no reason for a healthy seventy-two-year-old to want to be in a group paying the same premiums as someone with cancer or arthritis who can be expected to have continuing high medical expenses for many years. Elderly people often know much more about the potential cost of their health conditions than any insurance company can, and thus create adverse selection problems when allowed to purchase insurance individually. These difficulties are exacerbated by the need to save up early in one's career to pay for medical expenses that come after retirement. There must be a mechanism for transferring dollars from consumption at early ages toward old age. The Social Security Acts of 1965, which established the Medicare (Title XVI) program for the elderly and Medicaid (Title XVII) for the indigent, created the most fundamental changes to date in the U.S. health system, and made government a major partner in financing medical care. Adverse selection was no longer a problem for the elderly, because everyone over age 65 was insured. Poverty no longer excluded the indigent from health insurance, because the government made these benefits available at no cost.

4.8 INSURANCE, PRICE COMPETITION, AND THE STRUCTURE OF MEDICAL MARKETS _____

After a century of development, health care financing in the United States is still in flux, with a mixed public and private system in which government accounts for 44 percent of total funds, 36 percent is accounted for by private insurance (including Blue Cross/Blue Shield, self-funded employer plans, commercial insurance companies, and HMOs), 2 percent by charitable contributions, and the remaining 18 percent paid directly by patients and family members out-of-pocket. A sizable fraction of those out-of-pocket costs are for deductibles and coinsurance, and thus could in one sense be considered part of the third-party insurance payments. Among this variety of health insurance organizations, government—and Medicare in particular—is the dominant payer. During the 1950s Blue Cross set the tone and structure for insurance coverage, and Medicare copied the Blue Cross reimbursement system. However, subsequent reforms have changed the balance of power. No hospital can afford to be without a Medicare contract, and thus must make use of the complex and highly regulated Medicare cost and activity reporting scheme. It has become easier for other insurers to adapt the Medicare payment system than to develop their own. Since all of the other insurers follow the Medicare lead, the influence of Medicare is even greater than its percentage share of the market. A similar expansion of influence is occurring with regard to insurance coverage of physician services under the part B relative value system known as RBRVS (see discussion of physician payment in Chapter 5). However, the rapid growth of HMOs and other managed care plans (see Chapters 10 and 11) is currently changing the way medicine is contracted for, and may significantly modify the financial structure by the year 2000.

Health *insurance* markets are very price competitive, but prices do not play a large role in contracting for the underlying services. For a patient seeking medical care, quality rather than price is paramount. Medical care must be purchased at the time it is needed, often under great stress. Serious illness may strike at any moment, without warning, or a person may go for years without visiting the doctor or the hospital. Medical services must be performed on the person. The outcome of treatment is uncertain, and depends on the quality of care in a way that patients are usually not sufficiently knowledgeable to judge. Even though quality is the most important characteristic, it is also hard to measure, and even more difficult to translate into dollars so as to enable the patient to rationally consider whether or not a highly regarded physician is really worth an extra high fee. Indeed, in many cases, patients are not even sure exactly what is being done for them, so they can hardly be sure that they got their money's worth. Also, if a mistake has been made, no amount of money can readily compensate the patient for having been crippled or killed by poor quality. Experience in purchasing care for one illness may be of little help the next time you get sick, because it may be pneumonia instead of a broken leg. Insurance, on the other hand, is a very regular and routine product that is easy to buy in advance and for which small price differences are meaningful. Every year, people renew their insurance, and the choice can be planned and researched ahead of time. Insurance is not a direct personal service that must be performed in person; the check can be sent from anywhere. Insurance offers money, an absolutely standard and universal commodity, so that there is little quality variation (friendliness of service and amount of paperwork vary between insurance companies, but are these trivial compared to the variation between good and bad surgeons). If there was a mistake made by the insurance company, its effects could be entirely erased by sending another check. This is not to say that consumers have no problems in determining the value of their health insurance coverage and whether they got what they paid for, but that those information problems are orders of magnitude less formidable than the information problems faced in the purchase of medical care. Furthermore, the actual purchasing of insurance is carried out mostly by the group through a broker or full-time company benefits specialists, whereas consumers must go out and purchase medical care on their own.

WHY THE HEALTH INSURANCE MARKET IS HIGHLY PRICE-COMPETITIVE

Unlike medical care, which suffers many market failure problems from lack of consumer knowledge to variable incidence, the market for health insurance meets most of the conditions for a purely competitive goods.

1. It is a homogeneous product. It provides dollars in reimbursement, so there is little "quality" variation.
2. It can be bought far in advance, when there is no time pressure or illness.
3. It can be bought far from home, in a national market.
4. Purchasing is done by large and sophisticated buyers (firms, brokers) who can afford to compare and examine the contracts purchasers.

While the health insurance market itself is very competitive, *the existence of insurance tends to make price competition more difficult to maintain in the medical care market.* Insurance breaks the linkage between buyer and seller, splitting payment "for" services by patients from payments "for" services to providers. The reimbursement provided by an insurer to a hospital may have almost no relation to the bill that the patient receives, or to what the insurer would have reimbursed to the patient if the bill was paid out-of-pocket. In third-party transactions there is often no longer a single "price" in any meaningful sense, and the role of prices as information is seriously degraded. They can no longer communicate to suppliers what the value of services is to consumers, nor do they reflect the costs of inputs in production. By design, insurance removes the burden of medical costs from the patient. There is no longer any need to worry about whether or not it is worthwhile to go to the doctor, or if an extra visit is worth the additional cost. Insurance acts like a price subsidy by increasing demand and by removing the incentive to use less expensive substitutes. Once the insurance premiums are paid, everything costs the same. Price competition is replaced by quality competition, since prices no longer matter.

Insurance tends to distort production behavior as well. Under many reimbursement systems, hospitals and doctors are paid according to the cost of care, rather than the value of services (primarily because value is too hard to measure). Hence, there is little incentive to work hard for increased efficiency. Some additional costs will be incurred for no reason other than the fact that the insurance will pay for them. With revenues coming from insurance rather than from patients, the connection between consumer service and profits is eroded. It may become easier to make money by providing what the insurance company thinks is important (detailed bills with lots of documentation) rather than what patients want or need.

Control over health care is exercised by control over the money that goes to doctors and hospitals. Thus, *insurance and reimbursement rules, rather than legislation, have become the dominant regulatory force in health care.* The government does not need to pass a law telling hospitals to do or not to do something. If reimbursement rules are shifted so that only hospitals that meet certain standards get paid, then hospitals will do what the flow of money directs them to do. It is not necessary to exhort doctors to provide examinations. If the money is made available through insurance, the services will appear in the marketplace.

Medicine is a vital service with a broad public and professional interest. What that means in practice is that there is often a rhetorical cover blanketing the operation of self-interest by any party. Insurance companies, consumers, and providers all talk about the public interest while trying hard to maintain their own position, or to get ahead. The advice of economists as natural observers of the social scene is that following the path of dollars through the system will often tell a student more about what is really going on than reading the lawbooks or listening to the arguments presented in the newspapers and on TV. For physicians and hospitals (even nonprofit hospitals), money talks. For those willing to listen, it speaks loudly and clearly about how the health care system works.

SUGGESTIONS FOR FURTHER READING _____

Employee Benefit Research Institute, *Databook on Employee Benefits.* (serial publication).
William A. Glaser, *Health Insurance in Practice: International Variations in Financing, Benefits, and Problems.* San Francisco: Jossey-Bass, 1991.
Medicare and Market Change, the Winter 1995 issue of *Health Affairs.*
Health Insurance Institute of America. *Sourcebook of Health Insurance Data,* Washington, DC: HIAA (annual).

SUMMARY _____

1. The **government is the single largest insurer**, paying for 44 percent of all medical care. Medicare, which pays for the medical care of the elderly, is the largest and most influential government program, although the state/federal Medicaid program dominates long-term care reimbursement. Tax advantages have fostered the growth of health insurance as an employee benefit. Private health insurance covers 62 percent of the population, but pays only 35 percent of the total bills. About 18 percent is paid for out-of-pocket by patients or their families.

2. About 38 million Americans, 14 percent of the population, are **uninsured**. For many of them it is a rational decision to go without insurance based on their relative youth, good health, and/or low current earning power. For some, it is exclusion due to chronic disease, bad luck, or the size of the firm they happen to work for.

3. Insurance comes in a range of contractual forms, from pure insurance with fixed premiums, through various forms of risk sharing, to administered services only and self-insurance plans where the employer bears all the risk. Obtaining **tax benefits and exemption from state-mandated coverage** under ERISA has been a major reason for firms to self-insure.

4. Historically, the development of voluntary insurance plans in the United States was led by groups of hospitals and doctors who were interested in **assuring payment to providers** as well as protecting patients from losses.

5. **Markets for health insurance are more competitive** than for the underlying service, medical care, because insurance is (a) a homogenous product (dollars

to pay bills) with little quality variation, which is (b) bought in advance (c) on a geographically dispersed national market, and (d) often purchased by sophisticated corporate benefits managers who are well informed.

6. **Insurance distorts the market for medical care** since use of third-party payment breaks the link between buyer and seller. It acts like a price reduction or subsidy, making consumers less price-sensitive, fostering competition on the basis of quality rather than price, and necessitating special contracts to reimburse providers who do not collect much money directly from the patients they serve.

7. **Insurance rules**, by controlling the flow of money, act as the dominant regulatory force in the health care industry.

PROBLEMS _____

1. {*gains from trade*} Who benefits from a three-party transaction?

2. {*accounting, incidence*} How can a patient benefit if the premiums paid are more than the cost of the medical care received? How can an insurance company benefit if the medical care provided costs more than the premiums paid in?

3. {*calculation of benefits*} Your insurance:

    Blue Cross:

Hospital	in full
In-patient diagnostic	in full

    Blue Shield:

Gastrectomy	up to $840
Appendectomy	up to $250
X-ray (each - max 20)	up to $10 per X-ray
Visits (deductible of $8 for each visit)	up to $20 per visit

Your expenses:

(I)	(II)B
In-patient	In-patient
5 days × $400	1 day × $300
3 x-rays × $16	Appendectomy $275
Gastrectomy $950	2 visits × $15
Other	Other
4 visits post-op × $15	3 x-rays × $ 20
	5 office visits × $20

For (I), then for (II), calculate how much is paid by BC, by BS and by you.

B) How much would be paid in (I) if you had major medical that paid 80 percent of charges after $200? Under (II)?

4. {*marginal incentives*} Suppose a person had only one of the types of insurance described in problem 2, BC, BS, or major medical. Under which plan would there be the greatest incentive to:

a. choose a higher-quality (more expensive) hospital?

b. spend more days in the hospital?

    c. use more drugs?

    d. choose a higher-quality (more expensive) surgeon?

5. {*uninsured*} The law now gives a worker who becomes unemployed the right to buy continuing health insurance coverage after leaving the company. Why might it be rational for a factory worker who loses their job to give up this legal right to purchase coverage and be uninsured, even knowing that he or she is at risk for high medical expenditures?

6. {*competition*} Why are the markets for health insurance so much more price-competitive than the markets for medical care?

7. {*mandated benefits*} Prior to 1970, why was maternity usually treated differently than other medical expenses, either excluded entirely from coverage, or subject to flat lump-sum cash (indemnity) benefit? During the 1970s, 23 states mandated that treatment related to pregnancy be covered the same as any other type of treatment, and in 1978, such coverage became uniform throughout the United States. Would mandated maternity benefits make working in a salaried position more or less attractive to women? Would it make women of childbearing age more or less attractive as employees? Would it increase or decrease the number of births performed surgically by Cesarean section? Who do you think bore the expense of implementing this mandate? (For a discussion of these issues, see "The Incidence of Mandated Maternity Benefits" by Jonathan Gruber, *American Economic Review* April 1994 84:3, pp. 622–661.)

8. Why was it more common for railroads and timber companies to provide health insurance in the early 1900s than for textile mills or accounting firms?

9. {*ownership*} Who controlled Blue Cross when it was formed? Did this form of insurance generate profits for its owners?

10. {*adverse selection*} Which government insurance program is more affected by adverse selection, Medicare or Medicaid?

ENDNOTES _____

1. Insurance companies are regulated and taxed as large financial investment institutions, with underwriting gains and losses treated as secondary sources of income.
2. C. Rufus Rorem, "Sickness Insurance in the United States," *Bulletin of the American Hospital Association,* June 1932. Odin W. Anderson, *Health Services as a Growth Enterprise in the United States since 1875,* 2nd edition, Ann Arbor, Mich.: Health Administration Press, 1990.
3. Estimates of coverage are from the *Sourcebook of Health Insurance Data,* Health Insurance Association of America, Washington, D.C., 1994. Note, some people may have coverage from more than one source, so the number of insureds is greater than the number of people who have insurance.
4. Ibid.
5. National Health Accounts, Office of the Actuary, Health Care Financing Administration.
6. Estimates of the number of uninsured are always in flux and subject to dispute for a number or reasons. Some people are uncovered only temporarily, and may even be eligible for coverage should they need it. Some dependents remain uncounted, or get

double-counted because they are eligible under several plans. The uninsured are less likely to have regular jobs and residences, so are harder to track. A reasonable range of estimates, and some evidence about whether the number is growing or shrinking, is probably the best that can be obtained.

7. George A. Shipman, *Medical Service Corporations in the State of Washington: A Study of the Administration of Physician-Sponsored Pre-paid Medical Care.* Cambridge, Mass: Harvard University Press, 1962.

8. Howard S. Berliner and Sonia Delgada, "From DRGs to Deregulation: New Jersey Takes the Road Less Traveled," *Journal of American Health Policy,* 3:44–48, July/August 1993.

9. R. Munts, *Bargaining for Health: Labor Unions, Health Insurance and Medical Care,* Madison, Wisc.: University of Wisconsin Press, 1967.

10. William A. Glaser, *Health Insurance in Practice: International Variations in Financing, Benefits, and Problems,* San Francisco: Jossey-Bass, 1991.

11. Committee on the Costs of Medical Care. *Medical Care for the American People,* Chicago: University of Chicago Press, 1932.

12. Shipman, *op.cit.*

13. Institute of Medicine, *Employment and Health Benefits: A connection at Risk,* Washington, D.C.: National Academy Press, 1993, page 70.

14. Herman M. Somers and Anne R. Somers, *Medicare and the Hospitals: Issues and Prospects,* Washington, D.C.: The Brookings Institution, 1967.

CHAPTER 5

Physicians

QUESTIONS

1. *Which types of physicians earn the highest incomes?*
2. *How much does it cost to practice medicine?*
3. *Are rising malpractice premiums a major cause of higher doctor bills?*
4. *Why, and how, are doctors giving discounts on fees?*
5. *How are physicians paid?*
6. *Is medical care "sold" like other goods and services?*
7. *Is it doctors or patients who decide what hospital to use, what drugs to buy, and what specialist to see for a second opinion? In what sense is the doctor the patient's "agent?"*

At the center of medical practice stands the physician. Physicians direct the flow of patients through control over admissions, referrals, regulations, insurance reimbursements, and drug prescriptions. There is a very powerful and special bond between doctor and patient. This relationship is based on medical science—and ethics and emotions—as well as economics.[1] Even when a transaction does not directly involve a physician financially, they still play a dominant role.

5.1 PHYSICIAN PAYMENT: HOW FUNDS FLOW IN

While most of the labor force is employed and paid a salary by some large organization, most physicians are still independent entrepreneurs or partners running what are, in effect, small businesses.[2] The income of physicians in solo or group private practices mostly comes from **fee-for-service (FFS)** payments, a specified amount for each visit or procedure, although an increasing amount is coming from more complex negotiated third-party contracts. In the 1930s, physicians were essentially free to charge whatever they decided was appropriate, but often collected much less than what they charged. Today, 85 percent of physician revenues come from third-party payments[3] and most fees are subject to some form of external review or control (see Table 5.1).

It is important to distinguish between what the physician **charges,** that is, the amount that appears on the bill, and the actual payments made by insurance company, which may be considerably less. One of the initial steps in the evolution of physician payment in the United States was the development of **UCR,** "usual, customary and reasonable" fee screens. The Blue Shield plans, which then provided the largest portion of physician insurance and operated with the support of the local medical societies, collected information on all charges for each service for each physician in the area during the previous year. Then, when a physician submitted a bill, it was checked to see if it was above that doctor's median charge for the same service during the prior year (usual), above the 75th percentile of charges by all doctors in the area (customary), or was justifiably higher because of a complicating secondary illness in this particular patient's illness or some other acceptable reason (reasonable). When Medicare was implemented in 1966, it adopted the Blue Shield UCR method of paying physicians.

An effort to reduce payments, particularly for certain services, led insurers to promulgate **fee schedules.** A fee schedule is like a menu that specifies how much will be paid for each of a number of listed services. Fee schedules can be proposed by the sellers (physicians) to try to keep prices up, or by the buyers (Medicare, insurance companies) to try to keep prices down. A major difficulty with fee schedules is the amazingly large number of services that must be priced. It is easy to come up with a reasonable price for a coronary bypass or a normal birth, but what about oblique lateral pelvic X-rays, bilirubins, management of schizophrenia, potassium levels, or a host of other medical services?

To bring order to fee schedules, organizations have devised **relative value scales,** which give each service a point value. Usually some common service (standard office visit or hernia repair surgery) is given a weight of one point, and then all other services are given point values (e.g., 5 points, 0.2 points) relative to that

TABLE 5.1 Types of Physician Payment

Charges: The amount appearing on the bill, without adjustment.

Fee-for-service: A specified payment for each unit of service provided.

Fee Schedule: A set "menu" of prices for each service agreed upon in advance.

UCR: A method for denying bills that are out of line with the "usual, customary and reasonable" charges made by this and other physicians for the same service last year.

RVS: A schedule based on objective standards showing relative value points for each service compared to a common unit (i.e., regular office visit). Deciding a dollar value per point converts it into a fee schedule.

RBRVS: The relative value schedule set by Medicare for physician fees.

Capitation: A set payment per month regardless of the number of services used.

Salary: A paycheck from an employer.

standard unit of service. After the physician and insurance company agree on the value per point, payment for each service is determined (e.g., if value per point is $20, then a physician providing a 3.5 point service is paid 3.5 × $20 = $70). In 1992, implementation of the Medicare "resource-based relative value scale," **RBRVS**, was begun. A team of health economists and health services researchers led by William Hsiao of Harvard University studied the resources used in providing physician care to estimate a point value for each service based on (1) physician time, (2) intensity of effort, (3) practice costs, and (4) costs of advanced specialty training.[4] The Health Care Financing Administration, which administers the Medicare program, has set the dollars per point for 1995 at $36.382 for primary care physicians and $39.447 for surgeons, with adjustments for geographical variation in the costs of practice and for malpractice insurance.

The existence of the Medicare physician reimbursement system provides a kind of "public good" (see chapter 17) for the other insurance programs, a standard fee schedule that they can adopt or easily modify (by changing the dollar conversion factor or separating out certain categories), which is universally understood and practiced. The importance of the Medicare RBRVS extends beyond the elderly, since it often shapes the payments made Medicaid, Blue Cross and commercial insurance contracts that cover the other 87 percent of the population.

Copays, Assignment, and Balance-Billing

Medicare and other insurers' contracts state not only what they will pay the physician, but also often specify what the patient must pay. A **copayment** of $5 or $10 per visit is often required, both to reduce premiums and also, by forcing the patient to bear some costs, to reduce the number of services utilized. Some plans may also have a **deductible**, which requires the patient to pay out of pocket the first $100 or $500 per year or per illness. **Coinsurance**, with patients paying 10 percent or 20 percent of the bill, is a common part of major medical benefits. The contracts are sufficiently complex that it is often difficult for either the patient or the physician to know exactly who is responsible for what part of the bill. Two forms of payment can be distinguished, individual reimbursement and assignment. Under **individual reimbursement**, the patient is responsible for paying all the charges, sends copies of the bills to the insurer, and is reimbursed for the medical expenses that are covered. Under **assignment**, the physician sends the bill directly to the insurer. The patient is charged for the copayment, and may also be **balance-billed** for the difference if the physician's charges exceed the maximum fee allowed by the insurance contract. Under the Medicare participation agreement, a physician who accepts assignment also agrees not to balance bill for any charges over and above the Medicare payment. Patients like assignment, since it means they do not have to handle paperwork and are not stuck with additional fees. Physicians like the fact that they are paid directly and more rapidly, but do not like being denied the right to charge as much as they feel their services are worth. Indeed, the prohibition of balance-billing in Canada led to a national physician's strike in that country when the rule was first imposed. Under current U.S. Medicare rules, physicians are limited to an additional 15 percent above the Medicare fee for balance-billing if they choose not to accept assignment, and are also penalized by receiving only 95 percent of the regular fee schedule—in effect, Medicare has ruled out balance-billing by making it economically unattractive. Medicaid often has even more stringent rules and significantly lower payment rates, and that is why many physicians choose not to participate in the Medicaid program. Some physicians may choose not to participate in Medicare to avoid the payment limits imposed by the RBRVS system, but since 20 percent of all physician bills are paid for by Medicare, that is difficult to do unless the physician's practice is mostly dermatology or sports medicine or some other specialty in which they treat very few elderly clients.

Physician Payment in Managed Care Plans

As insurance companies have tried to control their costs by exercising market power, the passive payment of bills has given way to a system of **negotiated fees**. For some common and easily specified services purchased in large volume (intra-ocular lens implants, psychiatric evaluations for drug abuse), the insurance company can often obtain a low fixed price set in advance in return for guaranteeing the physician a certain number of patients or procedures. When individual fees are not negotiated, it is common for managed care contracts to specify **discounted fees**, offering, say, 75 percent of what the physician would ordinarily bill for other patients. The complexities of unit pricing are bypassed completely under **capitation,** a single, all-inclusive payment per month for any and all services. A **health maintenance organization (HMO)** using a capitation rate of $100 per month pays that amount to the physician for each of the HMO members enrolled with that physician whether the member visits the doctor's office once, twice, ten times or not at all. **Independent practice association (IPA-HMOs)** that contract with many physicians use capitation rates to pay physicians, but a staff HMO will hire the physician to work exclusively in that HMOs facility treating their patients, and will pay the physician a **salary,** with perhaps some bonus based on productivity or the profitability of the HMO. With this arrangement, the physician in effect becomes an employee of a large medical care firm (even though legally they may still be considered independent practitioners due to laws in many states prohibiting the corporate practice of medicine). Salaried physicians are also found in administrative posts and in research and teaching organizations. Although only about 10 percent of physicians are currently salaried employees, the number continues growing as health care organizations become larger and more complex. Chapters 10 and 11 present a more extensive discussion of managed care contracting.

Incentives: Why Differences in the Type of Payment Matter

The way that physicians are paid determines the incentives that they face to work harder, raise prices, or admit patients to the hospital. Under fee-for-service, a physician gets paid more for doing more. Under capitation, the payment is the same regardless of the number of services provided, so a physician may do less. Under a relative value scale, payment is based on the number of points, so physicians may push for a higher category (the ensuing gradual rise in points while number of services remains constant has become known as *code creep*). In an intriguing experiment, half of the doctors in a pediatric clinic were randomly selected to be paid on a fee-for-service basis, and half on salary.[5] The fees were set so that the average doctor seeing the average number of patients would have earned the same on either FFS or salary. In practice, the fee-for-service doctors saw more patients, recalled them for more visits, and generally exceeded the normal guidelines for amount of services, while the doctors who were on salary saw fewer patients, had them return less frequently, and were in less conformity with standard guidelines. This randomized control trial demonstrates that economic predictions regarding the incentive effects of different types of payment are borne out in a practice setting.

Payment type may affect patients' access to physician care as well. The Medicaid program has come under severe budgetary constraints, and thus tends to pay less well than Blue Shield, HMOs, or commercial insurance. Although physicians are constrained by ethics and law to provide high-quality care to all who need it, economic theory predicts that government imposition of mandatory price controls would lead to shortages. A group of experimenters called three hundred physician offices and requested an appointment, identifying their type of insurance as Medicaid.[6] Almost half of the physician offices said that they were not accepting new patients, and when the experimenters did get an appointment, the average wait was two weeks. The experimenters then called back, identifying themselves as having commercial insurance, and 78 percent of the doctor's offices gave them an appointment within two days. Physicians try hard to provide adequate care to the poor, but if the payment levels are consistently lower, then the level of service will be lower as well.

A Progression: From Prices to Reimbursement Mechanisms

As the system has moved away from fee-for-service and closer to salaried arrangements, the linkage between the flow of funds from patients and the flow of funds to physicians has been attenuated, and finally severed. While there may be some "price" attached to each service under Medicare RBRVS, it bears almost no resemblance to what that would mean in a normal market: the patient does not pay it, nor does it allow the supplier to match output to demand, since it is imposed externally by the government. In such an environment, equilibrating varied interests through individual decisions based on price is replaced by a collective political market. Who gets paid and how much is determined in part by concerns about how the elderly will vote in the next presidential election, or the effectiveness of insurance lobbies, or a need to find the least offensive way of balancing the budget. Tracking the flow of funds to and from physicians is further obscured by the use of medical terminology to refer to all payments as *reimbursement*, even though they do not "reimburse" costs (physician time is the bulk of the expense) and are more accurately termed *fees* or *net income* or *salary*.

Shift from prices to UCR   Change from one payment system to another will only take place when the change benefits one or more of the parties involved sufficiently to make it worth the effort. Thus it is appropriate for an economist to ask who benefits at each stage. The shift to UCR helped physicians as well as the Blue Shield insurance plans (which the county medical societies controlled at that time). Physicians faced competition from **contract practice**, a kind of precursor to HMOs in which a company would pay a doctor $X per week to provide a clinic caring for all their employees.[7] With UCR, those employees could have coverage and still be paying patients of the community physicians, who could still raise their prices (and indeed, could do so more easily, since insurance made bills less burdensome to patients). Blue Shield plans could maintain the information on all doctor's fees required for UCR, which commercial insurers with only a few policies in the area could not. Thus, average UCR rates were lower than average charges, allowing Blue Shield to price their health insurance lower than commercial companies and increase market share. Medicare adopted UCR (a) so it would not upset the physicians whose cooperation they needed to make the Medicare system work and (b) because it was there, and easy to implement—and could, in fact, be handed over to the Blue Shield plans to manage as fiscal intermediaries, so that they, too, benefited and were supportive. By 1990 continuing cost growth and wide payment disparities (two physicians might receive very different payments for the same service) had made the UCR system untenable.

Shift to RBRVS   RBRVS was implemented to place the government, not physicians or the fiscal intermediaries, in control. Since there was really nothing in RBRVS for most physicians except the anticipation of pain from future cost-cutting, the government promised "budget-neutrality" to keep payment rates high and growing—at least for a while.

Shift to Discounts and Capitation   The mutual benefits from managed care negotiations are clear: HMOs give selected physicians a larger volume of patients in return for a discount on per unit price. Of course, this system can only help physician A by taking those patients from physician B, but self-interest plays an increasing role when business begins to get scarce and supply of eager young entrants is increasing. With capitation, the HMO knows in advance exactly how much it will have to pay for physician services, and physicians know exactly how much they will receive. However, physicians must then manage the care of all their capitated patients to stay within this fixed budget (which often includes laboratory services and specialist referrals as well as care provided by the physician) and so bears the risk that too many patients will become ill. Capitation is still so new that many physician groups are having trouble estimating rates, and some are so seriously underbidding in order to win contracts that they are likely to lose money over time, and even go bankrupt. The real advantage of capitation is that it reduces all the paperwork and billing hassle. This is fine for patients, potentially beneficial for well run physician practices, and useful to insurance companies that are willing to capitate fairly so as to build a business in the long run.

5.2 PHYSICIAN INCOMES _____

Physicians are among the most highly trained, most respected, and well-compensated workers in the United States. The average physician had an income of $182,400 in 1994, six times the average worker's salary. Physician earnings have grown more rapidly than average workers' compensation for most of this century. During the period 1982–92 when the average worker's earnings were almost flat (up only 0.8% in ten years after adjustment for inflation), physician earnings rose about 2.2 percent each year, 24 percent over the ten-year span. To a large extent, these high earnings are attributable to the quality of those who enter the profession (almost all in the top quarter of college graduates), the long years of post-college training required, the extra effort (most physicians work about 50% more hours than the average salaried worker), and compensation for having to act as an entrepreneur and manage a medical business (self-employed physicians earn 50% more than those who choose to work on salary). However, even after adjusting for all these factors, there is still a premium for becoming a physician. Perhaps even more important than the average income is the implied "floor:" physicians virtually never face unemployment, and many accept "low-paid" (i.e., less than $100,000 a year) positions in order to follow their own special interests in helping the poor, working with children, traveling to exotic locations, or studying interesting diseases. Even during training in residency programs, physicians earn about $35,000 a year—which is more than the average worker, although certainly less than the opportunity cost of their time (see discussion of the costs of time and returns in chapter 6, section 2). As with most workers, physicians' earnings grow rapidly early in their careers, rise to a peak around age 50, and decline thereafter (see Table 5.2).

There is a marked difference in earnings by specialty. Generalists and family practitioners are at the low end, with pediatricians and psychiatrists only slightly above. The high end is made up of the surgeons, radiologists, and anesthesiologists. While numerous factors are involved, much of the difference in incomes between specialties can be explained as a function of the reimbursement system; physicians get paid more for "doing something" (e.g., reading an X-ray or performing an operation) than for caring or thinking (e.g., listening to a patient's history, deciding on which path of treatment to follow, or helping the family of a dying person). The reimbursement system is driven by the "billable event." Although a colleague or a manager might be able to assess all of the work that a physician does on behalf of patients, the financial system is not able to do so. A physician always finds it easier to get paid for a procedure, since it is observable

TABLE 5.2   Physician Characteristics and Incomes

670,336	total number of U.S. Physicians
550,448	active in patient care
87,051	residents in training programs

Average

56.7 hours	worked per week	$103 charge per new patient visit
107.6	visits per week	$59 charge established patient visit
4.4 hours	charity or uncompensated care per week	

Sources of Revenue

26% Medicare   30% Other Private Insurance
10% Medicaid   16% Patient copays, fees, etc.
18% Blue Cross/Blue Shield

Income		% of total
$182,400	*All Physicians*	100%
	Specialty	
$121,200	General/Family Practice	15%
$126,200	Pediatrics	8%
$128,500	Psychiatry	7%
$174,900	Internal Medicine	28%
$182,500	Pathology	3%
$200,400	Obstetrics/Gynecology	6%
$218,100	Anesthesiology	5%
$237,400	Radiology	5%
$255,200	Surgery	14%
	Type of Practice	
$158,400	Employee or contractor	33%
$210,200	Self-employed	67%
$178,900	Solo	49%
$211,300	2 physician partners	13%
$240,700	3 physician group	9%
$240,700	4 – 8 physician group	18%
$267,500	9+ physician group	11%
	Age	
$138,800	under 36 years	
$160,000	under 40 years	
$190,600	36 – 45	
$204,300	46 – 55	
$183,500	56 – 65	
$121,400	66 or more	

Source: AMA Socioeconomic Characteristics of Medical Practice, 1996, and other AMA surveys.

and has a standard billing code, than for a personal interaction or conceptual effort. A desire to rebalance incomes across specialties and provide more payment for thinking and caring was an important part of the design in the Medicare RBRVS system—which was only partially successful (see section 7.4). Health insurance was designed to protect individuals against potentially large but infrequent losses while minimizing moral hazard from excess purchase of discretionary services. While correct from a risk management perspective, in practice this meant that fees for some specialties were almost fully covered (e.g., surgery and anesthesia), leading to increased demand and higher incomes, while other specialties were subject to copayments and deductibles (e.g., pediatrics or psychiatry) that limited demand and incomes. The bottom line for the physician was that the income potential from choosing a particular specialty has had more to do with how the services of that specialty were treated by insurance than with the work or training involved.

5.3 PHYSICIAN COSTS: FUNDS OUT _____

Physician Practice Expenses

About half of all the funds flowing into physicians are taken up by the expenses of maintaining a practice. He must pay for all of the other medical professionals and assistants who help him to take care of patients, as well as taxes, rent, utilities, supplies, malpractice insurance, and so on. In addition to all of these ongoing expenses, it will usually take at least $50,000 in start-up capital to equip even the most basic doctor's office, and an elaborate suite housing an active practice in specialties such as plastic surgery could cost several million dollars. One reason for physicians to work together in group practices is to obtain economies of scale from sharing office space, equipment, and information systems. Only a large group can afford to have assistants that specialize in support functions as lab technicians, billing and appointment clerks, therapists, and so on. Yet Table 5.3 reveals an apparently anomalous finding: even though it would seem that a large group practice would make more efficient use of ancillary help and equipment, such expenses take a larger fraction of total revenues than for solo physicians who practice alone. To understand why a more efficient practice uses more, rather than less, nonphysician inputs, it is necessary to consider a basic result from the microeconomic analysis of firm production. In order to reduce costs, it is necessary to increase the use of those inputs where the output per dollar of input is higher, and/or reduce those inputs for which it is lower.[8] At the optimum, the ratio of marginal productivity to input price will be the same for all inputs.

TABLE 5.3 Physicians' Office Practice Costs

$183,100	Average Expenses of Self-Employed Physicians in 1994 (equal to 47% of Total Gross Revenues)

35%	Non-Physician Employee Wages (3.5 FTE per physician)
26%	Office Rent
8%	Medical Supplies
12%	Malpractice Liability Insurance
3%	Equipment
16%	Other Expenses

Source: AMA Socioeconomic Characteristics of Medical Practice, 1996.

Equilibrium Condition for Cost-Minimizing Use of Inputs in Production

$$\frac{\text{Marginal Productivity}_{\text{input A}}}{\text{Price}_{\text{input A}}} = \frac{\text{Marginal Productivity}_{\text{input B}}}{\text{Price}_{\text{input B}}} = \cdots$$

$$= \frac{\text{Marginal Productivity}_{\text{input Z}}}{\text{Price}_{\text{input Z}}}$$

A larger and more organized group is able to make better use of nonphysician inputs, raising their marginal productivity. Therefore, the group will use more of them relative to physician time. Efficiency is not defined as having the lowest amount of overhead, or even the highest number of patient visits per physician hour, but rather the lowest cost (physician and nonphysician) per visit. This raises the following question: what "price" should be applied to physician time?

The Labor–Leisure Choice

A physician-entrepreneur has an "income" of revenues less expenses, a flow that would be called *profit* by the IRS. Most of it is not economic "profit" but compensation for all of the hours of work put in. How should this time be valued? What is its opportunity cost? For a young physician starting out with relatively few patients, it is common to take on a temporary part-time "moonlighting" job in a hospital emergency room or for some well-established senior practice with excess work for wages of $75 to $150 per hour. Since doctors give up those jobs as their practice becomes established, their time must be worth more than that, but what forgone opportunity defines this higher hourly rate? What a busy physician gives up is leisure, time to be with family, to run and swim and watch television, or even to sleep. The more lucrative each hour of practice, and the more hours that the physician puts in, the more each hour of forgone leisure is worth. Most doctors work very hard, averaging more than fifty hours per week. Furthermore, once you are making $150,000 or $250,000 per year, a little time off may well be worth more than earning an extra $5,000 by working late. That is one reason why the supply of physician time is not very elastic—even doubling or quadrupling their income could not get them to double the number of hours worked. Indeed, it is even possible that for some physicians, supply is "backward bending"—higher income per hour may make them feel sufficiently rich that they work less rather than more hours.[9],* One difficulty physicians have in making the labor–leisure choice is that their income often depends crucially upon putting in many hours per week early in their careers when the rate of pay is low, or even zero. This is similar to the problem facing most college students—getting into the best business or law school and making partner depends on excess hours put in now to obtain future income. To fully analyze the trade-off between labor and leisure, it is necessary to recognize that some work is done more for its value as investment (in future earnings) than for current earnings.

---

*If this backward bending supply seems hard to understand, think about how much you would work if I paid you $100 per hour? $1,000 per hour? $100,000 per hour? Eventually you would decide to work little and enjoy it a lot because more money would not be worth all that much.

The Doctor's Workshop and Unpaid Hospital Inputs

Almost every doctor needs to use a hospital to provide patient care, and some specialties (anesthesiology, thoracic surgery, pathology) work almost entirely inside hospitals, and yet the physician does not pay the hospital for working there, nor are they usually an employee of the hospital. In terms of an influential model proposed by Mark Pauly and Michael Redisch, the hospital functions as the "doctor's workshop," and is a source of unpaid inputs in production.[10] Since the efforts of hospital nurses, laboratories, and recordkeeping do not "cost" the physician practice anything, they tend to be overused, and to supplant the use of similar inputs within the physician's office. For many physicians, the hospital medical staff, where they serve as volunteers, is the most important form of "management" and the only control over their professional activity. It is easy to see how physicians might favor a system of nonprofit hospitals supported by the community and government subsidy, since the value added to their practice far exceeds the hours they are expected to "give" to educational and administrative functions.

The hospital-based specialties of radiology and pathology form a special case, with high incomes that clearly depend on hospital practice. Since these specialties spend virtually all of their professional time within the hospital, have a regular flow of work, and do not meet individually with patients, it would appear that they might most readily be paid on salary—yet historically, radiologists have strongly opposed salaried practice, favoring fee-for-service, or contracts wherein they operate the diagnostic facility for a percentage of gross, or pay rent to the hospital. Their opposition was sufficient to force Medicare to separate the professional fee for reviewing X-rays and specimens from the hospital charges for producing them. The primary issue is control—over professional activity and over money. If the pathologist runs the lab, then they in effect "own" the captive block of business constituted by the hospital's patients. However, if the hospital runs the lab, then pathologists must compete on the basis of price (i.e., take a lower salary) and accept hospital direction over their working conditions. Consider the case of a sixty-year-old pathologist who has been head of the lab for twenty years and is friendly with most of the surgeons on staff. If it is his lab, he can bring in a junior partner to do the day-to-day work and semi-retire to play golf with the hospital administrator and his surgeon buddies. If it is the hospital's lab, and he is on salary, then the hospital can threaten to hire that junior pathologist and save money, unless he is willing to accept a cut in pay and work harder. This issue of who "owns" the patient's business will arise repeatedly in our examination of the organization of medicine, and is central to the managed care revolution currently taking place in the medical marketplace (see chapters 10 and 11).

Malpractice

One of the most contentious physician practice expenses is malpractice insurance. The rationale for allowing medical malpractice suits is that they improve incentives for safety by forcing doctors to behave more carefully when treating patients. Malpractice is not a good way of compensating patients for harm done to them, since it costs $1.20 in legal fees for every $1 a patient receives.[11] About one in twenty physicians will incur a malpractice claim in any given year, and two in five will be sued at least once during their careers. The premium for physician's malpractice insurance averages about $20,000 (3% of gross revenues), but ranges from just $5,000 or less for family practitioners to $100,000 and more for orthopedic and neurosurgeons. While malpractice premiums have risen rapidly in some years, virtually all of the additional costs are quickly passed on to the patients and their insurance companies in the form of higher fees.

Malpractice is a real problem, but the current malpractice system may not be the best solution. Studies have shown that there is a negligent iatrogenic (i.e., caused by the physician) injury approximately once for every one hundred hospital admissions. Only a tenth of those injured will ever file a claim, and less than half will gain compensation through the courts. At the same time, there will be a larger number of suits filed where there was no negligence, and some of these will win despite the lack of any physician error. The randomness of the legal process, as well as the fact that most physicians are rather fully insured for losses due to malpractice, limits the effectiveness of the system to change behavior. However, being sued is costly in terms of lost time and anxiety, and most physicians exercise extraordinary care in treating patients. After all, they became physicians because they wanted to care for patients, not because they wanted a job that was easy or did not take much effort. Although some physicians have claimed that the fear of being sued has raised medical costs by forcing them to practice "defensive medicine," studies have shown that higher levels of liability or greater numbers of suits do not lead to higher numbers of tests per patient, more admissions, or more prescriptions.[12] Since most suits are filed for some procedure that a doctor has done wrong, rather than for something not done, or for a diagnosis that was missed, the lack of excessive testing or other medical treatment attributable to malpractice is not surprising.

Does the malpractice system deter negligence by physicians? Only to a limited extent, and at considerable cost. Yet while the ability of malpractice suits to compensate patients for damages or to force doctors to practice better medicine has been roundly criticized with good reason, it has not been easy to find a solution that is clearly more efficient or acceptable to both doctors and patients.

5.4 UNCERTAINTY

In what is perhaps the most well-known and often-cited paper on health economics, Nobel laureate Kenneth Arrow stated that:

> . . . the special economic problems of medical care can be explained as adaptations to the existence of uncertainty in the incidence of disease and in the efficacy of treatment.[13]

As discussed earlier in chapter 3, uncertainty "in the incidence of disease" refers to the random occurrence of illness—one never knows when one will get sick, or how bad it will be. The problem of randomly occurring losses can be offset to some extent by pooling risks through insurance. The losses still occur and must be paid for, but the financial uncertainty is removed.

Uncertainty "in the efficacy of treatment" refers to the inability to know in ad-

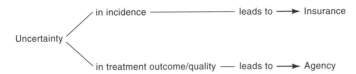

FIGURE 5.1 *Uncertainty in the incidence of illness can be ameliorated by the use of insurance. Uncertainty in the outcome and quality of treatment can be ameliorated by exchange using an agency relationship: licensure and trust in physicians, non-profit ownership, and government regulation.*

vance whether the treatment chosen will work. In theory, it might be possible to "insure" against such losses, but in the real world there are no meaningful guarantees for medical care. A cardiologist treating you for a heart attack does not guarantee that you will be able to run marathons again, nor does an oncologist claim that she can cure your cancer. The most either will promise is to provide you with everything modern medicine has to offer. Why can't they give a guarantee? First of all, because it is so hard to tell how ill you are in the first place, it is often impossible to tell if treatment has improved your health. Second, unlike a car or a house, there is no way to replace your body. While almost any ordinary loss can be fixed with sufficient compensation, a monetary guarantee is an empty promise if you are dead—and the appropriate dollar amount is quite hard to determine even for the loss of a limb.

The distinction between the two types of uncertainty, and the economic response to them, is shown in Figure 5.1. Note that in each case, there is a transfer of responsibility away from the patient. Under insurance, the responsibility for payment is transferred to the insurance company, relieving all actual and potential patients of the uncertainty of financial losses due to illness. Under agency, the responsibility for making a decision for the quality of care is transferred from the patient to the physician. Agency creates gains because it substitutes professional control for costly patient monitoring of quality. It is much cheaper for an experienced and highly educated physician to determine which treatment is best than for a patient to try to do so.

5.5   THE NATURE OF THE TRANSACTION BETWEEN DOCTOR AND PATIENT _____

The lack of good information is the central defect that prevents the exchange of medical care in ordinary market transactions. When patients show up at a doctor's office, they are apt to ask two questions: "What is wrong with me?" and "What should I do about it?" If told that they have a disease, most of time people will **trust** the doctor to perform the right diagnostic and therapeutic procedures, with little idea of what those might be or what the charges will add up to.[14] If a surgeon is called in, that surgeon is likely to be a complete stranger who will ask for thousands of dollars to make an evaluation and incision. Having been cut open, the patients will pray that in the long run it might do some good, since post-operative pain and possible mortality will make them worse off in the short run. Unlike a person shopping for a car, a suit or a haircut, the medical patient does not know what it is they need, what it should cost, or even, once paid for, how much good the treatment really did. Instead of a clear specification of what is to be expected from both parties, the patient must trust the doctor to do what is right and to bill fairly for the necessary care (which will mostly be paid for by insurance).

Asymmetric Information

While the physician's information is not perfect, it is much better than that of the patient, and the physician is also able to seek additional information required for treating an illness at much lower cost. This disparity is known as **information asymmetry.** When it is necessary to decide what test to do, which drug to prescribe, and whether or not to do surgery, all of these choices can be made better and at lower cost by a physician. An exchange relationship where one party makes choices on behalf of the other is known as **agency.**[15] Just as a purchasing agent buys supplies for a firm, or an actor's agent represents him in negotiations, a physician is the patient's agent deciding how to treat and what medical services to buy. The reason that agents act on behalf of another (the "principal") is that their information and transactions costs are lower.* It is cheaper for a physician to make health care choices rather than for the patients to go to medical school so that they themselves could choose as wisely, or to put up with the painful loss of welfare that would come from making decisions ignorantly or randomly.

While many goods and services are transacted under conditions of less than perfect information, it is the magnitude of the disparity that sets medical care apart. For example, while I may not know what my mechanic is doing, I can readily observe whether or not my automobile is working better when it comes back from the shop. Poor quality parts can be repaired or replaced. At most, I might ask for my money back. Bad surgery is not only hard to detect, it can be fatal. Once you are dead, repairs, replacements and even outrageously large malpractice settlements are irrelevant.

Market Transfer Points are Determined
by Information Costs

A good can be bought and sold in the marketplace at a price determined by supply and demand, but it can also be transferred internally within the firm, or between organizations through some nonmarket alternative (e.g., gift, favor, family, mutual understanding) in which there is no well-defined price. In the process of production from raw materials to final consumption, the steps along the way where market transactions are most apt to occur are those where the necessary in-

---

*The extensive economic analysis of agency has focused primarily on the manager of a firm who makes decisions on behalf of its shareholders. Many of these models are applicable, but since medical outcomes are not as readily measured as the profits of a firm, and since death has even more moral overtones than bankruptcy, the doctor–patient bond has important aspects above and beyond those which characterize the relationships of owner-to-shareholder or supervisor-to-employee.

formation is standardized and easy to obtain.[16] When an input is well-defined and inexpensive to transact (e.g., five thousand 250 mg tablets of acetaminophen, 50 486-DX66 computers, 100 gallons of 89 octane gasoline), it will be bought and sold in the market. Where measurement is difficult or dependent upon others (devising a strategic plan, monitoring quality), a nonmarket transfer carried out within an organization is more likely. For example, a doctor is often willing to use the market and contract out for billing or cleaning services, but not for nursing. Payments due and clean floors are easily monitored. Determining whether a nurse is competent, tolerant, dependable, able to maintain patient confidentiality, and understands the special demands of this particular doctor's practice, is not. Therefore doctors hire their "own" nurses rather than purchasing standard services from an impersonal marketplace vendor. Similarly, tests that are routine and easily separated out may be purchased independently (e.g., blood count, strep throat), while others that depend upon particular skills (e.g., listening to heartbeats, psychological evaluation) are not.

Health status is almost impossible to measure, and thus medical care carries no guarantee. Why can I get a guarantee on my car, but not on my body? First, consider who is and is not in a position to give me a guarantee on my car. At the time of purchase, the dealer offered me a guarantee for 6 years/100,000 at a cost of $823. They also offered to put in a stereo system for $960. After I bought the car, I went out and got an equivalent stereo system installed for less than $500. Why couldn't I also get a six-year guarantee for less by going to my local mechanic? It's because of information problems. If I went to my mechanic and tried to get a guarantee, the mechanic would be willing to guarantee only the work done, not the whole car (which might have been in a collision, or flawed from the start). The dealer knew that the car sold to me was in good shape, because it was new. An outside mechanic would have to spend lots of time to find out what shape it was in, and would still be reluctant to cover someone else's work. Even the dealer will guarantee only manufacturing defects and normal wear and tear, not driving abuse, accidents, and so on. A guarantee is a form of insurance against poor quality. If something cannot be measured, and it cannot be replaced, then there is no way to write a contract that will give an adequate guarantee against poor quality, and some nonmarket way of doing so must be found.[17]

Now, what about your body? Is it in good shape? Any latent cancer or heart disease or genetic defects? Has it been abused only during final exam week, or throughout the year? It would be impossible to determine exactly how healthy you are and how long you can expect to live with current technology. That is why medical malpractice is not a guarantee on your body, but only on the quality of the care you received. It pays off only when the physician's behavior can be shown to clearly deviate from normal standards of practice, not just because a patient ends up dead or crippled. If perfect information about a person's state of health and the effect of proposed treatments were easily and cheaply obtainable, then a person could go out and buy a guarantee on their next operation as easily as they can for a refrigerator, termite extermination, or fire damage. Things that can easily be measured and are used by many people are bought and sold in the marketplace. Things that are idiosyncratic and hard to measure are more likely to be provided through alternative, nonmarket economic organizations.

SUGGESTIONS FOR FURTHER READING _____

American Medical Association *Socioeconomic Characteristics of Medical Practice,* published annually.

Kenneth Arrow, "Uncertainty and the Welfare Economics of Medical Care." *Amer. Econ Review* 53(3):941–973, 1963.

Patricia M. Danzon, "Liability for Medical Malpractice." *Journal of Economic Perspectives* 5(3):51–69, 1991.

The Changing Character of the Medical Profession, Volume 66, supplement 2 of the Millbank Quarterly, 1988.

SUMMARY _____

1. **The relationship between doctor and patient stands at the center of the medical care system.** Although payments to physicians constitute only 19 percent of the total, the special characteristics of this exchange influence the organization and financing of all the other parts.

2. Over time, physician payment has changed from "fee-for-service" prices similar to prices of most other economic goods and services, to complex reimbursement schemes that depend on administrative formulas and negotiation. Increasingly, physicians are involved with managed care plans on a **capitation** (so much per member per month) or **discounted fee schedules** based on **relative value scales.**

3. Most physicians are owners or partners in small business rather than employees. They work long hours, but do not face much business risk. **On average, self-employed physicians earned $210,200 in 1994,** while the third that worked as employees, and were somewhat younger, earned $148,200. Cognitive and caring specialties (family practice, psychiatry, pediatrics, internal medicine) earned less than procedure-oriented specialties (surgery, Ob/Gyn, radiology).

4. The average office medical practice hired **3.5 allied health workers per physician,** and had overall expenses equal to 47 percent of gross patient revenues. While malpractice insurance is the expense category most frequently complained about, **malpractice takes only 3 to 6 percent of gross revenues** for most physician practices.

5. **Uncertainty** creates or exacerbates most of the information problems in medical care. While financial uncertainty due to the random occurrence of illness can be partially solved by insurance, the uncertainty about the quality of care and outcome of treatment cannot, and thus, collective agency mechanisms such as licensure and strong ethical traditions for physicians have been established.

6. **Information asymmetry** arises from the difference between the physician's knowledge of medical treatments and the patient's. Due to this disparity in the cost of knowledge, patients must trust physicians to act as their **agents** and make decisions on their behalf. In most economic exchanges, the point at

which goods and services are transacted is where information cost differentials are lowest. Since a low-cost valuation of well-defined goods is not possible in medicine, a trust relationship of agency has been established to ameliorate this potential market failure.

PROBLEMS _____

1. {*incentives*} Which type of payment would give a physician the most incentive to:
    a. Spend more time with each patient? Spend less?
    b. Provide more laboratory services to each patient? Less?
    c. Modify the listing of diagnoses to increase revenues? Be objective?
    d. Reduce hospital utilization? Increase use of hospitals?
    e. Ask patients to return frequently? Try to handle problems once and for all?

2. {*compensation*} Do you think that radiologists prefer to be compensated fee-for-service, by relative value scale, on salary, or as part of a capitated rate? Why? Why might different specialties prefer different forms of payment?

3. {*organization*} What organization provides the largest amount of payment to physicians in the United States? How do they choose to make these payments? Has the form of payment changed over time? Why?

4. {*earnings differentials*} What are some of the reasons that most pediatricians earn less than most neurosurgeons?

5. {*age earnings profile*} Generally, most physicians' incomes increase as they get older. Is the rate of earnings increase greater for some specialties than others? Why? Do you expect that male and female physicians have the same age-earnings profile? Why or why not?

6. {*earnings differentials*} Would you expect that physicians who earn significantly more than their peers have office practice costs that are above or below average? Are they more or less likely to hire other physicians?

7. {*price discrimination*} What is balance-billing? Who favors it: physicians, patients, or insurance companies? Is balance billing more likely to occur for doctors who have high or low demand? For patients who have high or low incomes?

8. {*valuation*} How are the values determined in setting up a relative value scale?

9. {*malpractice*} What are the objectives of the current medical malpractice system in the United States? How well does it work in achieving these objectives?

10. {*uncertainty*} If uncertainty with regard to the occurrence of losses can be dealt with through insurance markets, why can't uncertainty with regard to the outcome or quality of medical care be similarly priced and transferred?

11. {*agency*} What is an agent? How does employing an agent reduce the costs of making a transaction? Does employing an agent create any problems that would not occur if the consumer acted alone?

12. {*earnings differentials*} In any occupation, some professionals are better than others. Those who do the best job tend to earn more. Is the quality differential (i.e., percentage difference between top and mid-range) larger or smaller for physicians than other occupations (consider teachers, bus drivers, lawyers, basketball players, etc.)? Which medical specialties will have the largest variance in earnings? Are most or all of these differences in earning power due to differences in quality?

13. {*transactions costs*} The production of services in a modern economy is highly complex and involves thousands of organizations employing millions of workers and managers. What determines the point at which money will change hands? Give an example where conditions changed so that the way services were transacted changed.

ENDNOTES _____

1. Elliot Friedson, *Professional dominance: The Social Structure of Medical Care*, New York: Atherton Press, 1970. Victor R. Fuchs, *Who Shall Live? Health, Economics and Social Choice*, New York, Basic Books, 1983.

2. Most of the information here is from surveys done by the American Medical Association and reported in *Socioeconomic Characteristics of Medical Practice*, an (almost) annual monograph. A good sense of the entrepreneurial flavor of medical practice can be obtain by perusing several issues of the "Business Week" of physicians, *Medical Economics*.

3. Sally T. Burner and Daniel R. Waldo, "National Health Expenditure Projections, 1994-2005," *Health Care Financing Review,* 16(4):221–242, Summer 1995.

4. W. C. Hsiao, P. Braun, D. Dunn and E. R. Becker, "Resource-Based Relative Values: An Overview," *Journal of the American Medical Association,* 260(16):2347–53, 1988; William C. Hsiao, *et al.,* "Results and Impacts of the Resource-Based Relative Value Scale," *Medical Care,* 30(11 Supplement):NS61-79, 1992.

5. G. B. Hickson, W. A. Altmeier, and J. M. Perris, "Physician Reimbursement by Salary or Fee-For-Service: Effect on Physician Practice Behavior in a Randomized Prospective Study," *Pediatrics,* 80:344–350, 1987.

6. Medicaid Access Study Group. "Access of Medicaid Recipients to Outpatient Care," *New England Journal of Medicine,* 330:1426–1430, May 19, 1994.

7. George A. Shipman, *Medical Service Corporations in the State of Washington: A Study of the Administration of Physician-Sponsored Pre-paid Medical Care.* Cambridge, Mass: Harvard University Press, 1962.

8. Uwe Reinhardt, "A Production Function for Physician Services," *Review of Economics and Statistics,* 54(1):55–66, 1972.

9. Frank A. Sloan, "Physician Supply Behavior in the Short Run," *Industrial and Labor Relations Review,* 28:549–569, July 1975.

10. Mark V. Pauly and Michael Redisch, "The Not-For-Profit Hospital as a Physician Co-operative," *American Economic Review* 63(1):87–99, 1973.

11. Patricia Danzon, "Liability for Medical Malpractice," *Journal of Economic Perspectives* 5(3):51–69, 1991.

12. Peter A. Glassman, John E. Rolph, Laura P. Petersen, Melissa A. Bradley, Richard L. Kravitz, "Physician's Personal Malpractice Experiences Are Not Related to Defensive Clinical Practices," *Journal of Health Politics, Policy and Law,* 21(2):219–241, 1996.

13. Kenneth J. Arrow, "Uncertainty and the Welfare Economics of Medical Care." *American Economic Review* 53(3):941–973, 1963, page 942.

14. This special economic character of the "trust" relationship with doctors has long been noted, and is discussed in Adam Smith's seminal 1776 treatise, *The Wealth of Nations.*

15. Michael Jensen and William Meckling, "Agency Costs in the Firm." Michael C. Jensen and William H. Meckling, "Theory of the Firm: Managerial Behavior, Agency costs and Ownership Structure," *Journal of Financial Economics,* 3:305–360, 1976.

16. Yoram Barzel, "Measurement Cost and the Organization of Markets," *Journal of Law and Economics,* 25(1):24–48, 1982.

17. Mark V. Pauly, "Taxation, Health Insurance, and Market Failure in the Medical Economy," *Journal of Economic Literature,* 24(2):629–675, 1986.

CHAPTER 6

Medical Education and Licensure

QUESTIONS

1. *Is physician licensure a form of monopoly restriction intended to increase profits, or a form of public protection intended to assure quality?*

2. *How much is a year of medical education worth?*

3. *Are doctors more or less productive than they were twenty years ago?*

4. *Why are licensure restrictions more strongly enforced for some types of medical care than others?*

5. *Who controls the supply of physicians, the government or the AMA (American Medical Association)?*

6. *Is the AMA a professional society serving science, or a union serving the economic interests of its members?*

7. *Why are there more foreign doctors practicing in the United States than U.S. doctors practicing overseas if the needs are much greater there?*

8. *Are chiropractors a substitute for physicians, or a complement?*

6.1 LICENSURE: QUALITY OR PROFITS? ———

Licensure is a collective extension of the doctor–patient relationship of agency. Not only does the individual patient trust his or her physician to act as their personal agent, all of us together have collectively chosen to let the medical profession act as our public agent, deciding who is and is not qualified to practice medicine. Through the institution of **licensure**, the medical profession serves as a sort of quasi-governmental body making decisions of behalf of all consumers.[1] Consumers do not examine each doctor's credentials and legal records, they turn that responsibility over to licensure boards—it is cheaper for knowledgeable professionals to do it once for all consumers rather than having each patient individually try to determine if the person listed as a "doctor" in the phonebook is qualified to practice medicine. The government itself does not so much make laws regarding the practice of medicine, but rather, uses law to enforce the decisions made by voluntary and independent professional boards.

It has often been debated in newspapers and among economists whether licensure serves the interests of patients (by improving the quality of care) or of physicians (by raising prices and incomes).[2] Such a debate, framed in terms of one side or the other, misses the point: any public policy in a democracy is in fact a form of trade that must serve the interests of both parties if it is to be upheld. By the fundamental theorem of exchange, both physicians and patients must be made better off for licensure to work.

How Does Licensure Increase Physician Profits?

Licensure radically changes the market structure. A flexible supply curve is replaced by a fixed supply—diagrammatically, a vertical line, since quantity does not change as prices rise or fall (see Figure 6.1). To the extent that the supply of doctor services is reduced under licensure, prices are higher so that all doctors enjoy higher income (of course, this means that some persons who wished to become doctors are not allowed to do so). These profits are maximized if the profession acts as a monopoly in determining how many doctors are allowed to practice. Supply can also be reduced by work rules that control total productivity. For example, it has been common for dental practice acts to regulate how many assistants each dentist can supervise (and therefore the number of total patients that can be seen). Extending the training period also serves to reduce the effective doctor supply, since each graduate has fewer remaining years of productivity.

Thinking of the demand for physician services as derived demand suggests two further possibilities for raising income: 1) increasing the price of substitutes such as chiropractors and nurses, and 2) increasing demand for output. The price of many physician substitutes can be made infinite by prohibiting them from performing some acts (prescribing drugs, surgery, admitting a patient to the hospital). Less extreme, but also effective, are rules that limit health insurance to reimbursement for services performed by (or under the supervision of) a physician. Even if a substitute provider were willing to provide services at a much lower price, it would still cost the patient more since they would have to pay the whole bill out of pocket. Insurance has been the most important factor in increasing the overall demand for medical care. Physicians have played a major role in the

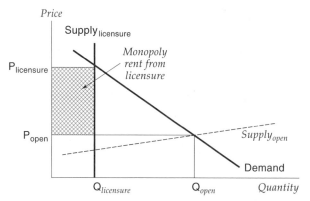

FIGURE 6.1 *Demand and Supply With Licensure.
Licensed supply is a vertical line because the number
of physicians in practice does not change as the price
rises or falls. The excess income due to restricting
supply and raising prices relative to open conditions
is the monopoly rent from licensure (shaded area).*

spread of insurance and the creation of payment systems rules, such as UCR
(usual, customary, and reasonable) and separate professional fees for radiologists
and pathologists, which all increase their economic power. Professional activities
also directly increase demand both through new medical discoveries, and by
monitoring and controlling quality so that patients are more willing to visit any licensed practitioner.

Supply and Demand Response in Licensed v. Unlicensed Professions

To illustrate the differences in market dynamics between licensed and unlicensed
labor supply, physicians are compared with health administrators in Figure 6.2.
Health administrators often take an MHA degree early in their career, but many
rise through the ranks without attending graduate school, and others obtain MBA
or MS degrees in schools of business, medicine, public health, public policy or
human services.[3] The crucial point is that there is no central control over the number of people who can enter the profession, no licensure or specific educational requirement, and no legal restriction on practice by outsiders. Administrators usually start at modest salaries ranging from $30,000 to $60,000, like most MBAs, and
work their way up the organizational ranks. While some administrators eventually earn large salaries, others tend to get stuck in the middle ranges, and some are
pushed out of the field entirely. Thus, administrator earnings are related to individual characteristics and experience, and hence rather variable. Physician earnings are in part monopoly rents shared by the profession as a whole, and thus are
not only higher, but are also more stable. While both physicians and administrators will see their earnings rise as they gain more experience, the growth is more
regular and virtually never interrupted by unemployment for physicians.

The comparative effects of an increase in demand are shown in Figure 6.2. For
physicians, who are licensed, virtually all of the increase in demand will go into

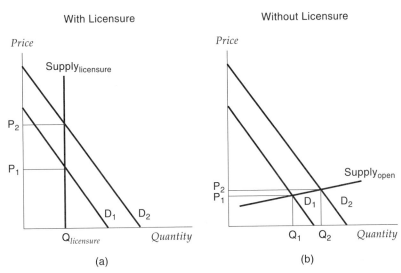

FIGURE 6.2 *Demand and Supply: Comparing Licensure With Open Markets. The effects of an increase in demand are shown in markets with licensed and unlicensed labor. In the licensed market, a, labor supply is fixed, and all of the demand increase goes into price increases. In the unlicensed market, b, part of the increase in demand is accommodated by an increase in the quantity of labor supplied, and therefore prices do not rise as much.*

higher incomes, since there is no flexibility for supply to increase. For unlicensed administrators, higher wages will attract more and better entrants, so that part of the increase in demand will go into an increase in the quantity of labor supplied, and only part into an increase in incomes. Although increased demand leads to more applicants for places in medical schools, there will not be any new medical schools built since numbers are controlled by the AMA (American Medical Association) and affiliated professional bodies. In contrast, increasing demand for health administrators has caused graduate programs to spring up around the country as universities compete to attract students.

How Does Licensure Improve Quality?

It is possible to improve quality by revoking the licenses of physicians whose medical practices are shown to be inferior, but in fact, such removals are quite rare.* The quality of physicians in practice depends much more on the initial selection of who will be allowed to enter the profession, the training they receive, and efforts by practicing physicians to monitor each other and impose informal sanctions (ostracism from professional groups, denial of hospital privileges, a re-

*Formal licensure actions against physicians are rather infrequent, and usually for misconduct (drug abuse, fraud, sexual advances) rather than poor quality of care, which has led some observers to conclude that the institution of licensure was never intended to improve quality. However, note that revoking of a driving license is similarly rare. The quality of daily driving is measured by a 15 minute test when a person is first licensed, but not thereafter, and revocation of driving licenses reflects a similar patter of egregious personal flaws rather than the traits associated with quality (vision, eye-hand coordination, etc.).

fusal to refer new patients or share business opportunities).[4] *The ability of sanctions and selection to improve quality would be greatly reduced if there were no monopoly profits.* Because licensure restrictions guarantee successful applications a career with high incomes and prestige, many outstanding students seek places in medical school. Having become doctors, they will work very hard not to lose that title. The money and power that come with being a physician, a form of monopoly profits, are too attractive to give up. If a doctor could earn more money and satisfaction working in a bank, an insurance company, or some other alternative career, why worry about losing a medical license? In fact, the opportunity cost of losing a license is so large that the mere threat is enough, and so it is rarely necessary for the profession to actually revoke a license and terminate a physician's right to practice.

The value of a license depends on the prestige of the medical profession as a whole, so each doctor has an incentive to maintain the professional franchise first by selecting only the best candidates to enter the profession, and then by continued efforts to make sure that all other doctors are as good as they can be at caring for patients so that demand remains high.* Choosing only the best candidates for admission means that the graduates will be superior regardless of how much they do or do not learn during medical school, and prestige and income plays a large part in attracting those outstanding students. The incentive to train long and hard is also related to the expectation of high incomes in the future. After graduation, the threat of losing those extraordinary returns to licensure provides an incentive to maintain competency. The existence of monopoly profits serves as a monetary performance bond that could be lost, a kind of collective collateral put up by the profession to assure good service on the part of all its members.

Observing that some specific restrictions on medical practice have no direct bearing on quality has made some economists question whether licensure boards are committed to protecting the public interest, or just the private economic interests of their own members. Application of the fundamental theorem of exchange indicates that there is no necessary conflict between the two objectives, and that they may reinforce each other. A particular restriction on medical practice may not directly improve quality, but removing it could cause quality to deteriorate by reducing the monopoly profits that provide incentives for the profession to police itself. A better test of whether or not licensure improves quality is to look at how the strength of licensure restrictions varies by type of medical practice—where and when the "licensure contract" is most apt to be approved by both patients and physicians.

A Test of the Quality Hypothesis: Strong versus Weak Licensure

The timing of licensure legislation suggests that until the level of a doctor's training can significantly affect quality and the (probable) outcome of treatment, effec-

---

*Unfortunately, the desire to maintain the value of physician licensure also provides an incentive to cover up cases of poor quality. Admitting that some licensed physicians were actually bad doctors would reduce demand, and thus diminish the value of all licenses. Therefore sometimes physicians will act to protect their own by hiding evidence of malpractice or other failures even when they strongly disapprove and wish they could get rid of the offender.

tive professional licensure is unlikely to occur, or will be very weakly enforced. Licensure was clearly desired by physicians in order to improve their economic status prior to 1900 as demonstrated by their vociferous support of such laws in state legislatures. Yet licensure laws could not get popular political support until medical science advanced to the point where knowledge made a real difference.[5] The strength of licensure was related not only to the increased effectiveness of new treatments, but also to the increased danger posed by the use of surgery and powerful drugs.

Some types of medical care, such as cardiac surgery, are inherently dangerous and demand great skill. Bad heart surgeons may have a mortality rate five times higher than good surgeons.[6] Given the great impact of measurable (by training, medical record review, and opinions of peers) physician quality indicators, we would expect licensure to be very strong for heart surgery (see Table 6.1). That is the case. Although legally a physician need only be licensed in order to perform heart surgery, in practice doctors are virtually prohibited from doing so unless they have completed residency, taken a fellowship in the subject, and been given special hospital privileges after a review by peers who have observed them acting as assistants on a number of operations. These additional mandatory checks make it evident that heart surgery has strong licensure restrictions. Conversely, there are other types of medical care that are much less dangerous and demanding, such as surgery to remove corns from the foot. While such surgery can clearly be practiced with greater or lesser skill, it is not likely to cost a life. One does not need a residency or hospital medical staff review to remove corns, and indeed corns are often removed by podiatrists who are not licensed medical doctors (although they are usually licensed DPMs). The lack of special medical staff restrictions, and the existence of alternative professional certification, show that care of the foot has weak licensure. Refractions to prescribe eyeglasses are similarly practiced by competing professions (M.D. ophthalmologists and O.D. optometrists) under weak licensure. Mental health is a specialty with a whole array of professionals—psychiatrists (M.D.), psychologists (Ph.D.), family therapists, counselors, and even psychics (palm readers, speakers for past lives, aura visionaries)—and such weak licensure that virtually anyone can offer to help you with your problems. There are substantial risks to life in mental health, and more people die of substance abuse and depression than many other conditions, but the professional does not necessarily have a great advantage over the patient in choosing the right therapist.

As the extent and value of the information asymmetry between patients and professionals increases, licensure becomes stronger. In types of care for which the

TABLE 6.1   Weak v. Strong Licensure

Weak	← Licensure →	Strong
consumers can choose		only trained professionals choose well
low risk		high risk
uncertainty small		information asymmetry high
Examples: *podiatry, eyeglasses*		Examples: *neurosurgery organ transplants*

differential is small, licensure is weak. For heart transplant, technical quality is paramount, and well evaluated by professional standards. Medical licensure is supplemented by hospital privilege review, insurance restrictions, and so on. For a broken heart, an M.D. psychiatrist may be no more effective than a sympathetic psychic whom the patient trusts, and for such counseling there are multiple forms of licensure, all rather weakly enforced.

6.2 MEDICAL EDUCATION _____

A select and hard-working group of 16,000 students will graduate with M.D. degrees from 1 of 126 U.S. medical schools this year.[7] For most of them it will be the middle of an arduous process that has compellingly taken over most of their life since high school, and will forever change the way that they view the world, and how the world views them. Many first thought about becoming doctors in elementary school, but some decided only after pursuing other careers. All had to take pre-med courses in chemistry, biology, and so on, and did rather well on average—almost half of them had an "A" average as undergraduates (GPA of 3.6 or better). Getting into medical school was serious business that took substantial effort, and many applied to ten or more schools. Much of the selection, however, was self-selection. Weaker students generally choose not to apply, and less than half of the applicants to medical school are rejected. Those who were admitted generally followed the path: 98% chose to enroll, and of those 95% graduated, almost all of whom then went into a hospital-based residency training program lasting three years or more before becoming a generalist family practitioner or a specialist in one of the other twenty-two recognized areas eligible for board certification.

Although much has been made of the cost of medical education, most of that cost is born indirectly by the government and the health insurance system. In 1994, just 4 percent of medical school costs were covered by tuition payments from students, whereas 46 percent came from patient fees and about 30 percent from research, and 20 percent from government appropriations and gifts.[8] Although the tuition might run as high as $35,000 per year, and 80 percent of medical students are left with debts from student loans when they graduate, the amount of those loans (which averaged $55,860 in 1992) is not very large in relation to the income a physician can expect, less than 1 percent of lifetime earnings.[9] Far more onerous than the monetary obligations are the years of toil spent in learning the practice of medicine.

Human Capital: Medical Education as Investment

We can use the **human capital** approach to evaluate whether going to medical school is a sacrifice, a sound investment, or both.[10] The returns on medical education are the increased annual earnings, relative to that persons' opportunity cost, that flow from the decision to go to medical school. The costs are all of the things that are given up, which of course includes tuition, but is mostly the forgone earnings and leisure from working eighty hours a week without pay in medical school, or for below-market wages during residency. Before evaluating medical education, let us first consider a hypothetical example, calculating the returns on a undergraduate college education. Bill pays tuition of $5,000 a year. He is also giving up a job that would pay him $20,000 a year (forgone wages). He also pays the university $6,000 a year for a dorm room and meal plan, but these costs should not be counted as part of the costs of his education. Thus the total cost of his degree is $4 \times \$20,000 + 4 \times \$5,000 = \$100,000$. After graduation he will be able to earn $27,000 a year instead of $20,000, for a gain of $7,000 a year. We will assume that although his earnings would increase with experience and inflation over time, the real differential will remain approximately the same. The returns on his college education are approximately $\$7,000/\$100,000 = 7\%$. Real returns after adjustment for inflation have historically been about 1 to 3 percent for savings accounts and treasury bonds, and 3 to 5 percent for stocks, which are a bit riskier, so the 7 percent return from investing in a college education compares quite favorably.

Empirical studies of rate of return on medical education get considerably more complex in practice, since one must adjust for the superior earning power of above-average students, the costs of the excess hours worked by physicians, and so forth. Also important is the fact that the returns from a medical education are much less risky than from a B.A., M.B.A., or J.D. degree, and so should be adjusted accordingly. In addition, becoming a doctor confers prestige and other valuable privileges. While all of these factors allow for a number of disagreements in detail, empirical studies in labor economics have reached consensus on some major conclusions. The return on investment in a college education clearly exceeds the market rate of return on financial assets, and the premium for being a college graduate is rising. Graduation from medical school, with real returns of 10 to 20 percent, is higher than for college and for most professional schools (returns on law school are estimated at 7%).[11] Returns on other graduate education, such as a Ph.D. in biology or sociology, are much lower, and in some fields the returns are effectively zero. Returns on residency training follow incomes; high for surgical specialties (20%), intermediate for internal medicine (10%), and low for pediatrics (2%).

6.3 THE ORIGINS OF LICENSURE AND LINKAGE TO MEDICAL EDUCATION _____

At the time of the American Revolution, there were about 3,500 established medical practitioners in what was to become the United States, but only 400 had received any formal training, and fewer than 200 held degrees. The ability to read and quote some Latin and an apprenticeship were considered sufficient qualifications for hanging out a shingle and calling one self a doctor. As late as 1830, the University of Virginia provided all its students with instruction in medicine. Yet before 1900, there was little scientific basis for the way most doctors practiced medicine, and indeed, the treatments prescribed were about as likely to harm health as to improve it. Since there was really no benefit from seeing a trained professional, there was no support for restricting the practice of medicine through licensure. Although state medical associations repeatedly pushed for licensure, and were sometimes temporarily successful, the lack of public benefit doomed such efforts. In New Jersey licensure laws were passed, and then repealed, at least 16 times between 1800 and 1900.[12] In other states, licensure laws were on the books, but did not mean much because they were not enforced. Two major technological breakthroughs radically changed the nature of medicine: anesthesiology (pain-killing) and antisepsis (germ-killing). Although surgery had been practiced since the dawn of mankind, the lack of anesthesia meant that most operations could last for only a few minutes, and even then many patients went into shock and died. The other problem was postsurgical infection, which claimed almost as many lives as the injuries that were treated. It is worth remembering that very few of the hundreds of thousands of soldiers who died during the Civil War were actually killed in battle: most died in hospitals days or weeks later. Today, most of those wounded soldiers could easily have been saved. Anesthesia and antiseptics changed surgery from a last resort for the desperate patient who would otherwise surely die into a routine procedure used in the treatment of many diseases. The very fact that twentieth-century surgery was more effective also paradoxically increased the risks. Patients who would never before have considered letting themselves be cut open now willingly went under the knife.

By the turn of the century, a confluence of factors had changed the political calculus sufficiently that the public was ready to accept and actively promote licensure for physicians. Science had advanced to the point where a university-trained physician was clearly superior to the home-grown practitioner. Yet, while these powerful new drugs and surgical techniques could cure, but they could also kill if used incompetently. Also, the start of the twentieth-century was a period of rapid scientific, economic, and political advance that favored active government intervention for reform. Regulation of child labor, sanitation, and workplace safety set the stage for the development of modern physician licensure.

In the absence of licensure, the public had come to measure quality by whether or not a physician had graduated from a medical school and obtained the M.D. degree. With the expansion of knowledge came a virtual explosion in the number medical schools. Yet many of these were little more than diploma mills, for-profit extensions of the apprenticeship programs run by senior physicians who were more interested in generating fees than modern training. Notable scandals included the report by a Chicago journalist that he had succeeded in getting his six-year-old daughter accepted by a local medical school simply by paying the application fee. This story was soon topped by the Cincinnati reporter who succeeded in enrolling his German shepherd. Leading universities pushed for reform of medical education. Following the more advanced European model, they advocated study in biology and chemistry as a prelude to supervised clinical practice, and requiring a high school diploma prior to admission. In 1876, twenty-two schools formed the American Association of Medical Colleges (AAMC). The organized practicing professionals represented by the AMA (founded in 1847) also supported these reforms, hoping to improve the image of physicians, and also to improve their incomes by gaining control of supply. In order to bring about higher standards, schools were evaluated for the quality of the education provided, and only half of the 160 then in existence were deemed acceptable. Some weaker schools closed, and others promised to substantially upgrade their teaching, libraries, and laboratories. To gather public attention and support of upgrading medical education, the AMA approached the Carnegie Foundation for the

Advancement of Teaching, which commissioned a study to be done by the notable educational researcher, Abraham Flexner.

The **Flexner report,** published in 1910, took the recently founded Johns Hopkins University as its standard for excellence. Their curriculum, built on science and direct observation of patients, emulated the German model of higher learning. The Flexner report advocated that all physicians receive at least a high-school education, followed by courses in chemistry and biology, and a year of training in a hospital. Flexner graded all medical schools as "A"(acceptable), "B" (doubtful) or "C" (unacceptable), giving only 20 of the 155 medical schools then in existence an acceptable grade of A, and proposing that soon all "C" schools be closed and all "B" schools upgrade their programs to meet higher standards, so that by 1930 only graduates of "A" schools would be allowed to practice medicine. Progress was rapid. Historian Rosemary Stevens notes that in 1905 only five schools had required any college preparation for admission, by 1915 eighty-five schools required one to two years of college, and by 1932 all medical schools required at least two years of college and some required a baccalaureate degree.[13] In Chicago, where there had been fifteen schools, the number was reduced to three. By 1920, seventy schools had been closed, and the remaining eighty-five had much higher standards—and of course, fewer graduates. By 1925, forty-six states had accepted the AMA–AAMC standards and would not recognize the low-grade schools in qualifying for state licensure exams.

Although legally the determination of physician supply depends on state licensure boards, control over supply is actually exercised by controlling the number of students allowed to enter medical school. Unlike lawyers, where many fail to graduate, or graduate and fail to pass the bar exam, or pass and then cannot find a job, almost all medical students graduate and practice medicine. There are exams in school and afterward, but almost everyone passes, and the limitation of numbers is sufficient to ensure that everyone who wants to can find a position practicing medicine. By the end of the Depression, the old laissez-faire system of unregulated physician practice with open entry had been entirely replaced by a modern system of medical licensure, with control over supply resting in the hands of the medical schools (who, in turn, were largely controlled by the joint AMA and AAMC Committee on Medical Education).

Some commentators have presumed that licensure was imposed on the public by fiat, a decree designed by physicians and then enforced by government. In fact, licensure was implemented by a local and consensual process across the United States during the 1920s and 1930s. In town after town, upgrading physician practice was proudly viewed by citizens as a public accomplishment in which they cooperated with the medical societies, not some restrictive legalism. The adverse economic consequences of a negative assessment by local medical societies (no referrals, restriction of hospital privileges, a declining reputation, and inability to attract new patients) was sufficient to drive most unqualified doctors out of business, and few practicing physicians ever had to be sanctioned by law.

A major practical difficulty in implementing licensure tied to Flexner's recommendations was how to handle all of the physicians then in practice who obviously had not received such an education. Although many were poorly trained and lacked ability, others were good physicians who had the respect of their communities and their colleagues. In order to allow these experienced doctors to continue to practice while upgrading standards for new entrants to the profession, they were *grandfathered* in. That is, a doctor could become licensed either by graduating from an acceptable medical school *or* by being an accepted member of the county medical society. Over time, the more highly qualified new graduates would replace the older cohort of non-university physicians. Analyzed in terms of property rights, the existing physicians owned the rights to vote on standards. It would not be in their self-interest to vote for higher standards that would put them out of a job, yet a higher quality standard would increase demand and benefit all physicians. The grandfather clause allowed them to reap the rewards from licensure reform, and in a sense became a form of payment for their property—control over the future of the profession. As usual, all parties, including the incumbents, must be made better off for a successful political exchange to occur.

AMA Controls Over Physician Supply, 1930–1965

With reform curtailing new entrants and forcing unqualified older practitioners out of business, physician supply declined steadily from its 1900 level of 173 MDs per 1,000 population to 133 MDs per 1,000 population in 1930 (Figure 6.3). The supply of physicians then held constant at this level for the next thirty-five years. Yet improvements in medicine greatly increased public demand, as did the rise in personal income over these four decades. With supply constant and demand increasing, earnings of physicians rose as depicted in Figure 6.1. Concern was voiced that not enough physicians were available, and that a shortage had arisen.[14]

There are several ways that this "shortage" could have been rectified. The steep price rise that did occur held quantity demanded in check and made physicians happy, but did little for the public. Supply could have been expanded by increasing the productivity of physicians, changing the organization of medical practice, and using more ancillary health workers, or some illnesses could have been treated by physician substitutes such as doctors of osteopathy or chiropractors, or

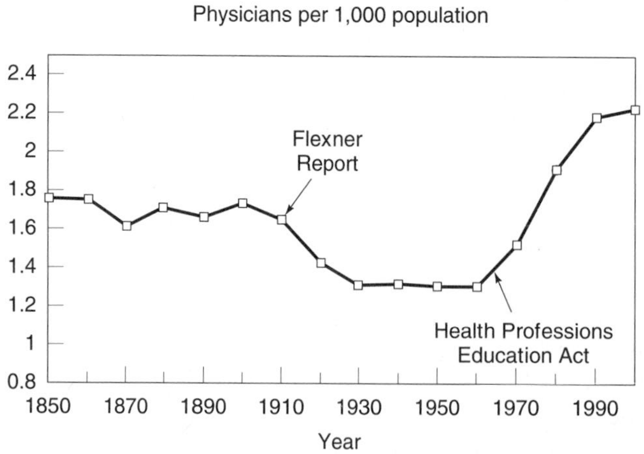

Physicians per 1,000 population

FIGURE 6.3 *Physician Supply Relative to Population, 1850 to 2000 (est).*
Sources: U.S. Census, AMA

physicians could have been imported from overseas. These alternatives would have undercut the control over physician supply and incomes by organized medicine, and were strongly resisted by the AMA. Productivity improvements and lower prices were most strongly identified with prepaid group practices such as the Kaiser Health Plan in California, or the Group Health Association in Washington D.C. Concerted opposition by local medical societies lead to the expulsion of group practice doctors and an obstinate denial of hospital privileges to physicians who were clearly qualified by education and experience.[15] In 1941, the Washington, D.C., Medical Society and the AMA were indicted, found guilty, and fined by the U.S. Department of Justice for having conspired to monopolize trade in physician services. This is but one of many in a string of cases across the country that left group practices bruised and hampered, but alive. Relations slowly improved, but opposition to prepaid group practice did not finally end until the 1970s.

The response of organized medicine to substitute providers took two forms: co-opting the competition and all-out war. Doctors of osteopathy (D.O.s) emphasized spinal manipulation in addition to standard medical practices and formed a separate type of care in 1900 with their own D.O. hospitals, but carried out many of the same Flexnerian educational reforms in those transitional years. Over time, M.D. and D.O. cooperation increased through sharing of hospital privileges, enrollment in each other's residency programs, and formation of joint political and social groups. D.O.s were tolerated by the AMA, and ultimately brought into the fold as a sort of slightly less polished M.D. Today, the differences between an M.D. and a D.O. degree are almost nonexistent, except that D.O.s are more likely to be general practitioners, and do not control any of the high prestige medical schools. In many states a single licensure board covers both types of physicians, and in California the M.D. and D.O. societies merged in 1961, although separate boards were later re-established. Throughout these years, the numbers of D.O.s relative to M.D.s has remained roughly constant at around 5 percent, and hence osteopathy has become more a partner to the AMA in controlling supply rather than a competitive threat.

Chiropractors, who often rely exclusively on spinal manipulation to treat disease and still train some practitioners in for-profit schools, have been severely and relentlessly attacked by the AMA.[17] Licensure acts explicitly exclude chiropractors from the practice of medicine, and this opposition has not changed even though the AMA has not been able to ban chiropractic practice, nor indeed to prevent some of their own members from referring to chiropractors. While some of the AMA opposition to chiropractic care is based on the lack of scientific foundations for manipulative treatments, much of it is motivated by economic concerns as well.

Foreign medical graduates, who ironically had been the standard for excellence in Flexner's reforms in 1910, came under increasing scrutiny. High incomes in the U.S. made emigration very attractive to physicians in war-torn Europe, and subsequently to the newly mobile populations of Asia. With licensure predicated on graduation from a U.S. or Canadian medical school, those who immigrated faced a much tougher set of exams and other regulatory barriers before they could practice medicine. Usually they were forced to take positions that the Americans doctors did not want: working in inner-city clinics, state mental hospitals, or becoming permanent "trainees" who supplemented the house medical staff with little opportunity of becoming self-employed.[18]

Under the control of the AMA and the medical schools, enough new M.D.s and D.O.s were being produced to keep pace with the numerical growth in the U.S. population (about 1% a year), but not with the increase in demand due to improved technology or higher disposable incomes. As the benefits of modern medicine became more evident, access to care was increasingly seen as a necessity in the rising American standard of living, and one that workers had already paid for through their health insurance premiums. The constraints on supply caused longer waits for an appointment, less time talking personally with an increasingly rushed physician, fewer old-style general practitioners willing to make house calls, and other deteriorations in service. The public was unhappy, and the politicians, who now provided most of the financing for the medical schools, were willing to do something to redress the balance.

Breaking the Contract: The Great Medical Student Expansion of 1970–1980

In essence, frustration with the inaction of the AMA led the government to unilaterally disrupt the old system. Congress passed the Health Professions Educational Assistance Act of 1963 forcing medical schools to admit more students and allowed more foreign physicians to immigrate to the United States. In response to the act and subsequent amendments, physician supply rose steadily to 161 physicians per 1,000 population in 1970, 202 in 1980, 244 in 1990, and a projected 280 before the year 2000—more than twice the level of supply that prevailed from 1930 through 1965 (see Figures 6.3. and 6.4). The number of entering students almost doubled in ten years, from 8,759 in 1965 to 15,351 in 1975. The government used two methods to bring about this increase.[19] First, it built more medical schools. Second, it offered additional funding on the condition that existing schools increase the number of students enrolled by at least 5 percent each year. At this time federal and state funding accounted for 63 percent of medical school

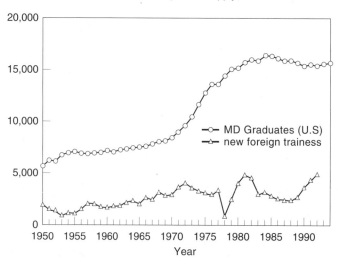

Additions to U.S. Physician Supply, 1950–1995

FIGURE 6.4   *Source: American Medical Association*

finances, and hence the schools were not in a good position to resist, even if they had wanted to. At the same time, changes in immigration rules were made to favor "shortage" occupations, including physicians. Foreign graduates made up just 6 percent of all the physicians in practice in 1960, but by 1965 that fraction had doubled to 12 percent, and further increased to 17 percent in 1970 and 20 percent in 1980. The tide of public opinion had turned by then. As the number of residents in training grew rapidly during the 1970s, it began to seem as if there were already plenty of physicians around, and that so many new entrants might create a surplus, or even unemployment. The flow of foreign graduates was severely restricted by changes in immigration law included in the Health Professions Educational Assistance Act of 1976. Moves were also made to reduce the rate of growth in the number of U.S. physicians. No more new schools were to be built. The number of first-year students peaked at 17,320 in 1981, and has been held below that number since then.

6.4 ADJUSTING PHYSICIAN SUPPLY _____

The Flow of New Entrants and the Stock of Physicians

Although the number of students entering medical school jumped by 50 percent between 1968 and 1973, this had no immediate effect on physician supply because these extra students were still in school for four years. Even then, the sudden increase in the number of new M.D.s caused only a gradual rise in the supply of physicians. It order to see why, it is necessary to trace the lifecycle of work, distinguishing the stock of physicians (the number available at any point in time) from the flow of entrants and retirees in and out of the labor force. Suppose that the average physician began practice at age 33 and retired at age 66. If the same number of physicians started work each year and retired after 33 years, then 1/33, or 3 percent, of all the physicians in practice would be leaving each year, and another 3 percent would be joining. The number of physicians in practice (the physician *stock*) would stay the same from year to year in this steady state. What would happen if the nation decided to double the physician supply by doubling the number of new graduates each year? In 33 years there would be twice as many, or 100 percent more, practicing physicians, but in the first year there would only be 3 percent more. The number of new additions is twice as much as before, or $2 \times 3\% = 6\%$ of the total, and the retirements are the same, 3 percent, so that net growth is 3 percent in the first year, 6 percent after two years, 9 percent after three years, and so on. The actual response is even slower, because there is a lag of eight years from the time new students are admitted until they complete their residency and become practicing physicians. The full effects of the 1965–1975 "Doctor Boom" will not be fully realized until this cohort of new physicians has moved through the professional ranks and completed their entire work life, sometime between the years 2000 and 2025 (see Figure 6.5).

Balancing Supply and Incomes: Tracing the Past and Projecting the Future

The development of the scientific medicine created the need for a new type of doctor in the twentieth century, and the history of physician supply and licensure

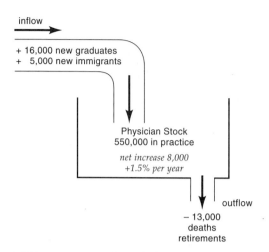

inflow

+ 16,000 new graduates
+ 5,000 new immigrants

Physician Stock
550,000 in practice
net increase 8,000
+1.5% per year

− 13,000
deaths
retirements

outflow

FIGURE 6.5 *Stock and Flow of Physicians.*
The total number of physicians in practice
(stock), changes only slowly as the inflow
(new graduates and foreign immigrants) and
outflow (deaths and retirements) change.

must be interpreted in that context. In order to raise the quality of the individuals who made up the profession (as well as their prestige and incomes), the reforms envisioned by the AMA leaders and the Flexner report required that most of the inadequately trained practitioners be forced out, thus reducing physician supply in a contraction that lasted from 1900–1930. From then until 1965, the number of new M.D.s graduating each year was held steady at about 4 percent of the total physician stock, numbers just sufficient to offset the 3 percent who retired each year and a 1 percent growth in the U.S. population, so that the physician : population ratio remained constant at about 133 : 10,000.

For a professional thinking technically in terms of medical "need" (a specific, fixed number of physicians required to treat a given number of illnesses), a constant physician-to-population ratio was sufficient to meet demand. From an economic perspective emphasizing responsiveness to prices and incomes, it is clear how inadequate both the concept and the numbers used by the medical profession were. Changing expectations, new technology and a rising standard of living meant that demand was increasing, and the 1 percent growth in physicians set to match the 1 percent increase was not enough to forestall market stress and public dissatisfaction. Since total physician supply only gradually rises as the number of new graduates is increased, a rapid increase in supply could only be obtained by "importing" physicians. The number of foreign medical graduates practicing in the United States doubled in just three years, going from 15,154 in 1960 to 30,925 in 1963, with 15,000 more arriving in the next four years. By 1968, the effects of building new U.S. medical schools and raising class size began to kick in. Subsequently, the AMA began to complain loudly about a potential surplus, and commissioned a number of studies to show that the U.S. was training an excess of physicians, and also that foreign immigrants were no longer needed. These arguments were successful in helping the profession reestablish control over supply in the 1980s. The number of entering medical students has steadily declined since then (even though total stock of practicing M.D.s, new and old, has risen and will continue to do so for at least the next ten years).[20]

What evidence does the market provide about the assertions that too many physicians were trained or allowed to immigrate? Pent up demand kept physician incomes from falling during the 1970s as supply rose. Although real earnings dipped in 1985, and again from 1989–1990, physicians have done much better than the average American worker over the last fifteen-years. However, fewer college students are applying to medical schools. About 2 percent of those admitted to medical school do not attend. While this fraction refusing the opportunity of a medical education is still quite small, it is fourfold above the rate between 1975 and 1985, when just 0.5 percent of those offered a place in medical school turned it down. While projecting the future is always to some extent speculative, it is possible to give a reasonable assessment of the economic situation and prospects of physicians from these trends. Becoming a doctor still offers above-average rates of return on post-college education. However, the very high earnings growth that physicians enjoyed during the 1960s and 1970s were a temporary historical aberration, brought about by rapid growth in demand due to new technology in the context of fixed supply. In the future, doctors will have high, but not such extraordinarily high, earnings. While still doing much better than most graduates from other fields, new physicians will face more competition as they enter the market, and thus will be more likely to become employees holding salaried jobs, and to hold on to such positions for longer in their careers. The few who become truly wealthy will be those who have worked their way up the ladder in large health care organizations, or who have taken substantial risks as entrepreneurs.

SUGGESTIONS FOR FURTHER READING _____

M. W. Raffel & N. K. Raffel, *The U.S. Health Care System: Origins and Function*, Delmar Press: Albany, 1994 (4th ed).

Richard Shryock, *Medical Licensing in America, 1650–1965*, Baltimore: Johns Hopkins University Press, 1967.

Paul Starr, *The Social Transformation of American Medicine*, New York: Basic Books, 1982.

SUMMARY _____

1. **Licensure is a collective extension of the doctor–patient relationship of agency.** It helps to solve the problems caused by uncertainty and information asymmetry.

2. **Licensure increases profits by restricting supply**, and thus changes the traditional supply and demand curve analysis. **The supply curve is fixed, or vertical**, and increases in demand do not bring about any increase in quantity, but increased profits for suppliers known by economists as **rents**.

3. **Licensure increases quality by;** (a) **selection** of only the best students to enter medical school, (b) **training** during three years of medical school, four years of residency, and periodical refresher courses thereafter, (c) having physicians

monitor each other. Note that all of these depend up having some excess profits or monopoly rents to serve as an incentive.

4. Licensure is **intended to both increase profits and to increase quality**. Like any law, it must **satisfy both parties (physicians and the public/patients)** to be a self-enforcing political exchange. The importance of quality concerns is evidenced by comparing the types of care for which licensure is strong (cardiac surgery, chemotherapy) with those for which it is weak (removing corns, prescribing eyeglasses, counseling).

5. About 16,000 M.D.s graduated from 126 medical schools in the United States in 1995. Since the bulk of the physician supply is constituted by those who have already been, and will continue to be, in practice for many years, **any changes in the number of new graduates will only slowly affect the supply of services**. The "physician baby boom" of the 1970s will move through the health care system creating strains and opportunities until the year 2020. The supply of physicians stayed roughly constant at around 1.4 physicians for each 1,000 population from the start of modern medical education in the 1920's until 1965, but has risen rapidly since then to 2.5 physicians per 1,000 population today.

6. Although medical school tuition is expensive, running as much as $30,000 per year, it is still a very good **investment in human capital**. The average medical student will graduate with a debt of about $55,000—but this is less than four months of the average physician's earnings. Overall, taking account of the tuition, years of training, extra hard work, and other factors, going to medical school provides an annual inflation-adjusted return of about 12 percent, three or four times what one could expect if one invested in financial assets rather than education, and about 1.5 to 2 times as much as one gains from most undergraduate and graduate education.

7. **Control over physician supply and licensure in the U.S. is actually exercised by control over the medical education**, a system that grew out of the Abraham **Flexner Report of 1910** to the Carnegie Commission supported by the American Medical Association. Three factors contributed to the development of medical licensure based on graduate training at this time: (a) advances in medical technology (surgery, anesthesia, radiology) that were powerful aids to healing, but could also be harmful if used improperly; (b) a scientific knowledge base that gave university educated physicians a real advantage over physicians who only learned by apprenticeships; and (c) a reformist political climate favoring regulation, combined with evidence that many doctors were not competently trained before entering practice.

8. **Competition for clients** in medical care is dominated by quality, not price. Physicians have used quality concerns and licensure laws to attempt to foreclose competition by graduates of foreign medical schools, osteopaths, chiropractors and other health practitioners.

9. **Control over supply** by the professional associations has increased the profits of physicians relative to other workers. While the physician:population ratio stayed constant from 1930 to 1960, demand was actually increasing due to new medical advances and an increasingly affluent society, creating a **physician**

shortage. The AMA was unwilling to increase the number of physicians (which would have meant lower incomes) but the public consensus was sufficiently strong to force the opening of new medical schools and revisions in immigration laws to make it easier for foreign doctors in the United States. As the increase in new graduates during the 1970s and 1980s relieved this pressure, the size of entering medical school classes was reduced and immigration was again restricted.

PROBLEMS _____

1. {*licensure*} Does licensure raise the quality of medical care, or does it just raise the profitability of medical practice?

2. {*information asymmetry*} How do agency and information asymmetry lead to licensure? Do agents get more or less of the gains from trade as the degree of information asymmetry increases? Explain why and how the strength of licensure is related to the extent of information asymmetry.

3. {*incidence*} Who pays the costs of medical education: the student, the patients, the insurance companies, or the taxpayers?

4. {*annualized returns*} If the rate of return on human capital is 15%, and the opportunity cost of time for a newly graduated physician is $60,000 per year, how large is the incremental increase in annual earnings that the physician should expect to obtain from a four-year post-graduate residency?

5. {*demand curves, derived demand*} Draw the demand and supply curves for two medical professions, one with licensure, and one without (e.g., physicians v. hospital administrators).
   a. Which would show the larger percentage increase in incomes for an equivalent shift in demand?
   b. What would be the effect of the government giving scholarships of $10,000 per year to all students entering the licensed profession as compared to the unlicensed profession?
   c. What would be the effect of the scholarships on tuition at the licensed and unlicensed professional schools? On the number of students applying?
   d. Would it make a difference if instead of giving scholarships to everyone, the government gave them to just 5,000 students?

6. {*price controls*} Some states have mandated Medicare "assignment." Assignment means that the doctor agrees to treat a patients and accept the fee Medicare sends as payment in full. Doctors not accepting assignment bill the patient (almost always for more than Medicare would pay) and the patient pays the doctor, sends in the bill, and gets reimbursed by Medicare. Typically 20% to 60% of physicians in an area accept Medicare assignment because patients prefer it and payment is assured. Other physicians want to bill for the extra money. How many doctors accept assignment depends on the rates Medicare is currently paying, local market conditions, how "full" the doctor's practice is, and so on. Draw demand and supply curves to show the effects of passing a state law mandating that all physicians accept Medicare assignment. What hap-

pens to price, quantity, demand, supply? Distinguish between the short-run and long-run effect. Describe what other effects you might expect.

7. {competition} Several politicians have proposed that the United States become more restrictive with regard to immigration, allowing fewer foreign-educated physicians to undergo training or establish practices in the United States. Would this increase or decrease the earning power of U.S.-educated physicians? Which specialties would be most affected?

8. {licensure} The state of New Jersey was unwilling to allow physicians to become licensed in 1850; what factors changed to make them willing to enact and enforce licensure restrictions in 1950?

9. {licensure, property rights} How did the reformers in the medical profession who wanted to impose higher standards obtain the consent of physicians who were educated under the old system? Did power get translated into money in the process?

10. {supply} What controls the supply of physicians in the United States? Distinguish between short- and long-run, and also between proximate and fundamental factors (i.e., the actual decision-making individuals and organizations versus the underlying economic and political forces).

11. {anti-trust} Has the AMA ever been sued for restraint of trade? Did it win or lose?

12. {competition} Are chiropractors substitutes or complements for physicians in the production of medical services? Podiatrists? Psychologists? Osteopaths? Homeopaths? Which professions are more competitive and which are more cooperative? Why?

13. {dynamics} How long does it take to become a doctor? How long does a doctor usually practice medicine? How long does it take for the supply of doctors to adjust to a change in the number of patients or a change in the availability of technology? Is the time required for adjustment different for a city than a state, or the country as a whole? What is the relevant geographic unit for measuring the market for physician services?

ENDNOTES _____

1. Richard Shryock, *Medical Licensing in America, 1650–1965*, Baltimore: Johns Hopkins University Press, 1967.
2. Elton Rayack, *Professional Power and American Medicine: The Economics of the American Medical Association*, Cleveland, Ohio: World Publishing, 1967.
3. U.S. Bureau of Labor Statistics, *Occupational Outlook*, BLS Bulletin 2450, Washington, D.C.: U.S. Government Printing Office, April 1994.
4. Eliott Friedson, *Professional Dominance: The Social Structure of Medical Care*, New York: Atherton, 1970; and *Professional Powers: A Study in the Institutionalization of Formal Knowledge*, Chicago: University of Chicago Press, 1986.
5. John Duffy, *From Humors to Medical Science: A History of American Medicine*, Urbana: University of Illinois Press, 1993.
6. *A Consumer Guide to Coronary Artery Bypass Graft Surgery*, Vol. IV, 1993 Data. PHC4, Pennsylvania Health Care Cost Containment Council: Harrisburg, PA, 1995.

7. Enrollments and other data are taken from the annual "Medical Education" issue of the *Journal of the American Medical Association*.

8. J. Ganem, J. Krakower, R. Beran, "Review of U.S. Medical School Finances, 1993–1994," *Journal of the American Medical Association*, 274(9):723–730, September 6, 1995.

9. J. Ganem, J. Krakower, R. Beran, "Review of U.S. Medical School Finances, 1992–1993," *Journal of the American Medical Association*, 272(9):705–711, 1994.

10. Gary S. Becker, *Human Capital*, Cambridge, Mass: Harvard University Press, 1975.

11. Roger Feldman and Richard Scheffler, "The Supply of Medical School Applicants and the Rate of Return of Training," *Quarterly Review of Economics and Business*, Spring, 1978; W. Lee Hansen, "Shortages and Investment in Health Manpower," in *The Economics of Health and Medical Care*, Ann Arbor, Mich. University of Michigan Press, 1965.

12. Richard Shryock; Rosemary Stevens, *American Medicine and the Public Interest*, New Haven, Conn.: Yale University Press, 1971.

13. Rosemary Stevens, *In Sickness and In Wealth: American Hospitals in the Twentieth Century*, New York: Basic Books, 1989.

14. Rashi Fein, *The Doctor Shortage: An Economic Diagnosis*, Washington: Brookings Institute, 1967.

15. Edward Berkowitz and Wendy Wolf, *Group Health Association: A Portrait of a Health Maintenance Organization*, Philadelphia: Temple University Press, 1988.

16. Erwin Blackstone, "The AMA and the Osteopaths: A Study of the Power of Organized Medicine," *Antitrust Bulletin*, Summer 1977.

17. Elton Rayack, "The Physicians Service Industry," Chapter 6 in Walter Adams (editor), *The Structure of American Industry*, 5th edition, New York: Macmillan, 1982, pp:407–408.

18. David Kindig, "Growth in International Physician Supply, 1950–1979," *Journal of the American Medical Association*, February 1984.

19. U.S. Department of Health and Human Services. *Fifth Report to the President and Congress on the Status of Health Personnel in the United States*, Washington, D.C.: U.S. Government Printing Office, 1984.

20. U.S. Department of Health and Human Services, Office of Graduate Medical Education. *Report of the Graduate Medical Education National Advisory Committee to the Secretary, Department of Health and Human Services*. Pub No. 81–651, Washington, D.C.: U.S. Government Printing Office, 1981. This became widely known as the "GMENAC Report."

CHAPTER 7

Physician Organization and Business Practices

QUESTIONS

1. *Do physicians trade patients? Are payments between doctors for referrals legal, ethical, or efficient?*

2. *Can medical groups advertise to attract more patients and increase market power?*

3. *Is price discrimination legal?*

4. *Are there economies of scale in physician practice?*

5. *Who sets the standards of practice to guide clinical decisions?*

6. *Why do patients in Boston get more surgical operations than patients in San Francisco?*

7. *Why are some patients charged more if the services they receive are no different?*

8. *How did medical specialties develop? What determines the boundaries between specialties?*

9. *Do physicians get compensated for technology, or for skill?*

7.1   GROUP PRACTICE: HOW ORGANIZATION AND TECHNOLOGY AFFECT TRANSACTIONS_____

Physicians who join together into groups have higher net earnings than those who practice alone: $178,900 for solo doctors, as compared to $211,300 for those in two-physician partnerships, $240,700 in three-physician groups, and $267,500 in groups where nine or more physicians practice together (see Table 5.2). It is also generally accepted that physicians in group practices have better lifestyles: more interaction with colleagues, more support services, and fewer nights spent handling patient emergencies.[1] Economists must ascertain what factors lead to greater efficiency and hence higher incomes for group practice, and conversely, what factors limit the attractiveness of groups so that one-third of all physicians still choose to practice alone. There are fundamentally three ways that group practices serve to increase net income:

1. Economies of scale raise the productivity of inputs, and hence lower costs.
2. Market gains bring in greater revenues.
3. Sharing spreads risks.

What does it mean to have **economies of scale** that make larger practices more efficient in the use of inputs? To a physician owner, it could mean either (a) that the cost of inputs required to produce a given amount of output has been reduced, or (b) that the output in visits per hour of physician time has been increased. Analysis of group practice expenditures shows that some of both occurs.[2] Equipment and office space comes in discrete units, and is therefore inefficiently used in small practices. An X-ray machine that can handle 10,000 patients may cost only 50 percent more than one that can handle 2,000, and even the smaller one is frequently idle for a doctor practicing alone. A large group can match equipment needs to the total patient volume of the group as a whole, and so achieve economies of scale. Similarly, each physician may need from one to four examining rooms at a time to maximize patient flow, and from two to six assistants. A solo doctor will compromise by having an office with three exam rooms and four assistants, and thus sometimes the ancillary inputs will be overcrowded and limit productivity, while at other times they sit idle and waste money. A group can plan for an average, since it is unlikely that all of the physicians will be busy or slack at the same time, and thus achieve a better match. Office rent takes up 12 percent of the gross revenues of solo practices, 10 percent of two-physician partnerships, and just 7 percent for large group practices.

On the other hand, labor costs and FTE (full-time equivalent) employees per physician increase as practice size increases. A large group can allow for more specialization in the use of labor, so that a ten-physician group can have a laboratory technician, billing specialists, receptionist, intake nurse, exam room assistant, and so on, while a solo practice must make do with general-purpose medical assistant or nurse. Increasing the productivity of an input can either decrease or increase its share of total expenditures depending upon the elasticity of substitution with other inputs. Office space apparently cannot be substituted for physician time; thus, as it becomes more productive per square foot, it takes up a smaller fraction of total practice expenditures. Ancillary labor can be substituted for physician time, and as it becomes more productive, physicians use more employees rather than less. It is worth paying more for helpers to save the physicians' time because their net profit per hour of work increases.

Risk sharing across the members of the group is a form of scale economy. Just as random variation in the number of examining rooms required by each doctor can be averaged out in a large group, so can other revenues and expenses, so that the group can collectively enjoy a smoother and more certain income stream. Perhaps even more importantly, the emergency calls that interrupt the home life of every doctor are much less disruptive when combined and redistributed in a group. A solo practitioner must be "on call" every night, or find someone else who is willing to cover. On Sunday, one emergency call might interrupt a football game, and then there might be no more until a sleep-shattering call at 3 A.M. For a group, it is usual for each doctor to accept all the calls for a single day. The group doctor might handle seven emergencies on a Sunday, but know that Friday night and Saturday are free, since any patients who need assistance will be handled by one of the partners. The burden of emergencies is not the time spent in caring for patients, but the uneven spacing. This is the risk that is shared, and thus effectively reduced, in a group.

Since it is obviously so much more efficient for a doctor to handle ten patients in one night than one to three patients each night per week, why don't solo doctor's contract with each other to do just that? For that matter, why can't independent physicians arrange to share office space, or nurses? To some extent they do, and to that extent, they start to become a group. As the contracts and sharing become more and more complete, and cover more aspects of practice, the doctors who trade with each other become a single firm—that is, a group practice. But, it is hard to share. All of the doctors must agree to standardize certain practices, to coordinate efforts, to pick a leader, and accept his or her ruling on disputes between them, and so on—in short, to be managed. It means being an employee or partner rather than the boss. Management is costly, and good physician managers, like all good managers, are rare and valuable commodities. Some studies of physician productivity overestimated economies of scale because they did not account for the time physicians must spend in management, and how that management time increases as the size of the practice increases.[3] For some physicians, it is cheaper (and more fun) to put up with some inefficiencies and lack of specialized inputs in order to call all of their own shots and not have to listen to, or give orders to, anyone else.

Contracting between many parties and managing larger operations create the costs that limit the attractiveness of group practice. Transactions costs are also the source of the economies of scale in marketing and revenue generation, which are often more important than production cost economies. Consider what happens when a successful older doctor combines his practice with that of a younger physician who is just starting out. The older physician has too many patients, and must turn some away or provide poor service. The young physician has too few patients, and must spend hours waiting for people to show up or moonlighting as an employee in hospital emergency rooms. By combining their practices, the successful doctor is, in effect, selling some patients to the younger doctor in return for a part of the younger doctor's income. In order for such a transfer to occur, patients must be convinced that the young doctor is as good as the senior one. The quality of the junior is guaranteed by the senior by the act of forming a partnership. In effect, Senior Doctor is saying "I trust this doctor; so should you." Transfer is also facilitated by arranging for the junior partner to take a disproportionate share of the night emergencies, the new patients who show up at the door for the first time, and those who do not want to wait weeks to see Senior. It is the patient's concerns about quality and trust that make the doctor–patient relationship special, and that make it hard to obtain economies of scale by treating patients en masse. In order for a group to act as a collective, the guarantee of quality must extend to all of the physicians in it. Just as all licensed physicians benefit from monitoring the quality of care provided by the profession and eliminating or reforming bad doctors, so a medical group practice benefits from increased demand to the extent that it can closely monitor and control the quality of all its members.[4] The Mayo clinic is a premier example of a medical group practice that acts as a "brand-name firm" and gains a marketing and revenue advantage from being perceived as a group with identifiable quality rather than just a random collection of individual physicians who happen to work in the same building.[5]

In medicine, as in most of commerce, market share is valuable, but hard to trade. HMOs must often seek care for thousands, even hundreds of thousands, of patients. It is much less costly to negotiate with one or two large groups of physicians than a multitude of solo practitioners, each of whom has a different billing form. A single specialty group may be able to exercise some monopoly power to raise prices and incomes. Even when there is competition between groups that limits price flexibility, a group can afford lawyers, business managers, and other representatives that cut costs and keep their members from being exploited, while a solo practitioner acting alone may be taken advantage of. As the medical care system becomes ever more complex, and as employers and insurance companies organize large blocks of patients for managed care, the contractual economies of scale become a crucial factor leading physicians to combine into group practices.

7.2 PRICE DISCRIMINATION

One of the characteristics of the medical markets first noted by economists was that different patients pay very different prices for the same service.[6] Some price differences are attributable to differences in cost or value: surgery by a board-certified specialist versus a new intern, midnight treatment in the emergency room versus a routine visit to the doctor's office. However, even after these factors are taken into account, there is still a sizable and systematic variation in charges. It is frequently noted that people who are well insured or have high incomes pay more, that laboratory and other minor services are overpriced, and services that patients "shop around" for such as eye exams, normal deliveries, and physical therapy, show less price variation than emergency medical care where immediate treatment is required.

A major reason for **price discrimination**, charging different prices for the same service to different types of patients or in different types of care, is that it increases total revenues. It is important to remember that the change in revenues, marginal revenue, depends on price elasticity as well as price. More formally,

$$\text{Marginal Revenue} = \text{Price}\left(1 + \frac{1}{\text{Elasticity}}\right)$$

In order to maximize revenues when providing two different types of care, the physicians should charge different prices even if their costs are the same, and should *charge the higher price where demand is least price sensitive* (i.e. where price elasticity is always negative, is smaller in magnitude). Conversely, where demand is very price sensitive, a reduction in price will bring in many more patients and increase revenues (see Figure 7.1). Pain, fear of dying, and wealth all serve to reduce price sensitivity. However, the most important factor making medical consumers less price sensitive is insurance (see Figure 7.2). Therefore, we would generally expect physicians to charge more for those services that are more fully insured, more life-threatening, more painful, and for which patients have the least ability to shop around. Some ancillary services (lab tests, X-rays, sonograms, etc.) are not very price sensitive even when insurance coverage is incomplete, because they are considered secondary and inevitable byproducts,

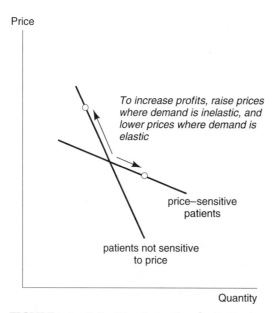

Price

To increase profits, raise prices where demand is inelastic, and lower prices where demand is elastic

price–sensitive patients

patients not sensitive to price

Quantity

FIGURE 7.1 *Price Discrimination by Patient Type*

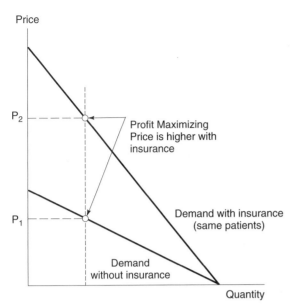

FIGURE 7.2 *Price Discrimination by Insurance Status*

and thus rarely receive the kind of scrutiny given to an operation or other major expense.*

There is an important empirical discrepancy at odds with the revenue maximization model of physician price discrimination: the lower price is sometimes clearly below the cost of providing services, and so must decrease rather than increase physician income; often, valuable care is provided entirely for free. Indeed, when queried about differential pricing, some physicians will respond angrily to the suggestion that they are maximizing profits, and assert that they act from a benevolent impulse, charging high prices to those who can afford to pay (or are well insured) so that they can take care of the destitute. Under closer examination, it becomes evident that there is a mixture of motivations that includes both charity and higher incomes in a blend that is not always clearly separated. Charging less to students clearly helps out a group that is poorer and might not get care if they had to pay full price—and also brings in more revenues for exactly the same reason. (Why do you think movie theaters and airlines give student discounts—is it a charitable impulse or a smart business practice to raise revenues, because they know you have little discretionary money and wouldn't come as often otherwise?) Price discrimination is pervasive in medicine, and well accepted by patients, the government, and insurance companies. If two people came into a shop and the second was charged twice as much for oil, food, or rent, the person charged extra would complain or threaten to sue. The unusual willingness of people to accept or even praise price discrimination in medicine is one of the factors that has convinced economists that health care markets differ in significant ways from markets for most other goods and services.

_____

* The same process of overcharging for less price-sensitive ancillary items is found when purchasing a car, as the dealer puts a higher mark-up on radios, air-bags, floor mats, and so on.

7.3   KICKBACKS, SELF-DEALING, AND SIDE PAYMENTS _____

". . . and if a doctor shall cheat his patient by overcharging for medicaments, then shall a finger of his left hand be cut off."

Code of Hammurabi, 2300 B.C.

From the beginning, the AMA code of medical ethics has dealt with economic issues, rightfully noting that doctors must put the health of patients above profits if people are to trust them. The agency relationship is most threatened in day-to-day business by the practice of paying "referral fees" or **kickbacks**. The agent is supposed to be, and is paid for, acting in the principal's (the patient's) best interest. When doctors accept a fee for referring patients to one hospital rather than another, or for giving a surgical case to Dr. B instead of Dr. A, they may be tempted to go with the one who will pay them the most, not the one who will provide the best care. In ordinary business dealings, such a payment would be termed a *bribe,* or a kickback. Corporate purchasing agents are sometimes caught accepting presents or kickbacks from suppliers in return for steering business their way. For suppliers to pay for business is not bad—they can give rebates, or provide customer treats, or price discounts. The problem is the distortion caused by directing a payment to the agent who is supposed to be making an objective choice, rather than the principal, who is supposed to get the benefits of any discounts. Before medicine became established as a profession, such practices were common. Surgeons in the large cities would advertise in rural newspapers their willingness to pay $100 or more for each case sent to them. While such behavior seems unthinkable now, kickbacks keep cropping up. Recently, the nation's largest chain of psychiatric hospitals was investigated and convicted for paying physicians and social workers who sent in clients. The kickback scheme had become so well established that there was a standard going rate of $70 for each patient day.[7]

Why do kickbacks continue to occur if everyone knows that they are bad and they are condemned by all of the official governing organizations? They continue because an agent's control over who gets the business is valuable property. To not make use of that value—that is, to act ethically and follow professional standards which puts the interests of patients first—forces a doctor to put aside his or her own narrow self-interest. In the short run it is easy to profit by betraying a trust to make a dollar. The violator hopes not to get caught. Even if an unethical physician does get caught, much of the punishment actually falls on other doctors, as the profession as a whole gets blamed for a lack of standards and suffers from a reduced demand and falling prices for services. Trust and agency build professional value, and taking a kickback is one way for a member to steal a part of that value, benefiting personally while harming others.

One of the major activities of physicians is to prescribe drugs. If drug companies made payments to physicians, those dollars could distort the physicians' choices on behalf of their patients, perhaps prescribing a drug that is less effective, or one that is effective but three times as expensive as all the substitute drugs that would work just as well. An even more difficult problem arises when the physician is not just prescribing the drug, but also selling it. Knowing that the patient is in pain and trusts the physician, physicians could fatten their profit margins by overcharging for drugs. That such a problem is not new is evidenced by the quote from the code of Hammurabi given at the beginning of this section. The potential for abuse is such that physicians in this country have been legally prohibited from selling drugs or owning pharmacies since 1934. When there is a pharmacy in a medical clinic, even that must be run as a separate business to avoid conflicts of interest. In Japan, where no such law exists, the government sets price controls to keep physicians from overcharging, but that does not stop them from over-prescribing: general-practice physicians in Japan get about a third of their net income from sales of pharmacy items, and their patients are prescribed twice as many drugs as similar patients in the United States.

In the quote from the code of Hammurabi, the prohibition is on overcharging for *medication*. Why isn't overcharging for service similarly condemned? The issue with kickbacks is not price, it is deceit. If Dr. Arnold says "I am better than the others, and I want $20 more for each visit," that is his privilege. Patients can agree or go somewhere else. There is no fraud. To prescribe a drug and accept a $20 rebate from the manufacturer, or to send a surgical case to Dr. Jones knowing that he will send a case of wine in return, is fraud. The patient is unknowingly paying (somebody has to pay for the wine—to Jones it is just a cost of doing business that he adds into the overhead for the surgical bill) and has an agent whose decisions may be based on maximizing kickbacks rather than patient welfare. If Dr. Arnold and Dr. Jones were partners in a large group practice, then a patient would expect to be sent to one of the surgeons in the group (Jones) and there would be no fraud. Also, Jones would have expected Dr. Arnold to send the case as a matter of routine, and there would be no kickback payment. The amount of money changing hands in the transaction might be the same, but the ethical and economic considerations are quite different. In essence, a patient of the group is buying "the group" and does not care how Dr. Arnold and Dr. Jones split the money. The patient going to Dr. Arnold, *and unaware that Dr. Arnold has any business arrangement with another doctor,* has a right to expect Dr. Arnold to choose objectively the surgeon who is best, and to negotiate the lowest price.

As medicine has become more complex, with more transactions involved in each episode of patient care, it has become ever more difficult to avoid conflicts of interest. Of particular concern in recent years have been the actions of for-profit companies providing ancillary services such as diagnostic radiology or home IV therapy, and then offering "investments" in these businesses in return for sending in patients.[8] So many abuses of this sort took place that in 1976 federal anti-kickback laws were passed prohibiting any payment to physicians based on the number using Medicare or Medicaid funds. The 1989 "Stark" law (named after its sponsor, California Congressman Fortney Stark) banned physicians from referring patients to a clinical laboratory in which they have a financial interest. The 1993 "Stark II" widened the ban to prohibit self-referrals to hospitals or radiology laboratories in which a physician has invested. It also prohibits bonus plans within group practices based on the volume of laboratory referrals. Only a minority (less than 10%) of physicians invest in businesses that raise conflict of interest problems from self-referral, and only a few engage in profiteering at the expense of the government and patients.* Yet the actions of these few are so troubling to a public already dismayed over the high cost of health care, that it is likely that further restrictions will be placed on independent diagnostic and therapeutic facilities owned by physicians. Eventually, physician ownership or partnership in ancillary facilities may be banned entirely, as ownership of pharmacies has been.

Balance Billing: Half a Reform May Be Worse Than None

Some physicians used to add to the net income of their practice by adding an extra charge on all tests sent to outside clinical labs. In order to prevent abuses, Medicare in 1987 banned such "balance billing" and decreed that clinical laboratories would henceforth bill the patient directly. Although the intent to avoid extra charges was clear, the effects of the rules were more complex. For some physicians, the changes led them to stop handling laboratory tests, and payments were reduced as surcharges disappeared and less expensive laboratories were sought out. Other physicians, denied the ability to take a profit on the lab test they sent out, simply expanded what had been a limited in-office laboratory to handle most testing, or built a new in-office laboratory if they did not already have one inefficiently making care more expensive just to gain more revenues.[9] Although occasionally an in-office laboratory is needed for immediate results or special tests, for the most part such small laboratories are very expensive and of low quality, since they lack the trained technicians, expert systems, economies of scale, and routine monitoring that is standard for large laboratories. Thus, the rule had the perverse and unintended effect of raising costs and lowering quality in many instances.

7.4 TECHNOLOGY AND THE DEVELOPMENT OF SPECIALTIES _____

The modern medical profession, with its requirements for higher education and licensure, grew out of scientific progress that promised more cures for the public, and more income and prestige for physicians. Yet the same advances in technology that led to an organized medical profession under the leadership of the AMA also created divisions among doctors. The span of knowledge in medicine became too large for a single person to master. In order to become truly expert, physicians had to limit their practice to a specific area, becoming specialists. Specialties were not arbitrary divisions of medicine, but instead grew up around technological innovations; with the discovery of X-rays came radiologists, anesthesia led to surgeons and anesthesiologists, the otolaryngiscope to ear, nose & throat specialists, and so on.[10] The divisions were not theoretical, but practical, involving the use of a particular piece of equipment in the treatment of disease.

The listing of physician specialties by income (see Table 5.2) shows that those specialties that are more technological (radiology, surgery, anesthesiology) are at

---

* Physicians are allowed to buy stocks and make other forms of investments in laboratories, hospitals and medical business, but they cannot be partners or get special treatment different from non-physicians who are not in a position to refer patients.

the high end of the income scale, while those that are not based on the use of equipment have far lower earning power (family practice, pediatrics, psychiatry). Family practice and pediatrics are perhaps better called *fields* than *specialties*, but psychiatry is clearly a specialized area of study, requiring years of training and mastery of a complex body of theory—but no piece of equipment. The major technological advance in psychiatric care has been the development of powerful drugs such as thorazine, lithium, valium, and other psychotropics. These drugs are used by all sorts of physicians who have not been given any special training. Thus, the psychiatrists do not have any unique technology to claim uniquely as their own, and no designated stream of earnings to defend. Surgeons, on the other hand, have control over a set of practices with powerful curative ability that they may exercise even in the absence of theory. A psychiatrist who discovers a brain defect will be paid modestly for his or her diagnostic capability and testing, but the neurosurgeon who operates will be well compensated for an hour of his time. Most physician reimbursement shows this pattern of "procedure bias," physicians get paid more for "doing something," and particularly for doing something that takes a lot of fancy equipment, than for observing a patient, thinking about their illness, or giving advice.

Why is it that *procedures are well paid, while thinking and caring are not?* The problem is one of measurement. Insurance must be based on some objectively defined event to be reimbursed, and procedures are much easier to count than other inputs into patient care. One physician may spend seventy minutes on a patient's initial visit, while another spends just ten. Basing payment on time does not solve the problem, because the kidney specialist who spent ten minutes might discover more in that time than the previous physician discovered in an hour, or may know of a better treatment. Such cognitive skills are by their very nature unobservable, and hence, difficult to compensate. Surgery, on the other hand, is obvious, fits well into thousands of neatly defined categories, and causes claims reviewers few problems. Even for internists (internal medicine specialists) who have always been known as the thinkers of medicine, higher incomes go to those who perform procedures using elaborate tools: the cardiologists doing catheterization, the colon expert using endoscopy.

Ophthalmology: Competition and the Creation of the First Specialty Board

A historical review shows that economic competition played a substantial role in shaping the organization of specialties, determining control over new technologies and the professional fees they generated.[11] The first specialty to create an official certifying body was ophthalmology in 1916. For many years some physicians had maintained a special interest in illnesses of the eye, just as others were interested in illnesses of the stomach, spine, or mind. It was an entirely separate group of nonmedical practitioners who undertook the making of eyeglasses to correct defects in vision. These lens grinders were considered master craftsmen, not medical doctors. The major technological advances were Helmholtz's discovery of the ophthalmoscope in 1851 and the work on refraction and fitting of spectacles by the Dutch physician Donder, translated into English in 1864. The ophthalmoscope gave ophthalmologists the technological edge that might define the boundaries of a specialty, but it could also be used by the nonmedical opticians. Although the advanced European specialists trained in Universities were primarily concerned with the pathology of the eye, and only peripherally in the use of lens for corrections, the more pragmatic and less theoretical American ophthalmologists were more interested in eyeglasses, which had gone from being a minor aid to a major industry. In 1911, one ophthalmologist observed that more glasses were then being bought in his city than had been in use in the entire world just sixty years before, with a commensurate increase in the potential for profits.

The making of eyeglasses was done by opticians, and ophthalmologists had little desire to compete for what they saw as manufacturing. *Dispensing opticians* made glasses to order based on a prescription from a physician. *Optometrists* or refracting opticians did their own eye examinations and wrote the prescriptions for the patients who visited them, as well as making the glasses. It was the latter that the physicians objected to, since they were a form of direct competition. The principals in the professional quarrel that led to the founding of rival societies were a leading optometrist, Charles F. Prentice, and a noted ophthalmologist, Henry Noyes, both of whom practiced in New York City. Prentice was a highly educated engineer and accomplished student of the eye. Initially, he and the physician Noyes were friends, and Noyes invited Prentice to lecture on his system of prism measurement at the New York Academy of Medicine in 1891. Prentice looked for cooperation between the more advanced opticians who wished to perform eye exams and their physician colleagues. However, in 1892 Noyes wrote to Prentice complaining that while it was perfectly all right for him to prescribe glasses, he should not charge for doing so, explaining that it was an issue of economic competition and "unjustly" misleading the public into thinking that Prentice had "the qualifications which entitle you to a fee for advice." Prentice replied that his patients were clearly informed that he was not a physician, that he always referred clients to physicians when he discovered any disease in the eye, that he and many of the other opticians were at least as well qualified as many of the M.D.s to perform eye examinations, that overcharging for glasses rather than making a separate charge for the eye exam was a form of fraud, and that he did not care to ease the physicians "ethical" concerns by using the deceptive practices of many New York optical firms who hired an untrained and poorly paid young physician merely to write out the prescriptions. The dispute might have been settled, except that Noyes passed Prentice's letter on to some members of the medical society, who then sent back to Prentice their opinion that he (Prentice) was violating the law and doing so merely to make more money. Prentice fought back, creating slogans such as "a lens is not a pill" and organizing the Optical Society of New York in 1896 to seek recognition and licensure as a profession. The dispensing opticians, who depended on physicians for referrals, refused to join. Prentice and the optometrists then referred to the combination of medical ophthalmologists and dispensing opticians as a form of collusion that created a concentrated monopoly dangerous to the public interest. At this point, there was little hope that the two groups could be reconciled.

The first optometry bill was passed by the Minnesota legislature in 1901, and by 1924 a separate profession of optometry had been recognized in every state. The M.D. ophthalmology specialists were put at a competitive disadvantage not only by the newly licensed optometrists, but also by a number of second-rate physicians who sought to enter this lucrative field by taking a short course and so becoming "six-week specialists." The public had no way of identifying who was really qualified, and who was just claiming to be an expert. Trapped between the optometrists and their own ill-qualified colleagues, the ophthalmologists had to act to enforce quality standards and maintain a professional distinction that would protect their incomes. In 1916, the American Board of Ophthalmic Examinations was created. It was to award a professional diploma following two years of graduate study and one year of supervised clinical practice in a hospital (usually one of the specialty eye hospitals) and passage of an exam. Thus, the pattern was set for all subsequent medical specialties: a voluntary certifying exam to be taken after an extended period of specialty training (residency) that a doctor could elect in order to obtain and publicly demonstrate special competence, but no "license," and thus no legal restrictions upon the practice of those physicians who chose not to be board certified. In the initial year, 120 certificates were awarded, although only 28 by examination, indicating how common the custom of grandfathering in experienced practitioners who lacked university educations was at that time. By 1925, 501 physicians had received diplomas. There were about 900 who limited their practice exclusively to the eye, and another 400 who gave it special attention; thus, between a third and a half of all the physicians who might call themselves ophthalmologists had become board certified.

   Science, money, and personalities all played a role in the creation of the first official medical specialty certification. Although surgical organizations had developed earlier (the American College of Surgeons was founded in 1812) and used more technology, there was no competing group of nonmedical professionals to force the issue. In radiology and pathology, nonmedical expert personnel were welcomed because they practiced only under the direction of, and at the discretion of, the physician specialists, and were not allowed to charge fees for their professional services, but instead increased the earning power of the physician in charge. Recognizing that economic competition shaped the organization of medicine does not imply that quality of care and the health of patients were not foremost in the minds of doctors, but merely an acceptance of the fact that self-interest must also be served if the interests of the public are to be taken on as a professional responsibility. Policy is always a form of exchange, not just a moral or scientific decision.

Producing Family Physicians: A Failure of Medical Economic Policy

The rise of specialties brought more expertise to bear on the patient's illness, but de-emphasized the patient as a person. As medicine fragmented into ever-more narrow fields of expertise, the patient was fragmented into a collection of body parts or illnesses: the emotions belonged to the psychiatrist, the skin to the dermatologist, the eye to the ophthalmologist, but the whole person was left to wander through an increasingly complex maze. As scientific medicine was advanced to a peak of prestige in the 1960s, concern was being raised not only about a shortage of physicians, but about a lack of caring. Both the public and health policy experts lamented the profession's emphasis on narrow specialization and the demise of the good old doctor who was a friend to the family and took care of everyone and everything. The modern hospital, with its laboratories, operating suites, and different specialty clinics requiring a chain of referrals and chart transfers, was seen as being technically better, but cold and impersonal, and inadequate for dealing with human needs. One response of the profession was to create an American Board of Family Practice so that generalists, too, could be board certified and recognized as "specialists." Yet by any objective assessment, it must be agreed that the policy was a failure. Most experts asserted that at least half of all physicians should be primary care generalists, but the fraction going into specialties rose from 17 percent in 1931, to 57 percent in 1960, 76 percent in 1969, and 85 percent in 1993. Although many students begin with a desire to become family practitioners, exposure during medical school changes their minds. And why not? Specialists make more money, have higher prestige, and often do not have to put up with the inferior compensation and lack of appreciation for being on call night after night. The technological imperative to learn more and earn more does not lead the best and the brightest to do general practice in rural settings, or in urban clinics, despite the clear findings that this is where the needs are greatest. The public has repeatedly asked to redirect medical education toward primary care, and the politicians have vociferously agreed, but the reimbursement system still favors specialists, as it has for the last fifty years. Money speaks louder than words, and the tale it tells is of a broad failure to bring payment systems in accord with public pronouncements. Only recently have the incomes of family practitioners risen relative to specialists, and shift in the career plans of graduating medical students shows that they have responded to market forces rather than rhetorical exhortations.[12]

7.5 PRACTICE VARIATIONS _____

The agency relationship arises because the patient trusts the physician to do what is right. What happens when the physician confronts a lack of information, or when medical science provides no clear guidelines on what to do? The professional concept of "need" that assumes there is a right way to treat an illness, and hence no necessity for examining trade-offs between costly alternatives, falters if the clinical pathway becomes ambiguous. The fact that some medical practices have been widely used with confidence that they were important cures, only to be later discarded as ineffective or harmful, fosters some doubts about the infallibility of medicine. In a 1934 study, the American Child Health Association chose 1,000 schoolchildren to be examined by physicians to determine whether or not they should have their tonsils removed.[13] Six hundred children had already had the procedure. The remaining 400 were examined, and the physicians recommended that 45 percent of them have a tonsillectomy. The 220 that remained after the first round were examined by another group of physicians who recommended that 46 percent of them have their tonsils out. A third exam by another set of physicians on the 118 who were left provided recommendations that 44 percent of them have their tonsils removed. After these three examinations, only 65 of the original 1,000 children had not had a tonsillectomy recommended for them! From this study, the experimenters concluded that the decision about whether or not a child needed a tonsillectomy was not primarily based on signs or symptoms or any objective evidence, but upon a generally held opinion among the doctors consulted that they should give tonsillectomies to one-third to one-half of all the children they treated in that age range.

Today, tonsillectomy is a much less commonly performed procedure, in part because of these pioneering epidemiological experiments (epidemiology is the study of the distribution of diseases in populations, applying statistical methods to groups rather than studying individual patients). However, the insights regarding the range of uncertainty in common diagnoses were essentially ignored during the glory years of medicine after World War II, when it seemed that science could diagnose and cure every ailment. This optimistic conviction that medical advances would be continuous and consistently beneficial faded as the Vietnam War, the Opec Oil Crisis and rising environmental concerns led to a more cautious and critical assessment of technology. In what was then (in 1973) a little-noticed study, John Wennberg and colleagues found that the rates of many common types of surgery varied widely across counties in Vermont, with difference as large as sixfold, and were not explainable by differences in insurance, availability of hospitals, or illness rates.[14] For tonsillectomies, the rate varied from as few as 8 per 10,000, to as many as 60 per 10,000. In a subsequent study, he found that the people of Boston, Massachusetts, had more hospital beds, more employees per bed, and paid 87 percent more on average for hospital care than the people of New Haven, Connecticut, yet in both cities the average health statistics were about the same, and most people receive high-quality medicine with many patients being treated in academic medical schools. Interestingly, Wennberg found that while the overall rate of surgery was higher in Boston, for some conditions, the rate of surgery was significantly higher in New Haven. Thus, it is not simply a question of more or less, but of a large degree of unexplainable variation (see Figure 7.3).

This phenomenon of **practice variation** or **small area variation** has now been confirmed by a number of researchers. It suggests that there is a large element of ambiguity that can make widely different treatment choices constitute acceptable medical practice. Those conditions for which indications are not so clear, or for which there are good alternative forms of treatment, show large variations (e.g., knee replacement, spinal surgery for back pain, tonsillectomy, psychoses). However, where there is a clear indication and a generally accepted treatment, the range of variation is much smaller (e.g., hernia repair, open-heart surgery, lung resection). Work is now underway to develop more formal **clinical pathways,** sets of instructions developed by the medical staff, based on verified results of scientifically validated studies. These clinical pathways suggest how a particular illness should be managed, including what tests to perform, what medications to give, how long to wait for symptoms to improve before surgery, and so on. Many doctors denigrate such efforts as "cookbook medicine," while others recognize that clinical pathways, although not able to replace the physician's personal judgment, can help to make treatment more efficient.[15] What is important to recognize is that repeated demonstrations of wide variations in practice patterns have called into question the role of the individual doctor as final arbiter of right and wrong.

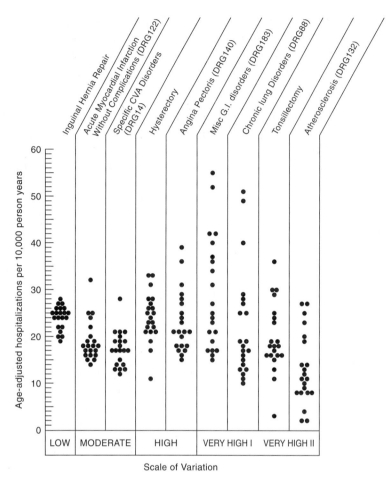

FIGURE 7.3 *Variation in age-adjusted rates of hospitalization for different diagnoses and procedures. Each dot represents one hospital market area.* Source: *J. Wennberg, K. McPherson & P. Caper,* New England Journal of Medicine *311:298, 1984.*

Impetus has been given to examining health policy on the basis of verifiable costs and outcomes of care, rather than accepting current practices as a standard, or relying on the public opinions expressed by professional associations.

Small area variation is one form of **population medicine,** which uses groups rather than individual patients to define quality of care. Although long used in public health (see chapter 17), it is only with the spread of managed care contracting for large numbers of people that population medicine has become recognized as a valuable tool for assessing the quality of physician practice. As hospitals become integrated into health care systems so as to organize and better manage the care they provide to the community, decisions regarding treatment will be shaped more by analysis of statistics on large numbers of patients, and less dependent on the experience of a single physician.

SUGGESTIONS FOR FURTHER READING_____

Rosemary Stevens, *American Medicine and the Public Interest,* New Haven, Conn.: Yale University Press, 1971.

John Wennberg and Alan Gittlesohn, "Variations in Medical Care Among Small Area," *Scientific American* 246:120-134, 1982.

Frederick Wolinsky and William Marder, *The Organization of Medical Practice and the Practice of Medicine,* Ann Arbor, Mich.: Health Administration Press, 1985.

Medical Economics (monthly), Medical Economics Publishing: Montvale, New Jersey.

SUMMARY_____

1. **Group practice**, increasing the scale of physician operations, requires more co-ordination and uses more ancillary help, but is able to increase output per physician, and to use physicians' informational advantages by having them monitor the quality of each other's practice. The ability to **trade patients** more efficiently is a major function of such economic organizations. However, such coordination also increases transaction costs and limits the autonomy of the individual physician, since they must now operate as part of a team.

2. **Price discrimination**, charging higher prices where demand is less elastic (due to insurance, high income, lack of information or alternatives) is common in medicine, although much of the motivation seems to be purely charitable and is officially sanctioned by the public. Even though there are many physicians in a city, each one is unique and patients are reluctant to switch. The reduced price sensitivity that arises from such "monopolistic competition" allows price differentials to endure.

3. The potential for **kickback payments on referrals and profits from related business may hamper the ability of physicians to act as the patient's agent**. Ownership of pharmacies and sale of drugs by physicians is prohibited outright in the United States (but not in Japan, where patients are prescribed more drugs for each visit and many physicians make a third of their income that way). Ownership of laboratories, physical therapy clinics, and diagnostic radiology facilities has been shown to lead to abuses of trust (excessive ordering of tests, excess charges) and is increasingly being discouraged and regulated by government payers.

4. The development of **new technology leads to the development of new medical specialties**. As medicine becomes more complex and specialized, the nature of the transactions changes. Because doing something (operations, X-rays, scans) is easier to see and count than the effort of thinking (diagnosis, psychiatric advice), specialists who do **procedures, particularly those that use elaborate equipment, tend to be better compensated than those whose time is spent primarily on thinking or caring**.

5. The first official U.S. **medical specialty certification** was established in 1916 for ophthalmology, at least in part to try and forestall economic competition from the nonmedical optometrists who wanted to do refractions and prescribe eye-

glasses. Optometrists gained the right to practice and became an alternative form of licensed practitioner, the O.D.

6. It has been public policy for many years to **increase the number of primary care generalists**, and reduce the number of specialist to better meet the needs and desires of patients. Yet specialists have increased from 17 percent of all physicians in 1931, to 85 percent in 1993. **This failure of public policy is largely attributable to inappropriate economic incentives**, as reimbursement for specialists has been and continues to be much greater than for generalists. Would most ambitious students choose less prestige and less money, just because the government says it might be nice to do so?

7. Physicians in some areas perform a specific operation, such as tonsillectomies, at a rate six times that of physicians in another area, even though both areas seem to be similar in all respects. Such unexplained **practice variations** call into question the idea that there is some well-defined need for medical care that can be objectively agreed upon by most physicians. Since such variations have been shown to occur, governments have started studies to examine more carefully how differences in treatment are related to outcomes, developing standard protocols known as **clinical pathways** and **practice standards**.

PROBLEMS

1. {*productivity*} Is the productivity of a medical practice determined primarily by the amount of capital employed or the number of people employed?

2. {*trade*} Do physicians pay each other for patients? Explain how.

3. {*industrial organization*} Why do physicians choose to practice together in groups? Is assembling physicians into groups any different from assembling employees together into a manufacturing firm, or lawyers in a legal firm, or baseball players into a team?

4. {*economies of scale*} What advantages does a large physician group have over a solo physician? What disadvantages?

5. {*input compensation*} Do physicians who use more high technology equipment to assist them get paid more or less? Give examples to support your answer. Is it always true, generally true, or does it vary with the type of technology and type of payment system?

6. {*industry organization*} What creates the boundaries between medical specialties? How do changes in the boundaries affect prices or incomes? In your answer distinguish between proximate and fundamental factors (i.e., the individuals and organizations who make specific decisions versus the underlying political and economic forces).

7. {*incentives*} What determines how many new graduates choose each medical specialty?

8. {*input compensation*} Is it possible for a physician to use ancillary inputs to increase profits without paying for those inputs? Give several different examples.

9. {*price discrimination*} When physicians choose to give a discount on fees, does it raise or lower their income? Will a profit maximizing physician charge higher prices for those services or groups of patients for which demand is *more elastic* or *less elastic*? Explain why, providing a numerical calculation to illustrate your point, and give several examples.

10. {*price controls*} In order to save money, the state of Idaho decides that Medicaid will pay only 75% of what private insurance pays. Will this cause a shortage? What kind of evidence might you look for?

11. {*transactions costs*} Why are kickbacks illegal?

12. {*practice variations*} What factors determine the number of knee surgeries in a state? Will the same factors determine the number of hip surgeries? Colon surgeries? Asthma admissions?

13. {*price discrimination*} *THE SAGA OF THE DOCTOR AND THE WANNABE.*

A. Dr. Jones is the only doctor in Calexico, a town composed of Anglos who mostly own farms and local businesses, work in schools, government, etc., and of Chicanos who mostly work in the farms growing lettuce. Dr. Jones obviously has a "monopoly" on medical care in Calexico. Rodrigo is a field worker. Everyone who knows him says he is very smart, *muy simpatico,* (very empathetic) and knows a lot about what makes people sick. His grandmother was a *Curandera,* or herb-doctor, and taught him a lot. He has also learned from other native curers and read medical books. He earned straight A's until he had to drop out and work in the fields to help support his family. At night and on weekends he acts as the "doctor" to many poor families. He asks them to "pay what they can" to help him and his invalid mother.

   One day in May a man dies who was seeing Rodrigo for "faintness." A Chicana who was in labor and being cared for by Dr. Jones also dies. A big fight follows. Rodrigo says, "Dr. Jones gets rich by charging big fees, while he butchers our people." Dr. Jones says, "This illiterate Mexican tries to pass himself off as a doctor and kept this man from coming to me for treatment that could have saved his life." Dr Jones also states, "I am the greatest friend the Chicano community has. I charge them less than half what I charge my other patients because I know they can't afford more."
   Comment briefly on Dr. Jones pricing and its relationship to his desire to help Chicanos.

B. The fight between Dr. Jones and Rodrigo is getting worse and threatens this once peaceful agricultural community. Anglo and Chicano are openly hostile to each other. But within each camp there is dissention. Some Chicanos say, "Dr. Jones did help a lot of our people, and when they couldn't pay, he didn't send the bill collector or take their car, as the department store did. Besides, although the mother died, he saved the baby—if not for him, both could have died." Some Anglos say, "That young upstart Rodrigo may be right. I've been going to Dr. Jones for eight years, he's made a bundle off of me, and my arthritis isn't any better." At the urging of the mayor, Dr. Jones and Rodrigo get together to talk about the problem. Afterward, each has a much different point of view. Rodrigo states, "Dr. Jones is an honest and hardworking doctor who has the best interests of the community in his heart. He actually loses money taking care of Chicanos and should be paid more. I will work with him in every case I can." Dr. Jones says, "Rodrigo is an exceptionally talented young man who knows more than any layman, and some doctors I have met, about the practice of medicine. We are in complete agreement about the tremendous need for better medical care in Calexico and will work together to solve this problem. Many Chicano patients who could not afford to see me on a regular basis can be treated just as well by Rodrigo after I have done any initial diagnosis and evaluation, and I will send them to him. Together we can provide better medical care for all."

—*Explain why this togetherness occurred among two who just last night claimed that the other was a "killer." In your answer assume that each was motivated solely by economic considerations. Why does Rodrigo say that Dr. Jones should raise his prices?*

C. One year later, Dr. Jones announces, "Working with Rodrigo has opened my eyes to the plight of Chicanos and the reluctance of Anglos to accept them as equal members of society. Furthermore, as I become older I face the inevitable diminution of my ability to meet the needs of our community, and as a doctor I face the responsibility of assuring that Calexico can continue to receive good medical care. Therefore, I have formed "La Raza de Calexico Scholarship Fund." Rodrigo will work as a staff member of my clinic part-time while he completes college and his medical education. He will, of course, continue to help those Chicanos who have always come to him, but he will also treat on an equal basis Anglo patients. This exceptional person should not waste time as a field-hand when he can so ably act to meet the medical needs of all citizens in Calexico. We have just signed a contract that will make him my junior partner the day he graduates from medical school, and that will turn over my full practice to him when I retire." *Given that both of them had a good deal with their cooperative arrangement, why take this further step?*

D. In 1985 Rodrigo said, "I can only be grateful to Dr. Jones and his unselfish commitment to helping Chicanos like myself." In 1991, after graduating from medical school, he condemns Dr. Jones as "a racist exploiter who sought to take advantage of me and the whole Chicano community to help himself alone" and seeks to void the 1985 contract, and to have Dr. Jones expelled from the County Medical Society. *Why might he do that?*

ENDNOTES _____

1. Frederick Wolinsky and William Marder, *The Organization of Medical Practice and the Practice of Medicine,* Ann Arbor, Mich.: Health Administration Press, 1985.
2. Uwe Reinhardt, *Physician Productivity and the Demand for Health Manpower,* Cambridge, Mass: Ballinger, 1974.
3. Joseph Newhouse, *The Economics of Medical Care,* Reading, Mass: Addison-Wesley, 1978, page 40.
4. Thomas Getzen, "A 'Brand Name' Firm Theory of Medical Group Practice," *Journal of Industrial Economics* 33(2):199–215, 1984.
5. Helen Clapesattle, *The Doctors Mayo,* Minneapolis: University of Minnesota Press, 1941.

6. Reuben Kessel, "Price Discrimination in Medicine," *Journal of Law and Economics* Vol 1 (2):20–53, October 1958.

7. Sandy Lutz, "Troubled Times for Psych Hospitals," *Modern Healthcare* 21(50):26–27, 30–33, December 16, 1991: and "NME Totals Costs of Psych Woes" 23(43):20, October 25, 1993.

8. Jean M. Mitchell and Jonathan H. Sunshine, "Consequences of Physician's Ownership of Health Care Facilities—Joint Ventures in Radiology," *New England Journal of Medicine* 327:1497–1501, 1992.

9. Herbert Hammond, *Assessment of Billing Practices and Utilization of Physician Laboratories*, Health Care Financing Administration Report, 1984.

10. Rosemary Stevens, *American Medicine and the Public Interest*, New Haven, Conn: Yale University Press, 1971.

11. This discussion of the formation of ophthalmology as a specialty follows the account presented in Chapter 5, pp. 98–114 of Rosemary Stevens, *American Medicine and the Public Interest*, New Haven, Conn: Yale University Press, 1971.

12. Esther Fein, "More Young Doctors Forsake Specialty for General Practice," *New York Times*, Monday October 16, 1995, pages A1, B2.

13. American Child Health Association, *Physical Defects: The Pathway to Correction*, 1934, pp:80–96, as cited in David Eddy, "Variations in Physician Practice: The Role of Uncertainty," *Health Affairs*, 1985, pp: 74–89.

14. John Wennberg, J. L. Freeman and W. J. Culp, "Are Hospital Services Rationed in New Haven or Over-Utilised in Boston?" *Lancet* I, May 23, 1987, pp:1185–1188; John Wennberg, Klim McPherson and Philip Caper, "Will Payment Based on Diagnosis-Related Groups Control Hospital Costs?" *New England Journal of Medicine* 311(5): 295–303, 1984.

15. Laura Johannes, "Meet the Doctor: A Computer That Knows a Few Things," *The Wall Street Journal*, December 18, 1995, p.B1.

CHAPTER **8**

Hospitals

QUESTIONS

1. *How do hospitals get paid? What do they pay for?*
2. *Why don't philanthropists give to hospitals like they used to?*
3. *Does it make a difference to hospitals that 95 percent of their funds come from third-party insurance rather than patients?*
4. *Who pays for medical research?*
5. *Does cost-shifting help the poor or the rich?*
6. *Does tax exemption help hospitals serve the public welfare?*
7. *Why did hospitals borrow so much and load up their balance sheets with debt during the 1980s?*
8. *Does reimbursement increase employment? Does it drive up costs?*
9. *Are hospitals still charitable institutions, or have they become instruments of corporate control?*
10. *Who owns a nonprofit hospital? Who gets the profits?*

8.1   FROM CHARITABLE INSTITUTION TO CORPORATE CHAINS: DEVELOPMENT OF THE MODERN HOSPITAL _____

The hospital as an institution for the care of the sick has a long and noble history. During the twentieth century, hospitals grew to become the dominant organizational force in health care, and the biggest user of health care funds. As the century draws to a close, they are being replaced or transformed into larger and more complex "health systems" that encompass different modes of care (inpatient, office ambulatory centers, home health, nursing homes) spanning multiple sites.[1]

As long as people have gotten sick, society has needed a place to care for them, both to provide special support, and also to isolate the ill from the rest of the community. In pre-scientific times, cure was often identified with casting out evil, and hospitals were religious structures. In classical Greece (B.C. 600 to 1 A.D.), temples known as *asclepia* took in the sick, especially those who were poor and lacked resources to be cared for at home.[2] Cities used taxes to support hospitals and dispensaries staffed by physicians, who also received fees from those who could afford to pay. The Romans, who created their large-scale hierarchical organizations to rule a vast empire, also found it necessary to provide hospitals for the slaves and gladiators who served on plantations or in the military. The word *hospital* was first used in the twelfth century to refer to a facility run by the church that housed and cared for the sick, the disabled and the insane, as well as providing lodging for pilgrims and other travelers, orphans, and the poor. Only those who had no homes stayed in hospitals, because everyone else, even if ill, preferred to remain with their family if they could. Economic changes, and the great epidemics that came with the expansion of trade, greatly increased the need for institutional care. By the end of the thirteenth century there were 19,000 hospitals scattered across Europe. The shift from religious care to scientific cures took place gradually over the next six hundred years, but came ever more rapidly toward the end of the nineteenth century. Florence Nightingale's work with the injured and sick British soldiers during the Crimean war became the basis for her two books, *Notes on Hospitals* (1858) and *Notes on Nursing* (1859), which significantly changed the shape of the hospital and are still influential today.[3]

Hospitals were founded in 1527 in Mexico and 1635 in Canada, but it was not until 1751 that a hospital was founded in the American colonies. The Pennsylvania hospital, which is still a major hospital today, was created by a bill passed in the Assembly with the support of Benjamin Franklin, which obligated the governor to provide £2,000 to match £2,000 in public donations for construction of a hospital.[4] Philadelphia already had an almshouse and quarantine hospitals (temporary housing for sailors and others with contagious diseases), but the new building was to be an altogether more grand and permanent edifice that would promote science as well as providing care. The six physicians who worked twice a week without pay had been selected because they were outstanding, and had mostly been trained abroad. Other notable early American hospitals were the New York hospital chartered by King George III in 1771 to provide care for the sick poor and instruction to medical students of the Columbia Medical School, and the Massachusetts General Hospital built in 1821 at a cost of over $100,000, an imposing structure superior to the European hospitals of that time and the first to have indoor plumbing. American hospitals were based on the model of the British and Continental voluntary hospitals. However, the American hospitals were more likely to have paying patients, who tended to be charged extra so as to subsidize care for the poor.[5]

These three important hospitals still exist, but the economics of hospital operations has changed drastically. In the eighteenth and nineteenth centuries most funding came from donations, with patient fees playing a minor role, and there was no insurance reimbursement. The major category of expenditure was food, and the work of the staff was supplemented by making patients labor alongside employees cleaning, cooking, and nursing. Today "hotel costs" (room, meals) account for less than 10 percent of hospital expenditures, and it is impossible to imagine making patients work alongside doctors and nurses. The colonial hospitals were similar to most modern hospitals in that they were nonprofit institutions run by volunteer governing boards, with medical care directed and carried out by a physician staff who were not paid by the hospital but were in private practice as independent businesses in the community.

The development of the modern hospital, like the development of medical specialties, was driven by the creation of new technology. With anesthesia and antiseptics making safe surgery possible, a clean and controlled operating suite with skilled assistants became a necessity. The discovery of X-rays made it necessary to acquire access to radiographic equipment. Advances in clinical pathology and chemistry made the laboratory vital for diagnosis. Major capital investment was required to obtain access to all these new technologies. A solo physician practicing by himself could not make full use of this new equipment, or manage all of the specialized technicians who operated it. It was necessary to bring all the patients of many physicians together under one roof to obtain funding, make effective use of the new technology, and hire a manager to coordinate the efforts of medical and ancillary staff. In brief, an organizational revolution had to take place.[6] Within the custodial institutions that had existed for centuries serving the disabled poor, there arose a new type of hospital, a modern organization with sophisticated and expensive equipment to provide scientific cures where middle-class patients wanted to be treated and were willing to pay. The large and uncertain monetary requirements caused a corresponding financial revolution (insurance reimbursement), which further increased demand and enabled the massive flow of funds required to support a technologically sophisticated system of intensive care costing thousands of dollars for each patient.

8.2 REVENUES: THE FLOW OF FUNDS INTO THE HOSPITAL _____

From the founding of The Pennsylvania Hospital in 1751 until the beginnings of Blue Cross in 1929, the primary source of hospital funding was philanthropy from the community, supplemented by patient fees. Since 1940 there has been incredibly rapid growth in hospital revenues, but philanthropy and patient fees have decreased drastically in relation to the total. Now the largest sources of payment are Medicare, government funding for the 60 percent of patient days used by the elderly, and managed care firms shopping for low prices and good information systems to control costs. Midway between the Great Depression and today, around 1960, the dominant payers were non-profit Blue Cross plans. At that time, these plans were affiliated with the various hospital associations. They were designed to reimburse the full cost of patient care, thus allowing hospitals to break-even while taking care of the indigent and undertaking whatever new treatments, diagnostic technology, or research they wanted. By 1995, several Blue Cross plans had fallen into bankruptcy. The survivors all started managed care plans to compete with (or complement) their traditional insurance plans. Some, such as the giant Blue Cross of California, have turned themselves into billion-dollar private for-profit firms.[7]

A new financing system had to be created, and recreated again and again, to provide all the new technology and services that Americans wanted. By 1995, two hundred times as much money was being transferred from the pockets of the public into hospital expenses as had been paid at the end of World War II, with an average increase of more than 10 percent a year. Revenue growth has slowed substantially since 1990 as managed care has taken hold, and more revenues are coming from outside the hospital in the form of outpatient services or new business ventures (ambulance, nutrition counseling, home health care, etc.). In 1995, the average community hospital had inpatient revenues around $40 million, receiving about $5,000 for each patient admitted ($1,000 per day, for an average five-day stay), and another $20 million for outpatient services. Table 8.1 lists the current sources of hospital revenue.[8]

The first thing to note from Table 8.1 is that it is unlikely and implausible that hospital behavior will be significantly shaped by consumers' decisions based on prices in this environment, as they would be in most markets, because over 95 percent of revenues comes from someone other than the recipient of services.* The second, and perhaps even more important, fact to notice, is that the "someone else" is likely to be the government, which accounts for 57 percent of all revenues. The next thing to realize is that these are complex contracts for hundreds of thousands, even millions of dollars. Although we may talk about "patient revenue" or the "price" of a laboratory test, to actually bring in revenue, a hospital chief fi-

TABLE 8.1   Sources of Community Hospital Revenues, 1995

Philanthropy, grants, & interest income	2%
Tax appropriations	2%
Patients self-pay	4%
Parking, gift shop, education, & other operations	4%
Blue Cross, HMOs & other insurance	33%
Medicaid	12%
Medicare	43%
Total Revenues per Hospital (average)	$60,000,000

Source: American Hospital Association, Hospital Statistics, 1995.

* Prices paid for service by patients are even less important than table 8.1 would suggest, since much of the 4% is actually deductibles, copayments and other charges that are in effect insurance premiums or taxes and not directly related to the prices of the services chosen.

nancial officer (CFO) has to enter an intricate legal relationship with Medicare, or a joint venture with a group of radiologists, or structure a risk-sharing arrangement with a consortium of community physicians. Such deals are quite different than retail sales added up at the cash register.

Sources of Revenue

Although a complete picture is beyond the scope of this book (and indeed beyond the grasp of most economists and accountants, and even experienced hospital financial managers—the details, exceptions, exclusions, covenants, and formulas go on forever), a brief overview of the major ways in which revenues flow into the hospital is helpful in grasping the financial incentives it faces (see Table 8.2).

Philanthropy and Grants Grants are funds that are donated for a specific purpose: to carry out cancer research, build a new operating pavilion, provide outreach programs for prenatal care, and so on. Donors want to make sure that funds are used for the purpose intended, but there is little direct pressure to compete on price or to control costs. The program director spends the budget, and, if sufficiently good results are achieved in public-relations terms, another grant will usually be forthcoming sometime in the future. This revenue flows from the belief of the donor that the task facing the hospital is important and socially valuable, and is not to make profits or even necessarily to show measurable effects. All nonprofit organizations must begin with a charitable grant. Tax appropriations are a form of grant, with the donor being the government. "Tax breaks" in the form of relief from property taxes and user fees are even more important to many hospitals these days, and have become increasingly controversial.*

Global Budgets A hospital operating under a global budget is getting a grant for all of its costs. This form of payment is typical for state mental hospitals, military hospitals and the VA, and other government entities, as well as a few specialized private institutions. Since a global budget is fixed, there are few incentives either

TABLE 8.2 Major Types of Hospital Reimbursement

Philanthropy and grants
Global budgets
Charges
per diem
Cost reimbursement
DRGs (per admission)
Capitation
Managed care contracts

* Some legislators argue that hospitals are no longer providing the charitable public services for which they were founded, and hence do not deserve help, and that public funds should be redirected toward community programs or inner-city hospitals. The City of Philadelphia, for example, has forced local hospitals to pay millions of dollars under its PILOTs/SILOTs program (Payments/Services In Lieu of Taxes). A hospital is assessed an amount equal to its tax liability, and then must document provision of services provided without compensation of an equal amount, or pay the city the difference.

to attract more patients or to reduce costs. In Canada, England, and most of the developed world outside of the United States, global budgets are the most common form of hospital payment.

Charges   Hospital charges would be known as "list prices" in most industries. A hospital, like a flower shop, can set its charges at whatever level it likes. It is rare for a patient, or an insurance company, to actually pay what it is "charged." However, these paper charges often form the basis for reimbursement under a system of "discounted charges" (e.g., 60% of list price), or under a cost reimbursement system as will be described shortly.

per diem   Latin for "per day," *per diem* payments were common when hospitals originated, and are increasingly favored in managed care contracts today, discussed later. Originally per diems were charges set by the hospital and usually exceeded costs to help subsidize nonpaying patients. Today per diems are often negotiated with managed care firms under very competitive conditions, and are sometimes set below average costs per day in order for a hospital to maintain or increase its market share.

Cost Reimbursement   Cost reimbursement sets the payment level to equal the hospital's audited costs. "Days" and "discharges" are poor measures of the hospital's "product" since they do not account for variations in quality, severity of illness, or use of new technology. Because the hospital's output is so difficult to define or measure, it may be more equitable and easier to reimburse for incurred costs, rather than to try and set appropriate prices. The Blue Cross (BC) plans, organized under the aegis of the American Hospital Association, wrote manuals describing how a nonprofit hospital could break even by setting charges so as to cover costs (including coverage of nonpaying patients and a prudent reserve), and designed a method of cost reimbursement designed to break even, known as **RCCAC** (ratio of cost-to-charges applied to charges). When Medicare was created in 1965, it adopted the RCCAC methodology, and so this form of cost reimbursement came to be the dominant method by which funds flowed into hospitals from the 1960s until the mid-1980s, and is still used to determine most hospital unit costs today. The RCCAC is calculated separately for each revenue-producing hospital department using this formula:

$$\textit{RCCAC Method} \text{ BC payment} = \frac{\text{Total Department Costs}_{\text{all payers}}}{\text{Total Department Charges}_{\text{all payers}}} \times \text{BC Charges}$$

Thus, if radiology costs were $6 million, and total charges to all payers (i.e., for every insurance company and self-pay patient) were $10 million, then the ratio of cost-to-charges would be .60, and if BC patients had a total of $3 million in charges, BC would send the hospital a check for .60 × $3 million = $1.8 million as payment for its share of the costs. Note that while the reimbursement calculation uses charges, the amount paid does not depend on the level of charges. If the hospital doubles its charges (to $20 million), then its RCC is cut in half (to .30), and even though the BC charges are doubled (to $6 million), the reimbursement stays the same.

The complicated RCCAC formula is needed because costs must be divided among different payers who are responsible for the costs of different patients. If there were only one payer, it would pay all costs, and cost reimbursement would be like an open-ended grant. With many payers, however, some way must be found to allocate the costs across patients, and the RCCAC method uses the hospital's billed charges to do so. The method worked very well for a number of years to reimburse hospitals for all their costs, so well that costs rose explosively, forcing a number of cutbacks and reforms. An argument between hospitals and Medicare arose over whether or not a return on invested capital should be included as an allowable cost for reimbursement. Another source of contention was who should pay for charity care and bad debt. After initially being accommodating, Medicare switched and in essence said, "We pay all our bills on time, and should not be responsible for those who don't." Originally, charity and bad debt were overhead costs distributed across all payers. If charges for charity and non-paying patients are included (or not deducted) in the RCCAC formula, the ratio declines, and Medicare pays less because it is not paying for charity. This helps the Medicare budget, but not the hospital, who must then increase charges to other payers to make up the difference.

Per Case "Diagnostically Related Groups" (DRGs)   DRGs are fixed payments made based on the patient's diagnosis at discharge and covering the complete hospital stay, including all ancillary services (but not surgery or other physician fees). To create this "Prospective Payment System (PPS)" for Medicare payments, the government split all illnesses into 473 diagnostically related groups (hence the acronym, DRG) and estimated the cost per case within each group (similar to the RBRVS payment system for physician services discussed in section 5.1). Adjustments are made for local wages in the area in which the hospital is located, for extremely long or short stays, for having large teaching programs, or for having a large proportion of indigent patients. In essence, DRGs are administered prices set by the government at what they think is a "fair" rate. It is called a *prospective* payment system because the DRG rates are set in advance, unlike the previous *retrospective* cost reimbursement payments that were continually adjusted to match any change in costs, so that the final amount was never set until long after the year ended. Under a charge system, the sellers (hospitals) have the power to set rates wherever they feel like—subject to the power of the market to refuse to buy. Under a retrospective cost system, there is no set rate, but rather, reimbursement of actual costs incurred, perhaps subject to some review. With DRG prospective payment system, the buyer (Medicare) has all the rate-setting power. In the first year of operation (1983), Medicare did little to force rates down, but in the years since, reimbursement has become progressively tighter, so that Medicare patients have become less and less profitable. Once Medicare's DRG system was in place, it was adopted by many other payers.*

---

* State Medicaid plans used the DRG system but generally paid fewer dollars for each patient. In time, this underpayment led to complaints, and a series of court suits. Temple University Hospital sued the state of Pennsylvania under the "Boren Amendment" to the Social Security Act, which obligated states to make payments sufficient to cover the cost of efficiently provided services, and eventually won—creating a precedent that hospitals around the country quickly followed (and that forced state budgets into deficits). Hence although in concept a charge system gives all the power to the seller, and an administered price system (like DRGs) gives all power to the buyer, in reality both are at least to some extent constrained by the political process and public opinion.

Capitation Capitation payments, previously discussed in Chapter 5, are relatively rare for hospitals, since a large and well-defined number of patients must be pooled to reduce risks and make actuarial projections. Once an organization agrees to accept payment on a capitation basis, it in effect becomes a risk-bearing insurer. Usually, when it is said that a hospital is setting up a capitation arrangement, what is really meant is that some larger organization, such as the corporation that controls a number of hospitals, is creating an insurance company/HMO to provide services on a capitated basis. Once the contract extends to multiple institutions and different kinds of care, it becomes a "health system" rather than a traditional community hospital.

Managed Care Contracts Blue Cross and most private insurance companies are shifting to "managed care contracts" with hospitals (see Chapters 10 and 11). In these arrangements, payment is usually made on the basis of per diems, discounted charges, or some negotiated fee schedule. The crucial difference that sets managed care contracts apart from cost reimbursement or payment of charges is the role of the *care manager*. Rather than just paying the bills, the insurance company has a specialized **utilization review** nurse or physician critically examine each case to see if hospitalization was justified, if a lower cost alternative (such as outpatient surgery) was available, if adequate documentation was provided for all laboratory tests, for example. By negotiating discounts, discouraging use, and denying payment for disallowed or undocumented charges, managed care firms can usually obtain medical care for their clients at a lower cost than traditional indemnity or cost reimbursement insurers, and so are taking over the market. Being constantly questioned and audited has not been easy or pleasant for the doctors who admit patients, or for those working in hospital financial departments. Patients also dislike having to justify and obtain approval for every additional service or extra day in the hospital, but are willing to put up with it if premiums are sufficiently reduced.

8.3 COSTS: THE FLOW OF FUNDS OUT OF THE HOSPITAL _____

Hospitals are personal care institutions, and labor accounts for the bulk of the costs (Table 8.3). In the early days, food and housing took up most of the hospital's budget, but today such "hotel functions" are relatively minor in comparison to the provision of medical care. Physician care, in both 1750 and in 1995, is paid for sep-

TABLE 8.3 Community Hospital Expenditures by Category, 1995

Payroll	54%
Professional Fees	4%
Supplies & Other	33%
Capital Depreciation & Interest	9%

Source: American Hospital Association, *Hospital Statistics 1995.*

arately and so is largely not included in the hospital budget. Very few physicians are employees of the hospital, although the services of contracted pathologists, radiologists, and emergency room doctors do show up under the category "professional fees." It might be thought that the acquisition of lithotripters, magnetic resonance imaging (MRI) scanners, and other expensive medical technology would make "equipment" a large category, yet the wages of the skilled people required to operate each new piece of equipment usually runs two or three times the cost of the machinery itself. Much of the category "other" takes the form of services, and thus also involves labor hired in the local market. Adding together payroll, professional fees, and local services, about 75 percent of a hospital's costs are labor. This fact makes it politically difficult to "cut costs," since the only real way to do so is to "cut" people, by reducing wages or laying off employees. Energy, raw materials, and other goods traded in competitive national or international markets are relatively unimportant in the hospital budget. Access to capital, however, has significantly shaped the growth of health care systems (see section 8.5).

8.4 FINANCIAL MANAGEMENT AND COST SHIFTING

Revenues must exceed expenses for an organization to survive, but there is no particular reason that the individuals for whom expenditures are incurred must be the same as those from whom revenues are obtained. While individual matching of benefits and payments is common to most consumer markets, in health care it almost never takes place. For the early hospitals, donations of the wealthy members of the community and general tax funds (paid mostly by landowners) were used to provide services to the sick and disabled poor. *Funding and benefits were matched at the level of the community, not the individual.* It was considered fair that those who had benefited most from the economy should give the most to help those who were in need. Paying patients who could afford it were usually charged a bit extra to help support the hospital's charitable mission. In effect, the excess of charges above costs constituted a "hospital tax" on the working-class and upper-class people who happened to get sick.

When hospitals took care of the poor who could not help themselves, it was obvious and necessary that the burden of financing would fall primarily on a different group of people who did have money: philanthropists and taxpayers. As technology advanced and hospital services became more generally desirable to all classes of people, it was inevitable that there would be a great increase in hospital expenditures, and that there would be more overlap between the people who paid and the people who received care. Insurance, pooling funds from the many so that a few could receive care, was a significant extension of financing that furthered the ability of the market to transfer the burden of payment away from the individual who was sick. One of the "expenses" that was factored into private insurance premiums was charity care; thus, insured patients were also paying for those who had no insurance.

The process of using revenues from one group of clients to subsidize another group is known in health care as **cost shifting.** Under philanthropic funding, all revenues are cost shifted—they are intended as donations to benefit others, not the giver. With insurance and cost reimbursement, the flows are more complex, but it is clear that somebody else must be paying for the nonpaying patients (bad debt and charity care), since they do not bring any revenue to the hospital. Several other functions, such as medical education, research, and community outreach, are usually supported through cost shifting, because they bring in very little revenues, certainly less than what they cost to provide.

Financial managers in the early days assumed that the hospital would be a losing proposition, and that their job was to find additional revenues—from donors, grants, or tax rebates—to cover the deficit. Indemnity insurance brought in more funds, but did not change the underlying rules. Hospitals were still nonprofit entities, but many now made an "excess" that could be used to fund growth or extra services. As cost reimbursement came to dominate payment systems, the financial manager's task became more complex, but also easier. A fully reimbursed hospital was guaranteed to break even, and thus could do all the research, education, and outreach that it wanted because all costs were fully covered retrospectively. Medicare and Medicaid fundamentally changed the economic status of the hospital by providing coverage for what had been previously charity. As of 1970, the typical hospital faced a reimbursement situation something like this: at the top, commercially insured patients paid full charges, bringing in about 20 percent more revenue per day than the cost-based Blue Cross and Medicare patients; the indigent Medicaid rate was usually lower; and uninsured working patients paid what they could, and charity cases brought in no revenues directly, but did help to bolster the hospital's image and its cost reimbursement.

Cost shifting applied to certain services as well as to certain patient groups. Hospitals needed to do autopsies to help improve the quality of care, but obviously could not bill the patient. Clinical pathologists found it easy to support this scientific need by charging separately for laboratory tests that had previously been included as part of the regular hospital per diem for services. Billing for labs met so little resistance that charges were pushed up and up, and by the 1970s it was not uncommon for a lab to charge ten times what a test cost, and to be a major source of excess revenues for subsidizing other parts of the hospital, such as the emergency room, which was a chronic loser. Research programs must do extensive tests, keep patients in the hospital for extra days, and carry out experimental surgeries that may be totally useless to perfect techniques and make new discoveries. Since these bills are paid just like any other patient care, research costs are shifted to the insurance company. Also, the bill for a day in the ICU is based on the average; thus, the easy cases (since they actually cost less) provide an implicit subsidy for the complex cases and research. Medical education is expensive, and usually carried out along with the research that keeps faculties on the cutting edge. Teaching salaries and research equipment are included when calculating the basis for cost reimbursement. Cost per day in a major university hospital is often two to three times that in a small community hospital. Since insurance cheerfully pays whether the patient gets a broken arm fixed in a local hospital at $800 or a university hospital at $2,000, they (or rather, the employed workers from whom premiums are taken) are paying for most of the research and education expenses.

Cost shifting and cross-subsidies are a pervasive and long-standing feature of medical care reimbursement. In general, hospitals had public support for taking revenues from a variety of sources and using them to fund not just basic care, but also outreach to indigents, community prevention, research, teaching, and other activities that were seen as being in the public interest. A number of forces have interacted over the last twenty years to cause that basic consensus on the purpose and funding of the hospital to crumble.

Net income to be used in support of research, education, or growth could be obtained either by increasing income or reducing expenses. Growth is hard to accomplish without increasing expenditures, and thus it is unlikely that managers will concentrate on cuts. Furthermore, there was also a general perception in the 1960s and 1970s that health care workers were already underpaid relative to the rest of the economy, and there is always a resistance to laying people off. Thus in the era after 1965, "financial management" came to mean "revenue maximization." The new cost reimbursement rules were very complex and often ambiguous. This left some room for the creative accountant to reclassify, amend, and adjust in such a way that more dollars flowed in. Such financial gamesmanship, along with their inherent expansionary tendencies of cost reimbursement, fueled rapid growth in expenses. Although the number of patients grew only slightly (less than 1% a year), the number of employees per patient (FTE per occupied bed) went from 1.1 in 1960 to 1.4 in 1965, 2.0 in 1970, 3.3 in 1980, and 5.2 in 1995.[9] Cost control was out, and revenue max was in.

The tremendous and unanticipated rise in expenditures for Medicare and Medicaid forced the government to try to modify the reimbursement system to cut costs. Payments for returns on equity capital to investors in for-profit hospitals were eliminated, as was a differential payment for nursing and a number of other minor elements. Yet the basic forces that led to explosive cost increases still remained. Also, while the government could change the rules, the hospital financial managers had gained experience in working around the rules, and also could call on the assistance of consultants from major accounting firms to help them find the most remunerative interpretation or allocation basis. After a series of legislative "cost controls" attempting to maintain the solvency of the Medicare program failed to work, unpopular premium and tax increases had to be pushed through Congress. Medicare, forced into a corner, began to refuse to pay for the cost of charity care. It claimed that it needed to be a "prudent buyer" and so reneged on the fundamental cost shifting premise.

On one hand, Medicare's decision not to fund indigent care and bad debt made sense. The bills of all Medicare patients were being paid in full and on time. Acting as an insurer of people over 65, this new interpretation certainly fulfilled its financial obligation to the hospital. On the other hand, hospitals had always charged everybody extra to make up for losses on charity care. Furthermore, it appears that if anyone should be taking responsibility for the poor, it is the government. Medicare, by taking a narrow interpretation of their contractual responsibilities, broke up the larger social contract based on cost shifting, which had been fundamental to the hospital as a caring community institution. As Medicare ratcheted down its rates, the hospital had to look elsewhere to make up the difference. And so, where charges to commercial insurance companies had been 10 to 15 percent above average cost, the breakdown of cost-shifting pushed these "overcharges" up to 20 to 30 percent above cost. The private insurance companies howled in protest as they were forced to pick up what had previously been paid for by general tax funds. The university hospitals, with large indigent populations and big research programs, were in even worse shape than the community hospitals. They had a much smaller fraction of revenues coming from commercial insurance, and to make up for losses, had to raise their commercial rates 50 to 100 percent. The federal and state governments argued that the provision of Medicare and Medicaid had reduced the hospitals' burden of bad debts and charity, but the large number of people seeking care who were still uninsured made hospitals skeptical.

Small price differentials and a shared sense of purpose were sufficient to allow the cross subsidies that made up a social contract for hospitals to continue. Big differentials and a hostile, "I'll pay for mine, and you pay for yours" attitude ruined this consensus. Market forces came into play. The outrageously high prices for tests done in hospital laboratories created a profit opportunity for commercial companies. They started providing services through doctors, cut prices in half, and still had large profit margins. Specialized psychiatric hospitals who treated only mild cases of mental disorder sprang up, able to make money at a pier diem far below that of the inner city psych wards filled with violent and chronically disturbed individuals, and staffed by residents more interested in research and understanding the causes of mental illness than in cost-effectiveness of care. Whenever prices are distorted by cross-subsidy, there is an opportunity for a firm to make extraordinary profits by **cream skimming,** providing only the services that are overpriced, and not the one that is more costly and subsidized. Tradition and expressions of disapproval were able to limit the extent to which profits were drained from the system by cream skimming prior to 1970. Since then, the margins have become too large, and the ideology of health care too fragmented, to keep the old system afloat.

Founded initially on the premise that government and the wealthy would provide for the poor and support research, the social contract of the hospitals was so pervasive and unexamined that it is likely that the people who initially brought it under attack had no idea what those efforts might lead to. However, it has subsequently become clear that hospital financial managers, by taking advantage of the system, and Medicare, by refusing to take responsibility for all of America's needy, contributed to the demise of cost shifting. Rapidly rising per diem costs and distortionary cross-subsidies eventually led to stringent managed care systems where an insured employee group contracts to pay only for the services its members use. The public understands that it is not possible to "pay your own way" for hospital care, and that risk pooling through insurance is required. The collapse of cost shifting forces us to now confront the question of who will pay for the poor and who will pay for medical research. Although there is a general recognition that caring for the poor and paying for research will cost something, the public seriously underestimates how large that bill will be because of the cost shifting that has gone on for so many years. Most of the income in the United States is earned by employed people between the ages of 30 and 60. This healthy group, whose wealth is increasing, makes up less than a third of the population. Paying for the other two-thirds, and for all of the medical advances that working people want, will require transfers of billions and billions of dollars. We are in the process of giving up on the old system for transferring funds, but have not been able to find and agree upon a new one.[10]

8.5 CAPITAL FINANCING _____

Revenues for an organization must not only exceed current expenses, they must also be sufficiently above operating costs to compensate those who have invested capital. If a hospital borrows $10 million for construction it must pay back the principal over time *and* also pay interest on the loan each year. For a philanthropist making a donation, the returns on capital take the form of social services rather than interest or dividends. Having a nonprofit organization that is supposed to make a loss each year, with the difference made up out of endowment or contributions, tends to blur the line between capital and operating funds. However, the conceptual requirement for a return on capital is clear. The philanthropist could always invest the money in financial assets and make a donation each year from the interest if that were a more efficient way to achieve their charitable purpose than providing a lump-sum capital donation.

The start up capital for most hospitals came from some combination of philanthropy and local government funds. Land and buildings were often donated. At the turn of the century there were also a number of doctors' hospitals, usually started in a portion of the doctor's house, or in a converted dwelling nearby. The capital financing for these small, private hospitals came from the doctor's own savings, or from family members. Hospitals grew because they were successful in attracting funds, or because they were successful in attracting paying patients and could build up reserves (which would be called "retained earnings" in a for-profit organization). In World War II millions of servicemen had seen first-hand the benefits of modern medical technology. The power of antibiotics and new surgical techniques to heal impressed many, especially those from rural areas. This created a desire to spread hospitals across the land.[11] Yet only a few hospitals had been able to build up reserves during the Great Depression or the war that followed, and those that had conserved money wanted to expand their own operations, not to help rural communities. The success of the New Deal and the victories of the military made it seem natural to mobilize government resources to meet this need. In 1946 the "Hill-Burton Act" was passed, making construction funds available to new hospitals in areas that had less than 4 beds per 1,000. As a form of "repayment" the hospitals receiving these funds were to give an equal or greater value in free care to indigent persons. City and suburban hospitals were envious of the easy access rural areas had to capital and, since power tends to accrue to those who already have it (ie., existing hospitals), and not necessarily to those who need it, subsequent changes were made to allow Hill-Burton funds to also be used for expansion and renovation projects, as well as new construction.

Hill-Burton, retained earnings, and philanthropic fund drives provided most capital financing until the enactment of Medicare and Medicaid in 1965. Hospitals, which had chronically suffered operating losses, suddenly had steady revenue streams guaranteed by the government. They could meet the demand for new construction by borrowing against that promise, and they proceeded to do so. Borrowing went from under $100 million in 1960 to $200 million in 1970, $1,215 million in 1975, and $2.6 billion by 1977.[12] Three factors combined to make debt so quickly become the dominant form of hospital capital:

- Guaranteed revenues from Medicare and Medicaid that assured investors of repayment.
- Tax exemption as municipal bonds that made it cheap for non-profit hospitals to borrow.
- Cost reimbursement for interest expenses.

Medicare and Medicaid totally changed the financial picture of hospitals, from social organizations that had to beg each year, to solidly funded services backed by the government. For a time, it was virtually impossible for most hospitals to go bankrupt, and hence for investors not to get repaid. States and localities created "health care financing authorities" that allowed nonprofit hospitals to qualify as municipal borrowers, so that investors did not have to pay federal, state, or local taxes on the interest they received. This reduced the cost of borrowing by a third, making it possible for a hospital to issue bonds at 5 percent and invest at 7 percent while waiting to use the money for construction. Such arbitrage generated millions of dollars to astute hospital financial managers before being outlawed. The shift to cost reimbursement also favored borrowing. A hospital that used its own reserves to construct a new building could get reimbursed for depreciation, but the hospital that issued debt to do the same thing got reimbursed for interest expenses as well as depreciation.

In this environment with tax-exempt debt, willing investors, and cost reimbursement, it is not surprising that hospitals went on a borrowing spree, loading up with more than $10 billion in debt by 1980. However, any business that takes on lots of debt is more likely to come under financial pressure. Despite being organized as nonprofit organizations, hospitals were no exception. With millions of dollars of interest payments to make each year, hospital managers had to become more and more bottom-line oriented. As the threat of bankruptcy became more real, the social welfare and community benefit orientation that had prevailed since the turn of the century increasingly gave way to a business orientation.

Hospital borrowing rose so rapidly that it had to lose steam eventually. Too many new beds were built, and debt loads became insupportable. Also, pressures on the Medicare budget led to tighter and tighter reimbursement. In 1985, the first bond defaults began to occur. Investors quickly revised their expectations, and treated hospital debt as risky, and hence requiring a higher rate of interest. Municipalities were less and less pleased about the loss of property and income taxes, and calls were made to limit the use of tax-exempt revenue bonds such as those issued by hospital financing authorities. Access to capital became more difficult. Old and decrepit facilities could not tap the bond market, and were acquired by for-profit hospital chains that could use the stock market to quickly raise equity, refurbish the physical plant, and make money. Many towns were willing to sell off their hospital for nothing, even provide special subsidies and tax breaks, rather than let it go bankrupt and disappear. The environment had also changed, so that more hospitals felt it necessary to become part of a system covering all types of care over a broad geographic area. In order to do so, strong hospitals wanted to merge with or buy up weaker ones, and also to buy nursing homes, home health agencies, physician practices, and medical office buildings. In most cases, it would not be legal to use tax-exempt debt to do so, nor could the hospitals borrow the hundreds of millions of dollars necessary in the corporate (taxable) market.

The stand-alone community hospital was a good structure for creating a social contract.[13] Business leaders, citizens of the town, and the poor all participated in a visible symbol of community responsibility that was governed by a local board of directors. The move toward larger and more integrated health care systems has shown that this structure is inflexible and increasingly outmoded. People no longer identify primarily with a "community" or look to voluntary action to provide health care, and the solo hospital has no way to move capital from where the funds are (in wealthy suburbs) to where the needs are (in distressed urban and rural areas, in providing assistance to the disabled elderly). Creating a chain of hospitals is one way of regionalizing and rationalizing the allocation of capital. Recently there has been a spurt of acquisitions and conversions to for-profit status, although it is still unclear how far this trend will go, and to what extent the government, as the primary payer for hospital care, will let it go. What has become clear is that private equity markets have far outstripped private philanthropy as a source of capital for meeting the demands for new services and new construction in the twenty-first century.

8.6 ORGANIZATION: WHO CONTROLS THE HOSPITAL, AND FOR WHAT ENDS? _____

The standard model firm in a microeconomics textbook is an organization created by the owners, who invest time and money, in order to make a profit. To do so, the firm must meet the needs of customers who pay for the firms' products, and also meet the needs of employees and other vendors who get paid by the firm to supply inputs. By the fundamental theorem of exchange, each party must benefit for the organization to continue to exist. The customers get consumers' surplus from purchasing products they prefer in terms of price or quality to those of other firms, the employees get jobs they prefer in terms of wages or conditions, and the owners take home as profits the value added by organizing a firm. The owners are known as the "residual claimants" because they get what is left over, profits (or losses) being a net residual difference between revenues and expenses. A firm operates as a rational economic organization because the owners who make the decisions must bear the consequences, be they good (profits) or bad (losses). The linkages between owners, employees, and customers usually have some slack in the real world, which gets assumed away in textbook models of perfect competition. Corporate "agency theory" deals with the implications of raising capital through the stock market, which separates ownership (stockholders) from control (managers).[14] To the extent that managers are not perfect agents of the owners, they may dissipate or capture some of the firm's profits by purchasing inputs from favored relatives, having big offices, not taking enough risks, or not working hard enough. Such deviations from profit maximization may change the firm's behavior, as can taxes, regulations, social conditions, ideology, culture, and political constraints.

Hospitals differ from the standard firm in three significant ways: 1) *patients do not pay,* due to insurance or charity; 2) *ownership is usually unclear,* due to nonprofit voluntary or governmental organization; and 3) *medical care is largely controlled by doctors who neither pay nor receive any money from the hospital,* and therefore have no direct connection from a flow-of-funds perspective. Doctors are neither customers nor employees nor owners, but since in practice they are the dominant voice in hospital operations, they sometimes look like they are all three. This structure, combining power, money, and service with no direct line of control or financial accountability, is a unique form of economic organization that makes it difficult to model or predict the behavior of hospitals. A hospital does not do anything, except at the direction of a physician; only doctors are allowed to admit patients, perform surgery, or prescribe drugs. The hospital "organizes" a medical staff, but some would claim that the reality is the other way around, that the medical staff "organizes" a hospital as their workshop. This is the basis of Mark Pauly's model of the hospital as the doctor's workshop, which hypothesizes that the hospital will behave so as to maximize the profits of the doctors who are on staff, rather than maximizing the profits of the organization.[15] Joseph Newhouse has pointed out that the hospital is a nonprofit organization and has no owners who can claim the profits, and suggests that hospitals and other nonprofit organizations get run for the benefit of managers.[16] They want their hospital to be the biggest and the best, which, not incidentally, would justify the highest managerial salaries, and hence, maximize some combination of quantity and quality of services, rather than profits or doctors' incomes. Employees are also important stakeholders, but since their importance derives from being input suppliers, it does not seem that employees influence on the behavior of the hospital should be too different from their role in other organizations. Most hospital mission statements claim that their primary concern is patient care, yet this sort of general assertion does not address how prices are set, the trade-off between one group of patients and another (e.g., surgery or immunization, abortion or family planning clinics), or the trade-offs between employees and doctors. The American Hospital Association maintains that hospitals are, in essence, public institutions whose purpose is to benefit the community. From a flow-of-funds perspective, this would make sense, because most of the capital investment in a voluntary hospital comes from the community in the form of charitable donations and taxes. The problem is, how is community benefit defined, and who, exactly, exercises control?[17] The board, although in theory representing the community, is often deferential to the medical staff and depends on the information provided by the administration to make decisions (see Table 8.4).

TABLE 8.4 Who Gets the Profits from a Nonprofit Hospital?

- Doctors?
- Administrators?
- Employees?
- Patients?
- Community?

Despite a considerable amount of theoretical and empirical work by economists, and a clear recognition that insurance, nonprofit status, and medical control over admissions and treatment make hospitals quite different, no really satisfactory theory of the hospital as a distinct type of organization has been developed. In part, this may be due to the fact that competition and the pressure to survive forces a hospital to maximize revenues and minimize costs very much like a for-profit firm. The greater the amount of debt, the more pressure a hospital faces, and any deviation from profit-maximizing behavior becomes a threat to survival. Most of the research to date shows little difference between for-profit and not-for-profit hospitals.[18] This might be due to competitive pressures forcing nonprofits to behave in a profit-maximizing manner, but it might also be a result of social expectations that force for-profit hospitals to meet the standards of community benefit and medical professionalism in order to attract patients. Most of the differences that have sometimes been observed are in the direction that economic theory leads one to expect. For-profit hospitals are more aggressive in pricing services to maximize revenues, and respond more quickly to changes in reimbursement rules that could affect profits. They are sometimes less likely to provide charity care to indigents, chose to build in geographic areas of highest need, or promote immunization, prenatal care, and other uncompensated services. The large hospitals that do most of the teaching and research are almost always nonprofit institutions. Although all general acute hospitals seem to behave in basically similar ways, it is possible to discern a continuum with for-profits at one end being more aggressive and quick to respond to incentives, and government hospitals at the other end being a bit more inflexible and committed to public services. However, the range of behavior due to differences in ownership category does not appear to be very wide, and is probably narrowing over time as all hospitals confront rising patient expectations for service and technology, managed care, and reductions in funding due to cost pressures and the federal deficit.

SUGGESTIONS FOR FURTHER READING _____

Modern Healthcare and *Hospitals* are biweekly magazines covering the hospital industry in depth.

American Hospital Association, *Hospital Statistics* and *Hospital Guide*, is published annually.

Joseph Newhouse,"Toward a Theory of Nonprofit Institutions: An Economic Model of a Hospital," *American Economic Review* 60:64–74, 1970.

Mark Pauly and Michael Redisch, "The Not-for-Profit Hospital as a Physician's Cooperative," *American Economic Review* 63:87–99, 1973.

Rosemary Stevens, *In Sickness and In Wealth: American Hospitals in the Twentieth Century,* NY: Basic Books, 1989.

Burton Weisbrod, *The Nonprofit Economy,* Cambridge Mass.: Harvard University Press, 1988, and "Rewarding Performance that is Hard to Measure: The Private Non-Profit Sector," *Science* (May 5, 1989), pp 541–546.

SUMMARY _____

1. The Pennsylvania Hospital, founded in 1751, was the first hospital in the United States. Like most **early hospitals**, it was **funded primarily by charita-**

ble donations and government tax appropriations, and **housed the sick and disabled poor**, although some paying patients were admitted.

2. The development of **new technology** created the need for a central facility where the **capital cost** of equipment could be **shared by many doctors** and where dangerous surgical procedures could be carried out in a more controlled and supportive environment.

3. **Over 95 percent of all hospital revenues come from third parties**, with **more than half coming from government** through the Medicare and Medicaid programs. Patients pay so little of the hospital bill that **charges are virtually irrelevant** in decision making. Although cost-based reimbursement using the RCCAC (ratio of costs-to-charges applied to charges) formulated by Blue Cross plans under the aegis of the American Hospital Association was the major form of payment from 1965 to 1985, since then the prospective DRG per case payments and a variety of managed care plans have become the main sources of revenues. Approximately one-third of hospital revenues come from outpatient services, and an increasing amount comes from home health, long-term care, and other related services.

4. Hospitals may obtain revenues in a variety of ways, including **philanthropy** and grants, **global budgets**, billed **charges, per day** (diem) payments, per case (**DRG**) payments, cost reimbursement, or managed care contracts.

5. **Labor** is the largest category of health care expenditure. Including the employees of local service firms, personnel accounts for more than 75 percent of a hospital's costs. Therefore the only real way to cut costs is to reduce wages or reduce employment, neither of which is politically popular. Doctors are usually **independent contractors paid separately** by the patient, and thus do not show up as a large item on hospital budgets, even though they play a dominant role in providing and directing care.

6. **Cost shifting** is the process of charging one group (i.e., commercially insured patients) more to cover the loss due to undercharging another group (indigent patients or Medicaid). The pervasiveness of cost shifting and insurance coverage gave financial managers far more room to raise revenues as a means of supporting the hospital, and little incentives to find efficiencies that would reduce costs. **Cream skimming** is the action of taking on only the profitable patients for whom services are priced considerably above unit costs, while avoiding the loss-making patients with heavy care needs. Changes in Medicare reimbursement and the advent of managed care firms that shop to obtain hospital services at the lowest possible price have eroded the ability of hospitals to cross-subsidize and made it difficult to support research, teaching, or charity.

7. Although accounting for just 9 percent of operating costs, **access to capital** has been crucial in shaping the growth of hospitals. **Philanthropy** was first replaced by **government** construction grants through the **Hill-Burton** legislation enacted in 1946, and subsequently by **tax-free municipal revenue bonds** in the 1970s. **Equity** financing through the stock market is becoming increasing important as hospitals try to acquire nursing homes, physician practices, and other hospitals to form integrated health care systems.

8. Hospitals differ from most firms in that they are largely **paid for by third parties**, most commonly **nonprofit organizations** directed by volunteer boards rather than owners, and **dominated by doctors, independent professionals** who work for themselves with no direct financial ties to the hospital. Despite much research and lots of theoretical expectations, there appear to be only slight differences between voluntary not-for-profit, government, and private for-profit hospitals. In general, for-profits appear to be somewhat less likely to take on charity care, research, teaching and outreach, and to react more quickly to changes in reimbursement regulations, with government hospitals at the other extreme and voluntary hospitals falling in the middle, but any differences are small, and occur only sometimes.

PROBLEMS _____

1. {*industrial organization*} What technological, organizational, and financial innovations caused the rise of the hospitals in the twentieth century?

2. {*incidence*} Who pays for most of the care in hospitals? Are the people who pay the bills the same as the people who receive the care?

4. {*flow of funds*} Which input accounts for the largest portion of hospital costs? Which input is responsible for most of the growth in hospital cost per patient day?

5. {*payment methodology*} Both hospital A and hospital B are paid by Medicare using the DRG methodology. If hospital A has an average case-mix index of 1.62 and admits 24 patients who use stay in the hospital a total of 192 days, while hospital B has an average case-mix of 0.95 and admits 34 patients who stay in the hospital a total of 238 days, which hospital gets paid more? Which hospital gets paid more per case? Which hospital gets paid more per diem? Which hospital gets paid more for an appendectomy?

6. {*flow of funds*} Over the past hundred years, the major source of hospital revenues has changed three times. Name these types of payments, and explain why each one gave way to the next.

7. {*payment*} If a hospital decides to raise prices because it needs more money, what effect does this have on:
   a. Patients who pay their own bills.
   b. Patients whose bills are paid by an insurance company.
   c. Insurance contracts reimbursed on the basis of costs.
   d. Previously negotiated per diem contracts with HMOs.

8. {*cost shifting*} Is the mark-up (ratio of prices to direct per-unit costs) relatively constant across different types of hospitals? Are mark-ups the same for different services or departments within a hospital?

9. {*cost shifting*} How do hospitals pay for medical research?

10. {*ownership*} Are doctors usually employees, owners, or managers of hospitals?

11. {*ownership*} Who owns most hospitals? Who gets the profit when a nonprofit hospital makes money? Can nonprofit hospitals be bought and sold?

12. {*capital financing*} Are the ways hospitals obtain capital different than the ways that doctors obtain capital? Why?

13. {*rate of return, incidence*} How does a philanthropist who donates funds to a hospital get "returns on capital?" How are these returns measured, as a dollar amount, as an annualized percentage rate, or by some other method?

14. {*ownership, non-profit, capital financing*} Hospitals received special treatment from the government and were able to borrow subsidized capital using tax-free municipal bonds. During the 1970s and 1980s, billions of dollars of tax-free capital flowed into nonprofit hospitals. Did this make them more or less like for-profit firms?

15. {*financial reporting*} Which is more important in determining the type of financial reports a hospital must prepare, the type of ownership, or the major sources of funding? If capital is attracted from different sources, are different types of financial reports required?

16. {*cost shifting*} What does it mean for Medicare to act as a "prudent buyer" of hospital services? Does doing so strengthen or weaken Medicare as a social insurance program?

17. {*cost shifting*} What adjustments would a hospital have to make if it began to serve a larger number of indigent patients? Would most of the adjustments come on the revenue side or the expenditure side?

18. {*cost shifting*} Who benefits from cost shifting, the poor or the rich? Do any health care workers benefit from cost shifting?

ENDNOTES _____

1. Paul Starr, *The Social Transformation of American Medicine*, New York: Basic Books, 1992. Rosemary Stevens, *In Sickness and in Wealth: American Hospitals in the Twentieth Century*, New York: Basic Books, 1989.
2. George Rosen, *A History of Public Health*, New York: MD Publications, 1958.
3. Florence Nightingale, *Notes on Nursing: What It Is, and What It Is Not*, New York: D. Appleton-Century, 1938.
4. Charles Lawrence, *History of the Philadelphia Almshouses and Hospitals from the Beginning of the Eighteenth to the Ending of the Nineteenth Centuries*, Philadelphia: C. Lawrence, 1905.
5. Marshall K. Raffel and Norma K. Raffel, *The U.S. Health System: Origins and Functions*, 4th edition, Albany, NY: Delmar Publisher, 1994.
6. An illustrative case study is found in the history of the Mayo clinic. See, Helen Clapesattle, *The Doctors Mayo*, Minneapolis: University of Minnesota Press, 1941; Gunther W. Nagel, *The Mayo Legacy*, Springfield, Ill.: Charles C. Thomas, 1966; and compare with an annual report of the Mayo Clinic (now operating in Arizona and Florida as well as Minnesota) in the 1990s.
7. J. Hermann, "Blue Cross of California goes for the Gold—Wellpoint Health Networks," *Health Systems Review* 26(3):14–19, May/June, 1993; T. Kertesz, "California Blue Cross Tries Again With Bigger Foundation Plan," *Modern Healthcare* 25(16):2–3, April 17, 1995.
8. American Hospital Association, *Hospital Statistics*, Chicago: American Hospital Association, 1995.
9. American Hospital Association, *Hospital Statistics*, various years.

10. Henry J. Aaron and Robert D. Reischauer, "The Medicare Reform Debate: What is the Next Step?" *Health Affairs,* 14(4):8–30, Winter 1995.
11. Odin W. Anderson, *Health Services as a Growth Enterprise in the United States Since 1875,* Ann Arbor, Mich.: Health Administration Press, 1990.
12. Jonathan Betz Brown, *Health Capital Financing,* Ann Arbor, Mich.: Health Administration Press, 1988, pp. 14–18.
13. Robert Sigmond, "From Charity Care to Community Benefit," *Hospitals & Health Services Administration,* Summer 1994.
14. Michael C. Jensen and William H. Meckling, "Theory of the Firm: Managerial Behavior, Agency Costs and Ownership Structure," *Journal of Financial Economics,* 3:305–360, 1976.
15. Mark V. Pauly, *Doctors and Their Workshops: Economic Models of Physician Behavior,* Chicago: University of Chicago Press, 1980.
16. Joseph Newhouse, "How Do Hospitals make Choices?" in *The Economics of Medical Care,* Reading, Mass: Addison-Wesley, 1978, pp. 68–73.
17. Robert Sigmond and J. David Seay, "Community Benefit Standards for Hospitals: Perceptions and Performance," in "The Future of Tax-Exempt Status for Hospitals" issue of *Frontiers of Health Services Management,* Spring 1989.
18. E. R. Becker and Frank Sloan, "Hospital Ownership and Performance," *Economic Inquiry* 23(1):21–36, 1985; Deborah Freund et al., "Analysis of Length-Of-Stay Differences Between Investor-Owned and Voluntary Hospitals," *Inquiry* 22(1):33–44, 1985; Mark Schlesinger, Theodore Marmor and R. Smithey, "Non-Profit and For-Profit Medical Care," *Journal of Health Politics, Policy and Law* 12(3):427–457, 1987.

CHAPTER 9

Management and Regulation of Hospital Costs

QUESTIONS

1. *Why do some hospitals cost more than others?*
2. *If hospitals are not-for-profit, then what do they compete for?*
3. *The number of patients has gone down, and the number of days each patient spends in the hospital has gone down, so why have hospital costs continued to go up faster than any other aspect of health care?*
4. *Are large hospitals expensive because they suffer from diseconomies of scale, or because they treat the most difficult patients?*
5. *Why would a hospital want to buy a new MRI scanner if the hospital next door already has such a machine, and is only able to find enough patients to keep it busy half of the time?*
6. *Will computers and other new technology improve efficiency, and hence reduce costs, or improve quality, and hence raise costs?*
7. *Has regulation cut costs, or cut competition?*

9.1 WHY DO SOME HOSPITALS COST MORE THAN OTHERS?

The cost of a day in the hospital can be as little as $300, or more than $1,500. What factors could account for such a large range of variation? It is not surprising if it costs $1,500 for a critically wounded trauma patient in an intensive care unit (ICU) and just $300 for someone resting up after breaking a leg while skiing.[1] The ICU patient is much sicker, and requires more complex services. It is also understandable that being in one of the nation's top research and teaching hospitals under the care of famous doctors can cost more than a bed in a small rural facility with limited equipment and staff.[2] The hospital bill itself can be a misleading guide to costs. One hospital may charge more, but give every patient a discount, while another sticks to list prices. Or, one hospital could be charging $400 just for the bed, with extra charges for medication, lab tests, physical therapy, and so on, while another hospital charging $500 includes all of the above, and so is less expensive (see Table 9.1).

It is often assumed that when one hospital has a lower cost per patient day that it is more "efficient," but such a conclusion is only justified if the two hospitals are providing the same services to similar patients under similar conditions. Unless this *ceteris paribus* (all other things constant) assumption is valid, and it rarely is, efforts must be made to adjust for all of the other factors listed in Table 9.1 in order to compare costs. Of course patients (or their insurance companies) would prefer a cheaper stay in the hospital to a more expensive one if all other factors were constant, but when they are not, the more relevant question is: Is a hospital that costs 10 percent more (or 20%, or 400%) really worth that much more? While this relative value question is more meaningful, it is also much more difficult to answer, and depends on the patient's values as well as on calculations of technical efficiency. Therefore, it is useful to look first at the simpler and more standard question of variations in costs for the same unit of service.

9.2 HOW MANAGEMENT CONTROLS COSTS

Short-Run Versus Long-Run Cost Functions

What can management do to change the costs of production? If a hospital should receive fewer admissions than expected this morning, and try to reduce its costs by the afternoon, there really is not much that can be done. People have already shown up for work, meals have been prepared, ambulances and wheelchair transport arranged, and so on, so that *in the short run almost all costs are fixed.* Any reduction in the number of patients will therefore cause the average cost per patient to be higher than usual. If the reduction in admissions continues, and management is given enough time to respond, the hospital may shut down a wing, refrain from some new hires, and maybe even lay off some employees. This is but one case of a very general rule—as more time is allowed for adjustment, more changes can be made, and as more changes are made, costs per unit become lower.

**TABLE 9.1   Reasons for Differences in
Hospital Costs**

Severity of patient's illness
Quality of care
Intensity of services (e.g., number of nursing hours or lab tests)
Cost shifting to pay for research and teaching
Differences in billing
Prices of labor and other inputs
Efficiency

In the very long run, almost all costs become variable. The director can train new management, hire appropriate clinical staff, and rewrite treatment protocols, replace the existing building with a new one, pave some grounds for parking, even move the whole facility to a more efficiently located site near a freeway. This ability to plan and choose the optimal scale and combination of inputs allows management to minimize the costs of production for any desired level of output. If management expects to average only 100 patients per day, they would build a small hospital, hire fewer people, and incur lower fixed costs; if they expected 175 patients a day, they would build a medium-sized hospital; and for 300 patients a day, they would build a large hospital with a dedicated computer system, pneumatic transport tubes to speed laboratory samples between floors, and other equipment (Figure 9.1).

For any given (expected) level of output, management would choose the cost-minimizing size of building and number of permanent employees. In geometric

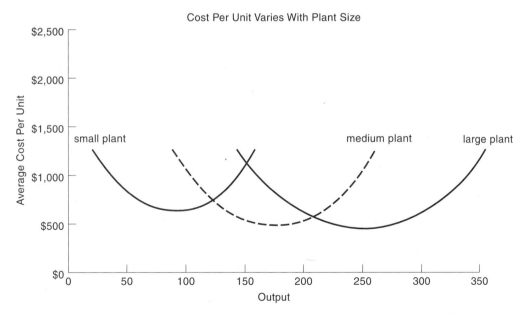

FIGURE 9.1   *The average cost per unit depends on the amount produced and the size of the plant. At low output (50 − 125 units in this example), a small plant can produce at lowest cost. At intermediate output levels, a medium-sized plant is more efficient. For high output (250 + units), a large plant has lowest costs.*

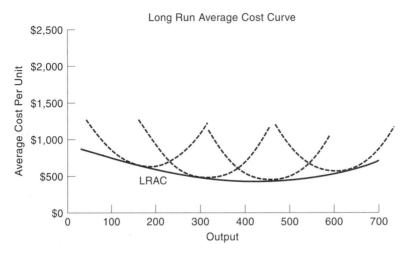

FIGURE 9.2 *With plenty of time to plan and perfect knowledge of the future, a firm can pick the optimal size of plant for any anticipated level of output. This long-run average cost curve, LRAC, is the "envelope" of all the short-run average cost curves.*

terms, the long-run average cost curve (LRAC) is an "envelope" that traces out a minimum, just touching all the possible short-run average cost curves (SRAC), as shown in Figure 9.2. Logically, no SRAC can fall below the LRAC because if there were some short-run cost function that had lower costs, then management would choose that production configuration instead, so that it became part of the long-run function. Whether a particular cost is fixed or variable is determined by the time frame for decision making. Decisions regarding temporary agency nurses can be made on a day-to-day basis, and thus are fixed for only 24 hours or so. Permanent employees take a while to train, or to terminate when no longer needed, and are thus fixed for at least several months. Reducing the number of vice-presidents is so traumatic it may take several years. Construction is a fixed cost once it is completed, but is a variable cost during the planning stage.

Uncertainty and Budgeting

A director must deal with two kinds of variation in the level of output—foreseeable and unknown. Expansion to accommodate a growing population in the suburbs, closing maternity beds in response to declining fertility, and opening a cardiac rehabilitation unit to serve an aging community, are all examples of foreseeable long-run changes. The lower number of hospital admissions on Saturday and Sunday, Christmas and New Year's day, and during August, are examples of foreseeable short-run changes. Foreseeable changes can be planned for in advance. Hiring and training can be accomplished efficiently over a reasonable period of time, space and building modifications carried out on a schedule, and so on, so that the path and pace of adjustment reflect conscious decisions by management to minimize costs. Random variations, on the other hand, must be accommodated in the operations of the organization, but cannot be known in advance. There may be sixteen admissions on Monday, twelve on Tuesday, twenty-two on Wednesday, only thirteen on Thursday, eighteen on Friday, and fifteen on Saturday. There is twice as much work for the admitting office to do on Wednesday as on Tuesday, with the same amount of staff and equipment. The staff are likely to do only what is necessary that day, and perhaps even work late, while putting off until tomorrow some of the routine tasks, such as filing charts, checking documentation, and entering data into forms. Long-run unknown changes in output might occur because a new factory is built nearby, so that many new families move to the area, or because an epidemic such as AIDS increases the demand for care, or because a competing hospital is built, taking away some of the demand. Such major changes will often force the hospital to change its long-run strategy (see Figure 9.3).

How do managers go about controlling costs? Primarily through the use of a budget, which is a plan stated in dollars.[3] A budget that does not change with volume is called a **fixed budget** (or sometimes, a standard budget), and a budget that changes with volume is known as a **flexible budget**. Typically, a hospital or medical group practice will create an **operating budget** that projects all the anticipated expenses for the next year. For example, if labor expenses rose 7 percent in 1991, and 9 percent in 1992, they may project an increase of 8 percent in labor costs for 1993. A reasonable definition of *short run* used by many managers is "any change that occurs during the current budget period." Long-run changes and plans are incorporated in a **strategic budget** (sometimes also known as the long-run capital budget) that focuses on trends in the number of patients and capital renovations and expansions (new buildings or equipment, adding partners). These will often be accompanied by financial projections, or *pro forma* **financial statements** of incomes, assets and fund balances that will cover the next three or five or even twenty years in summary format. Only infrequently are detailed budgets prepared for more than one year in advance. The definition of *long run* is often taken to be "any change occurring more than one year in the future," but some managers will designate the next two to five years as *intermediate run*. In any analysis, the terms are relative, and so any definition is somewhat arbitrary. The important points to gain from economic theory are that short-run adjustment is always more costly than long-run adjustment, and that as the time perspective changes, so does the focus of management attention on cost control.

Known short-run variations are dealt with by making limited changes in the num-

	Planned (known)	**Random** (uncertain)
Short Run	Scheduling Weekly budget Part-timers	Overtime, temps Inventory Maintain excess capacity
Long Run	Capital budgeting Change plant size Facility conversion	Hold financial reserves Encroachment by or on competitors Bankruptcy

FIGURE 9.3 *How organizations deal with change.*

ber of staff scheduled. Fewer nurses are working on Sundays, and at 3:00 A.M. However, the percentage change in staff is less than the percentage change in patient load, because all units must still have a head nurse, tech support, and so on, even though they are only partially full. Changes in plant capacity are prohibitively expensive in the short-run. Although there might be fifty beds empty in the hospital on Sunday night, not all of them would be in wing 7-East. To close that unit down, many patients would have to be transferred to clear out that floor, and then transferred back on Monday when patient occupancy increased again. The savings from not having had a head nurse on 7-East would be more than offset by all the transfers, so that it would actually end up costing more to try and shut down one unit for the sake of "efficiency." Therefore, most units will be underutilized on the weekends, and most staff will have an easy day.

A known long-run change, such as declining trend in admissions due to the closure of local manufacturing plant, calls for a permanent reduction in capacity. Unit 7-East can be converted into storage, or nursing home beds, or leased to a group of physical therapists. Furthermore, staffing should be reduced proportionately to the long-run decline in patients so that every employee is carrying a regular workload, rather than the partial adjustments made on nights and weekends.

Random short-run fluctuations are dealt with primarily by building in some excess reserve capacity, making the staff work faster or slower, and allocating less immediate tasks to the slower days. Suppose that admissions are as suggested earlier: Monday 16, Tuesday 12, Wednesday 22, Thursday 13, Friday 18, Saturday 15. The manager does not care about the cost of care on Monday or the cost on Tuesday, but wishes to minimize the cost for the week as a whole. There is no reason to yell at the manager for having too many nurses on duty Thursday, since there was no way to tell that admissions would be light until the shift actually started. Also, while management might be able to get the staff to work hard and stay overtime on Wednesday to accommodate the influx of patients, the staff will not stay if they are abused with continual overloads—they will quit and go to work at another hospital, raising labor cost, since the manager would then have to use temporaries and retrain frequently. If the hospital has a range of ten to twenty-five admissions per weekday, with an average of sixteen, then it can staff for sixteen plus a bit of reserve. However, if another hospital had less random variation, and always got fourteen to eighteen admissions per day, it could match staffing more exactly to the number of patients and would need less reserve capacity and have lower average cost per unit for the same average number of patients. This is but one example of the general principle that dealing with uncertainty is costly, and the greater the range of uncertainty, the greater the cost.

Unforeseen long-run changes in output are what really provide the test of the organization's ability to control costs. Here, tactical attention to detail is not enough—the hospital must make a strategic gamble based on some specific expectation of the future (population will grow older and increase demand, or people will move to Florida, reducing demand; major competitor will go bankrupt, giving us a great opportunity, or will go all out trying to survive by stealing our patients). The hospital could build in flexibility by making investments to cover both alternatives, but would then incur higher costs per unit, whichever happens.

9.3 CONFLICT BETWEEN ECONOMIC THEORY AND ACCOUNTING MEASURES OF PER UNIT COST _____

Timing

In Table 9.2, the "cost" per patient admitted is examined from two perspectives: direct accounting costs and a full economic cost that includes the hidden cost of dealing with disruptions (burnt-out staff, mistakes, overtime, etc.). In this example, the budgeted fixed costs are $5,000 per day and the variable costs are $300 per admission. The direct cost on Monday, when the expected number of patients (16) were admitted, is $5,000 + 16 × $300 = $9,800, so the cost per admission is $9,800 ÷ 16 = $613. On Wednesday, more patients were admitted (22) than the staff expected. Calculated average cost per patient is $11,600 ÷ 22 = $527. It appears that the hospital benefited from its "mistake" in planning for too small a number of patients. Why not increase the advantage by planning for only 15 admissions instead of 16? Then everyone would work even harder and faster, and if that is not good enough, the hospital could just plan for 12 or 10 or 6 admissions, and keep pushing the staff to become more and more efficient. Taking the example to an extreme highlights the flaw in the reasoning. The accounting measure does not accurately capture all the costs. Let's consider what really happens. To work so hard on Wednesday, the staff must put off some of their ordinary tasks until Thursday, and they also expect some extra consideration from management on Friday when they ask to go home early. Once these costs of catching up afterward are factored in, the surge of patients of Wednesday is seen to have been very costly, not inexpensive. If everything went according to plan, then 16 admissions each day would cost $9,800, for an average cost per admission of $613. Yet extra admissions mean disrupting the plan. To allow for the costs of making sudden adjustments, an "adjustment cost" must be added in the amount of $100 × (actual − expected admissions)^2, i.e., for deviating from the plan by one admission, the costs of adjustment are $100, for two, $400, for 3, $900 and so on. The actual economic costs (with adjustments) are $15,200 for 22 admissions, an average of $681 per admission rather than $613. Of course it would be cheaper if a hospital could get patients to come in evenly spaced out, exactly 16 each day, all between the hours of 9:00 A.M. and 4:00 P.M. so that workload could be exactly matched to staff and equipment. Yet illness does not go according to plan and the flow of admissions is never smooth. Health care managers have learned that such disruptions are costly, that *every deviation from the planned level of operations raises costs.*

In accountants' terms, the per-unit cost in row 3 of Table 9.2 is calculated on a cash basis (when spent), rather than allocating costs to different days on an accrual basis (when actually earned or obligated). In practice, accrual and all other adjustments made to the cost accounting system are inevitably incomplete and imperfect. The advantage of using economic theory is that the contradiction of the general principle, "short-run costs must logically always exceed long-run costs," let us know immediately that something was wrong with the analysis, and therefore that these cost-accounting figures, no matter how precise they might seem, did not reflect reality. It also explains why the budgeted $613 per admission was less than the actual expenses of $681—because random fluctuations forced the payment of overtime, hiring of temps, rush ordering of exhausted supplies and all of the other daily crises that managers are hired to work out.

Careful examination of Table 9.2 shows that cost per admission was not minimized on Monday, when the expected number of patients were admitted, but was actually lower on Friday when "too many" patients came in, even after including adjustment costs (see Figure 9.4). Why is it not more efficient to increase output or downsize the facility so that the lowest cost per unit came at the expected level of output? The reason is that *the manager must minimize not the cost on the day when output hits the expected level, but the average cost per unit over all the days, with their randomly varying levels of output.* If the average number of admissions had been 18 instead of 16, then 24 admissions might have shown up on the heavy Wednesday, so far exceeding capacity limits that an additional $2,800 in costs would be incurred. Having some extra reserve capacity is expensive, but not so expensive as not having it when you need it. In general, managers need to be able to accom-

TABLE 9.2   Accounting vs. Economic Costs per Unit with Short-Run Fluctuations

	Monday	Tues	Wed	Thur	Fri	Sat	average
Admissions	16	12	22	13	18	15	16
Direct Cost	$9,800	$8,600	$11,600	$8,900	$10,400	$9,500	$9,800
Accounting "Cost" per admission	$613	$717	$527	$685	$578	$633	$613
Adjustment Cost	$0	$1,600	$3,600	$900	$400	$100	
Total Cost	$9,800	$10,200	$15,200	$9,800	$10,400	$9,600	$10,900
Economic "Cost" per admission (AC curve)	$613	$850	$691	$754	$600	$640	$681

Table 9.2: Accounting per costs per admission are lower for days with many admissions, even though economic costs are larger. In this hypothetical example, a hospital has planned for 16 admissions each day, and has fixed costs of $5,000 plus $300 per admission. Deviations from the plan disrupt operations, reducing efficiency by a cost of $100 × (deviation squared), i.e., being 1 admission above or below the planned amount reduces efficiency by $100, 2 admissions off by $400, 3 by $900, and so on.

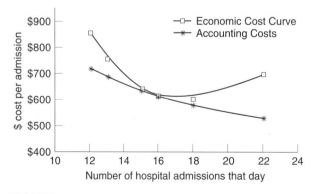

FIGURE 9.4   *Accounting vs. Economic Costs.*

modate the usual fluctuations in volume without major disruptions, to have "flexibility" that minimizes cost over a range. It is possible to have a highly routinized production process that is very efficient at a set level of output, but becomes very inefficient if it has to be speeded up or slowed down. Such fixed-output mass production may work well for cars or lightbulbs, but is not well adapted to services such as medical care, where constant adjustments and varying demand are the norm. Managers are willing to pay a bit extra in fixed costs to increase flexibility (see Figure 9.5). Building a facility that is very efficient when exactly the expected number of patients show up, but cannot easily accommodate changes in the level of demand (dark line), is less efficient in the long run than a more flexible facility (dotted line) that has slightly higher costs at the expected level of output but is able to smoothly maintain average costs per unit at a low level over a wider range.

Whose Costs?

The displacement of costs in time is only one of the mistakes that can be made. Attempts to increase efficiency lead to many management practices that are clearly wrong, yet persist for years because of an inability to count all of the costs. For example, many public clinics provide services free to indigent patients. They try hard to produce these services at the lowest cost to maximize the number of clients they can serve (and to keep taxes down). One way that public clinics can produce services at lower costs is to bring patients in early and keep them waiting so that the doctor's flow of work is never delayed because a patient was late or an appointment is broken. Such "block booking" or "clinic appointments" maximize the number of patients that can be seen by the physician, but they make patients unhappy because they have to spend so many hours waiting. If the cost of

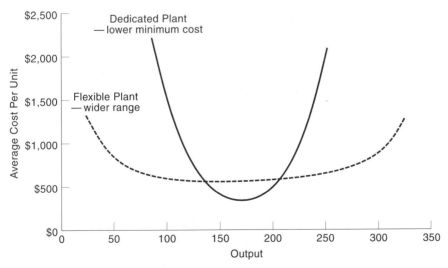

FIGURE 9.5   *A specialized plant has lower cost within a narrow range, but the flexible plant has wider range.*

the patient's time is included, it becomes apparent that block booking is not really efficient; it only seems to be so because the clinic budget counts only direct costs.

How can economists tell that block booking is inefficient? If block booking were truly efficient, then some paying patients would choose to patronize doctors who block-booked, putting up with extra long waits in order to save a little money (i.e., choosing to pay $30 for a block-booked visit rather than $35 for care by appointment). The fact that doctors in the medical marketplace cannot attract patients by block booking is evidence that the extra patient waiting time would be more valuable than the small $5 savings in doctor's time. Indigent patients must put up with inefficiency because they cannot obtain the convenience of an appointment by paying just the marginal $5 cost differential, but instead must forego free care entirely and pay the whole $35 private market price in order to obtain care by appointment. Although one might argue that the indigent patient has a lower cost of time and thus are more willing to put up with longer waits than most paying patients, the fact that even physicians in low-income neighborhoods have to provide appointments suggest that it is the large gap between marginal amenity cost ($5) and average per visit cost ($35), not lower value per hour of patient time, which allows free clinics to continue block-booking.

Time, pain, and other non-market costs borne by patients do not show up on the hospital bill. Yet it is precisely these issues—suffering, fear of death, a need for caring and respect—that distinguish the economics of medical care. That is one reason this textbook began with a broader perspective on optimization using the techniques of cost–benefit analysis (chapter 2) rather than a narrow look at minimizing cash outlays. Some of the common mistakes made in accounting for the true costs of medical care are:

1. Provider costs misallocated (displaced in time, overhead, wrong department)
2. Patient costs not counted (wait time, transportation, family care)
3. Emotional costs not counted (pride, fear, pain, lack of respect)

9.4 ECONOMIES OF SCALE _____

Hospitals exist to allow a large number of doctors to share expensive capital equipment and cooperate in the care of many patients. Since many of these costs are fixed, hospitals should show **economies of scale** (i.e., average cost per patient day falling as more patients are treated).[4] It appears that basic hospital services for routine care are most efficiently delivered when organized and staffed in units of twenty to forty beds, usually known as a *floor* or *wing*. The need to accommodate random fluctuations in the number of admissions, and to preserve some buffer of empty beds for emergencies, creates economies of scale. Admissions to a 40-bed hospital might fluctuate by ± 10, so that only 30 beds could be occupied on average. In a 400 bed hospital, excess admissions to one unit are likely to offset a lack of admission in another, so that the overall fluctuation might be ± 25, which is larger in absolute numbers, but much smaller as a percentage. Thus, percentage occupancy rates can be higher, and per unit costs lower, in a large facility that is more able to smooth out the patient flow. The greater division of labor in a large hospital that allows staff to become more specialized and efficient at a particular function also creates economies of scale.

There is good evidence that economies of scale are important in hospital services. Hospitals with fewer than a hundred beds are usually too small to offer a full range of services, are unable to fully utilize operating suites, CAT scanners, and other diagnostic equipment, and cannot allow staff to specialize. Very small hospitals clearly have higher costs per day, although this is somewhat obscured because they tend to offer fewer of the expensive and technologically advanced services. A better indication that hospitals below a hundred beds suffer from their lack of scale economies is that a disproportionate number of them have gone bankrupt or been absorbed by larger institutions over the last twenty years. Only in rural areas have small general hospitals been able to thrive, and even here their numbers are falling as better highways and helicopter transport have reduced travel time.

Diseconomies of scale arise from the difficulties of coordinating and managing a larger and larger institution. There are relatively few hospitals larger than five-hundred beds, good evidence that costly administrative and transportation difficulties arise when this size is exceeded. Patients increasingly complain about "getting lost in the system" and being part of a "factory" rather than a caring institution. It is also clear from Table 9.3 that costs per day are clearly rising long before the 500 bed size limit is reached. How, can such hospitals continue to exist in a competitive environment?

The Hospital is a Multi-Product Firm

Hospitals are complex institutions, and different parts of the hospital actually produce very different products. The "average" is made up of some basic services for routine admissions, along with some very specialized units such as heart transplant, oncology, and respiratory intensive care. Although it might take only twenty beds to create an efficient-sized cardiac care unit, only a large hospital will have enough cardiac admissions to fill such a specialized unit. Most 400-bed university hospitals are, in fact, composites, with perhaps 100 beds providing general care, 20 dedicated to oncology, 15 to nephrology and kidney transplant, 20 to cardiology, 40 to pediatrics, and so on. Thus, although the efficient size for any one product is just twenty patients, the more specialized types of care a hospital provides, the larger it must be to reach efficient scale. Indeed, it is clear that a hospital large enough to produce heart transplants and nuclear medicine efficiently is

TABLE 9.3 Average Cost per Patient Day by Hospital Size

6–24 beds	$ 634
25–49	604
50–99	576
100–199	690
200–299	784
300–399	894
400–499	876
500 or more	1004

Source: AHA *Hospital Statistics*, 1994, Table 5A.

already too large to produce basic routine hospital care for broken bones and pneumonia, and so suffers from diseconomies of scale with regard to these less-specialized services.

One solution to the conflict between economies and diseconomies of scale is to have patients with uncomplicated illnesses treated at local community hospitals of relatively modest size (100 to 150 beds) with few specialized services, while difficult patients whose treatment demands sophisticated technology and expertise are referred to "tertiary" institutions that are quite large and usually affiliated with universities. However, just as increasing hospital size causes diseconomies of scale by making management communications and coordination more difficult, so does the process of transferring patients back and forth between community and specialty hospitals. The savings from triaging patients so that their illnesses are treated in the most efficient size of hospital are to some extent offset and eventually reversed by the increase in the number of transfers required, since each transfer requires some extra documentation, management oversight, duplication of tests, and so on.

Contracting Out

Some services show economies of scale even at sizes far larger than any hospital in existence. Laboratory testing, for example, has become so automated that costs are minimized in facilities that process hundreds of thousands of tests per day. The equipment, information systems, and technical expertise that constitute the core of a good laboratory are largely a fixed cost, so that overhead per unit continues to decline even when millions of samples are being processed. In order to take advantage of such economies of scale, many hospitals are contracting out such services. Rather than have their own laboratory for routine tests, these are sent out to a reference laboratory that may service hundreds of hospitals. Food services, security, and even emergency rooms are now contracted out to allow hospitals access to economies of scale through contractual relationships.

9.5 QUALITY AND COST _____

Technology: Cutting Costs or Enhancing Quality?

What does it mean when it is said that technological improvements have made the production process "better?" It may mean that the same product can now be produced at a lower cost per unit. It may also mean that a better product can be produced, regardless of cost. Medicine has been dominated by the latter type of technological change. The tremendous value of any increase in cure rates is certainly one factor biasing researchers toward discoveries that have the effect of increasing cost. Yet quality enhancements have occurred rapidly in other areas of technology, such as computing, while still reducing unit costs. Why have such developments been so notably absent in medicine? Quite simply, it has been much more profitable to discover a new cure than to find a method to cut costs.

Insurance and cost reimbursement virtually eliminated price competition in hospital care. Without it, there was no incentive for research laboratories to seek innovations that reduced costs, or for hospitals to switch to cheaper versions of existing equipment. The process of trading off a small reduction in speed or accuracy for a large reduction in price that occurs in most markets has rarely taken place in health care.

Improved Efficiency May Raise Total Spending

It is important to recognize that improved production efficiency always causes the true, quality-adjusted cost function to fall, even though the amount spent and cost per unit may rise because high quality is so much more affordable than before. This is illustrated in Table 9.4. Suppose, for example, that in 1950 a person had a heart attack (myocardial infarction, or MI) and faced the choice of taking medication costing $150 that gave a 30 percent chance of not having another, fatal, MI within five years (70% mortality), or a new, experimental operation costing $25,000 that gave a slightly better chance of survival, with 68 percent mortality. It would be quite rational to take the medication rather than to give up $24,850 additional dollars for such a slight improvement in one's chances. In 1990, much better medication might more than double the chance of survival, with only 29 percent mortality, and cost only $75. However, research and practice has also improved surgery to the point where it has only a 14 percent five-year mortality and is reduced in cost to $15,000. The 1990 option of giving up $14,925 in order to cut the risk of dying in half is very attractive. Thus, even though technological advances reduced the cost of both options, the amount spent on medical care would rise. Improvements in the medical production function frequently create this type of response. Even though 1950s medicine can be produced now for less than it cost in 1950, patients choose to spend more to get high quality 1990s medicine that would have been impossible or prohibitively expensive to obtain in 1950.

Quality costs money, and the drive for higher quality is one of the defining characteristics of modern medicine. While we cannot always even agree on exactly what quality is, we know that more quality is always preferred to less, and that the cost–quality trade-off is usually more important in understanding the economics of medical practice than the cost–volume trade-off. Before making a comparison on the basis of cost per unit, it is first necessary to ask, "What is the product?" If the product is defined as "a day in the hospital," a top-flight research center may seem very expensive. If the product is "an increase in my chance of survival to age 75," then that same institution's $2,500 per day charges might seem like a bargain.

TABLE 9.4   Total Spending May Rise Even As Greater Efficiency Reduces Costs Per Unit

1950	1990
Medication cost $150	Medication cost $75
post-MI mortality = 70%	*post-MI mortality = 29%*
Surgery costs $25,000	Surgery costs $15,000
post-MI mortality = 68%	*post-MI mortality = 14%*
Decision:	Decision:
Take medication for $150	Have surgery for $15,000

9.6 HOW DO HOSPITALS COMPETE? _____

The flow of revenues into a hospital follows the flow of patients. In some cases, such as emergency room or outpatient clinic visits, patients themselves decide where to go, and for these types of care hospitals compete directly by trying to attract patients. However, for most care the decision regarding hospitalization is made by the physician. The agency relationship changes the nature of transaction, so that the patient follows the advice of the physician, and therefore the hospitals compete for doctors.[5] If the ability to decide on hospitalization is taken out of the doctor's hands by the insurance company, as it increasingly is under managed care (see chapter 10), then the hospitals must compete for contracts and appeal to payers—which usually forces the hospital to put more emphasis on lowering prices. The important point is that the hospital must compete for the party that has the power to make the revenues come to them, not necessarily the patient.

Quality is the most important aspect of medical care, and hospitals such as Johns Hopkins or Massachusetts General Hospital have an edge over the competition because of their reputation for outstanding care and scientific prowess. Regardless of whether the final decision-making power lies in the hands of the patient, the physician, or the payer, the other parties must be satisfied, and quality is usually the most important concern. It is very hard to convince patients to go to a hospital they have never heard of, or for doctors to give up control by transferring patients to a specialized facility where they are not on the medical staff, or for insurers to pay extra for admission to a facility where they do not have a contract guaranteeing discounts—yet each of these accommodations become easier to justify when the hospital is "the best."

Competing for Patients

The types of care for which patients make their own decisions are also those where they are able to judge important aspects of quality and where they bear a large share of cost directly from their own pockets. Maternity care is a good example. Mothers want to have their babies close to home, have strong preferences regarding patient services (natural childbirth, religious orientation, attitude of staff), and can get good information for comparing hospitals by talking to other mothers in the neighborhood who have already had babies. Since the need for a delivery is known months in advance, potential parents can do the kind of comparison shopping for births that are impossible for accidents or heart attacks. Also, the fact that births are planned in advance means that they are not "risks" in the insurance sense and therefore frequently are reimbursed on a shared or fixed-price basis that leaves much of the marginal cost to the parents. For all of these reasons, hospitals must actively compete for patients on the basis of price and services. Casual investigation will reveal a number of special deals on offer, from free baby clothes, gourmet meals and a post-partum vacation, to cut-rate "fixed-price packages," not unlike the competition for selling cars or houses. Outpatient clinics, where patients are more likely to self-refer than for inpatient admission, and where cost-sharing is usually higher, also use marketing strategies such as nice waiting rooms, receptionists who call to make or remind patients about appointments, offers of free transportation to the clinic, and waiver of deductibles or copayments. The rise of "preferred provider" plans (see chapter 10) that provide full coverage only for a limited group of hospitals has also increased the importance of direct marketing to patients.

Competing for Physicians

The agency relationship and control over admissions has meant that most hospital competition was over doctors rather than patients. Recruitment incentives are a very visible sign of such competition. Income guarantees (e.g., if you come to hospital X, and your income in the first year is less than $125,000, we will make up the difference), relocation assistance, and promises of referrals from other doctors on the medical staff are common contractual provisions, and sometimes there is even a "signing bonus" such as a professional athlete might receive. As Pauly's "Doctor's Workshop" model would suggest, hospitals also compete by assisting physicians to earn more money in their private practices: free or subsidized office space, secretarial, phone, and billing services, setting aside ten beds for nephrology so that the kidney specialist will always be able to admit a patient, and so on.[6] Reducing practice costs or work effort is a limited competitive tool. Far more important is helping a physician to build his practice by a hospital's reputation for quality and the technological sophistication of services offered.[7] A cardiologist is able to attract more patients if that doctor is the only cardiologist in town who has access to a catheterization lab that does stent, or PCTA, or whatever the newest development in vein obstruction removal is. In some instances, such competition can lead to a sort of "medical arms race," where nearby hospitals each try to be the first with the most, and respond strategically: if one gets an MR Scanner, then the other gets one that is bigger; if one gets a lithotripter, then the other gets one that has more settings and finer resolution; and so on. It is possible that competing on the basis of who has the most new technology can lead to inefficiencies and escalating costs, with the two scanners and two lithotripters both sitting empty half of the time because there are only enough patients in the market to keep one piece of equipment operating at full capacity. This points up one of the major problems of hospital markets structured on the basis of competing for physicians in order to increase patient flow. A hospital has an incentive to subsidize office space to attract physicians, not to reduce charges, change billing practices, or make trade-offs that would lead to overall reductions in the cost of medical care. The competition for physicians does not necessarily push hospitals toward an efficient use of inputs or mix of services.

Competing for Contracts

The scale upon which medical practice is carried out is increasing. When organized on the basis of atomistic transactions between individuals, the choice of hospital fell to the doctors acting as agents for the patients under their care. However, it has become more and more common for payers to make contracts directly with hospitals, negotiating a fixed or discounted price, and limiting patients only to hospitals with which they have a contract. They can direct patient flow even when they are not fully binding. Although Medicare has a contract with every hospital, it will allow heart transplants only in certain approved facilities, and in its request for bids to become an approved provider, price is a factor. HMOs can be even more aggressive, sometimes threatening a hospital that they will transfer a large group of patients to a rival facility unless negotiations result in a substantial discount, or making approval conditional upon assurances that they will receive the lowest price the hospital gives to any contractor.

Although managed care contracting at this level is a relatively recent development, structurally it bears a resemblance to the original social contract between the hospital and the community, and to the agreements under which hospitals receive tax subsidy and other favorable treatment from the government. In each of these contracts, there are two parties; the hospital and a representative of consumers as a group (community, insurance plan, taxpayers). Such large-scale arrangements are inevitably less accommodating to the needs of individual patients and the professional autonomy of physicians. However, any attempt to implement public accountability and successful cost-control will have to make compromises. Trade-offs are necessary in any system that takes seriously its broader social responsibilities, and are the core concept for creating economic efficiency in health care (see Table 9.5).

Measuring Competitive Success

How can it be determined which hospitals are more successful in the competition for patients? A firm that has failed by going out of business is clearly not successful, and economists have used "survivor analysis" to measure competitive success by counting the number of new entrants or exits (bankruptcy, takeover) within different categories. Survivor analysis has been used to show that hospitals below 100 or above 500 beds appear to be inefficient and less able to compete.[8] It has also shown that for-profit hospitals are not necessarily more efficient or better competitors than nonprofits (the fraction of hospitals that are for-profit has fluctuated up and down but stayed around 10 to 20 percent of total bed supply throughout this century, indicating competitive performance that is about average). A hospital that has grown relative to its competitors is clearly more successful, and such traditional measures as total assets, market share, and geographic spread have been used as indicators. With 90 percent of hospitals being either voluntary or governmental organizations, profits are less useful as a measure of success than in other industries. However, the excess of revenues over expenditures is available to fund growth, and is necessary to avoid bankruptcy, and can thus be a useful indicator. In the current environment, with many hospitals trying to form chains or acquire physician practices in order to cover a larger area and offer a full line of services for managed care contracting, strong earnings and large financial reserves clearly provide a competitive advantage.

TABLE 9.5 Competition Between Hospitals

Hospitals Compete for:	On the Basis of Quality and:
Patients	amenities, out-of-pocket $$
Doctors	technology, practice assistance
Contracts	price, information systems

What has proven almost impossible to measure is the success of a hospital in achieving its goals as a provider of health care to the community. Although charity care, participation in outreach programs, and mortality rates are often monitored and commented on, there is general agreement that these are incomplete and inadequate measures at best, and are frequently misleading. Efforts are being made to assess community benefit in more comprehensive and objective ways, but there is as yet no reason to believe that these will be any more convincing than previous attempts.[9] Economists and other policy makers are in the awkward position of recognizing that they know what dimensions are most important (quality, compassion, technological advance), but not how to gauge them numerically, or even how to make a fair comparison between hospitals.

Measuring the Competitiveness of Markets

Competition can be a significant factor in forcing hospitals to become more efficient and provide better services. However, a single hospital in a rural area, or a chain that controls almost all of the hospitals in an urban market, is not constrained by competition. The potential loss of consumer welfare due to a merger or acquisition that reduces the amount of competition is the central concern of the Federal Trade Commission and a source of much litigation under antitrust law, as well as giving rise to many consulting projects for economists called in to testify as expert witnesses on how competitive a particular market is or will be. Competition is usually measured by the number of hospitals or concentration of market share in a geographic area (e.g., within a 15-mile radius, or within a city, county, or metropolitan statistical area), or by the overlap between hospital services (how many patients use both hospitals). Although the complexities of antitrust law and the economic assessment of competition policy are beyond the scope of this text, it is worth noting that all hospitals are multiproduct firms, so that the relevant market for some services (liver transplant, residential psychiatric treatment, abortion) covers a much larger area than others (kidney dialysis, outpatient psychiatry, prenatal care), and that after decades of being exempt or ignored, have come under increasing scrutiny by the FTC, and antitrust enforcement is now looked upon as an important alternative to regulation as a means of controlling costs.

9.7 CONTROLLING HOSPITAL COSTS THROUGH REGULATION _____

Hospital costs have risen steadily throughout the modern postwar era, going from $9 per day in 1946, to $41 in 1965, then rising 600 percent in the next fifteen years, to $244 in 1980, $682 in 1990 and surpassing $1,000 in 1995.[10] Hospital costs have grown about 10 percent a year over the last fifty years. Even after adjusting for inflation, the increase in cost per day is still an astounding 1,500 percent from 1946 to 1995 (an average of 6% per year). By and large, the public has wanted the additional care and new technology, and is not displeased with the billions of dollars expended. However, after the passage of Medicare and Medicaid in 1965, costs became a problem for public policy for two reasons: (1) the influx of government money caused costs to rise much more rapidly than before, and (2) the costs were now being paid by the government (that is, taxpayers) rather than the mutually agreed-upon private transactions of individuals or employer-paid insurance, and thus caused state and federal budget deficits (see Table 9.6 and Figure 9.6).

In the immediate postwar period, the Hill-Burton Act of 1946 funded the building of more hospitals and the Health Professions Educational Assistance Act of 1963 increased the number of doctors. The early 1960s were boom years when it seemed that the economy could continue to grow robustly "forever," and it was this continuing desire to spend that enabled Congress to create Medicare and

TABLE 9.6   Hospital Costs per Patient Day, 1946–1995

Year	Cost Per Day	Cost Per Day (1995 $$)
1946	$ 9	$ 69
1950	14	92
1955	21	120
1960	29	147
1965	41	186
1970	74	274
1971	83	293
1972	95	318
1973	102	322
1974	113	329
1975	133	353
1976	152	380
1977	173	405
1978	194	420
1979	216	430
1980	244	445
1981	284	470
1982	327	509
1983	368	551
1984	410	587
1985	460	636
1986	499	672
1987	537	701
1988	581	730
1989	631	758
1990	682	786
1991	745	826
1992	816	881
1992	893	943
1994	968	1002
1995	1050	1050

Table 9.6: Hospital cost per adjusted patient day in nominal current dollars, and adjusted to 1995 dollars using the GDP deflator.

Sources: AHA Hospital Statistics, 1994, and HCIA. 1946–1960 and 1993–1995 adjustments extrapolated from data tables.

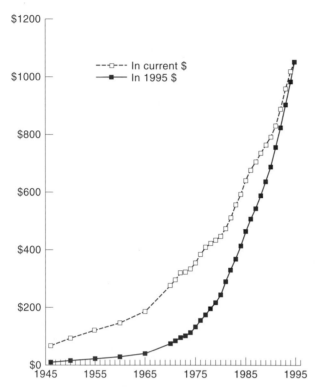

FIGURE 9.6 *Hospital Costs per patient day 1946–1995.*
Source: American Hospital Association, Hospital
Statistics, *various years.*

Medicaid as entitlement programs in 1965. However, by 1975 the U.S was trapped in a global recession, federal and state expenditures had escalated far beyond even the most outlandish budget projections, and the need for cost-cutting was clear. It was thought that the system efficiencies could be generated through better planning, and so a number of initiatives were funded to promote "regional medical programs" and create planning boards for oversight. Evaluations showing that planning alone could not affect costs, and the obvious excess capacity created by the Hill-Burton construction boom, led to the idea that a forced reduction in the growth of hospital beds could reduce the rate of growth in hospital costs.

Certificate-of-need (CON) legislation required that a planning body do a study and approve any capital project that would increase the number of hospital beds in the region.[11] In a path-breaking study of the economics of hospital regulation, David Salkever and Thomas Bice showed that although CON legislation reduced the number of new beds built, hospitals increased the amount of capital equipment for each bed, so that capital spending continued to rise at the same rate.[12] In discussing their findings, Salkever and Bice argued that *CON regulation is like pushing on a balloon;* forcing costs down in one dimension just caused them to bulge out in another dimension. Similar dynamics have been demonstrated in other studies of many different regulatory initiatives over the years; the type of cost subject to regulation declines, but any savings are canceled out by an overflow in another area, so that total health care costs are unchanged. An unintended side-effect of CON and most other regulations is that they create barriers making it harder for new organizations to enter the market, thus protecting existing hospitals and retarding the evolution of the health care system toward more efficient configurations. Studies of CON in operation confirmed the economists' version of the golden rule ("them that has the gold makes the rules"): almost every well-established, wealthy and politically connected hospital that applied for certification eventually got it, while denials fell disproportionately on outsiders that threatened the status quo or weaker institutions that lacked a constituency. The death knell for CON came in the form of a Supreme Court ruling that discriminatory reimbursement of a hospital chain that refused to apply for a CON (which they knew would be denied because of opposition from existing local hospitals) constituted an illegal restraint of trade under antitrust laws and harmed consumers by restricting competition (see Table 9.7).

The attempt to impose controls over other dimensions moved on to utilization review (UR), a process that was to eliminate unnecessary surgery and other service by having a panel of doctors and nurses in a Professional Standards Review Organization (PSRO) review patients' charts to find cases of inappropriate care. The PSRO or other agency would then be empowered to order the doctor to change improper behavior and, failing that, to deny payment. In practice, the process proved cumbersome and ineffective, although the current managed care review, which does appear to work better (see chapter 10), developed from the experience with UR. Rapid inflation and an unwillingness to accept the lessons of history, led the Nixon administration to impose **price controls** in 1971. Although removed for most sectors of the economy in 1973, they were maintained in hospitals for an extra year. Rate-setting through **budgetary review** was a much more labor-intensive process, involving the line-by-line examination of spending plans. The most notable example was that for the state of Washington, which was passed in 1973 when a severe local recession crimped the state's ability to raise tax revenues, and lasted, albeit in weaker and weaker form, for ten years. Perhaps the most far-reaching cost-control regulation was the replacement of Medicare's open-ended system of retrospective cost-reimbursement by the **prospective payment system** (PPS) in 1984 to use diagnostically related groups **(DRGs)** for setting federally **administered prices** per discharge covering the entire patient stay. However, the demonstrable reductions in cost per inpatient admission were more than offset by rapid increases in outpatient charges, so that overall Medicare costs have continued to rise just as rapidly as before—another example of a regulation pushing on one side of the balloon.

**TABLE 9.7 Types of Regulation to
Control Hospital Costs**

Certificate of Need (CON)
Utilization Review (UR, PSRO)
Budgetary Review
Price Controls (ESPN)
Administered Prices (DRGs, PPS)

The experience with price controls, state rate regulation, and PPS is examined more carefully in chapter 18, showing that whatever successes might be attributed to cost-control regulation have been quite limited and short-lived.[13] The failure of this kind of government price regulation to control costs should not come as a surprise since the central difficulty in medical care transactions is the inability to specify what the product is. Special market adaptations, such as nonprofit status and the agency relationships between physicians and patients, are signals that any attempts to set prices or to quantify quality and other important attributes are likely to be exercises in futility. A government official sitting in the state capital, or Washington, D.C., is not going to be able to specify a detailed contract in advance to purchase something that the participants have trouble measuring even after the fact. It would be easy to cut spending on Medicare and Medicaid in a number of ways (set global budget caps, eliminate services, deny eligibility), except that there is not sufficient public consensus or political willpower to do so. Managed care and new regulations may bring some relief, but the macroeconomic cost pressures examined in chapters 14 to 18 will eventually force the public to face these hard choices, and force politicians to deal with the fallout.

SUGGESTIONS FOR FURTHER READING ___

Howard Berman and Louis Weeks, *The Financial Management of Hospitals,* 5th edition, Ann Arbor, Mich.: Health Administration Press, 1990.

Joskow, Paul, *Controlling Hospital Costs: The Role of Government Regulation,* Cambridge, Mass.: MIT Press, 1981.

SUMMARY ___

1. Managers plan to produce efficiently, so that any deviation from the plan (more or fewer patients, shifting wage rates) tends to increase average cost per unit, particularly in the short run. Since management can more fully adapt operations over the long run, the short-run average cost curve always lies at or above the long-run average cost curve. The primary way **managers control hospital costs is through the budget process**. Often extra capacity and flexibility is built in so that uncertainty and changes are not so difficult to deal with.

2. **Economies of scale** are said to exist when increasing the level of output causes average cost per unit to fall. Gains from the **specialization of labor and spreading the fixed costs of capital equipment** over more volume are the major factors creating economies of scale. **Diseconomies of scale**, with rising costs per unit eventually set in, are primarily due to the **difficulty of managing and coordinating ever larger operations**. Hospitals appear to show economies of scale up to a size of about 200 beds, and diseconomies of scale after reaching a size of about 500 beds. For simple services, rather small sizes appear to be relatively efficient, but only a large hospital has enough patients of a particular type (e.g., brain cancer) to run a specialized service at an effi-

cient volume. Thus, a hospital may be both too big to deliver some services efficiently, and too small to deliver others efficiently.

3. **Cost per day in the hospital varies for many reasons**; differences in quality and type of services offered, cost shifting to pay for research and teaching, billing practices, severity of patient illness, prices of labor and other inputs, and differences in productive efficiency. **Hospitals are multiproduct firms**, providing many different types of care, so that comparisons of cost per day or per case may not be very meaningful indicators of how efficiently a hospital is producing care.

4. **Accounting costs often do not measure true economic costs**. A larger-than-expected number of patients may make average costs appear lower, but actually the overcrowding and staff stress tend to increase costs. Patient time, pain, and worry are other costs that are often not counted.

5. **Technology** has tended to increase total spending in health care because generous insurance payments and cost reimbursement have given little incentive to develop cost-reducing techniques, or to give up a little quality for a large reduction in cost. An increase in capability to improve health will often make more spending worthwhile.

6. **Hospitals compete for physicians**, because it is physicians who control the flow of patients (and hence, revenues). Unlike most businesses, hospitals do not compete directly for "customers" because their customers (a) do not pay their own bills, and (b) do not make their own choices, but are directed by physicians who act as their agents. Only for some patient-initiated or relatively uninsured services is direct competition for patients important (plastic surgery, births). Larger scale and cost pressures are causing hospitals to compete for contracts, trying to attract employers, HMOs, or insurance companies directly; and to do so, they must now compete more and more on the basis of price rather than quality.

7. While able to switch cost from one part of health care to another (pushing on a balloon), **regulation** has not succeeded in controlling the overall cost of health care. Certificate-of-need (CON) regulation to control construction, and prospective payment systems (DRGs) to control prices, have forced hospitals to respond in a number of ways, but total spending has continued to soar. Government is responsible for most of a hospital's patients (66% of inpatient days are accounted for by Medicare and Medicaid), but is unable or unwilling to pay the price, forcing the health care system toward a crisis point. The cost shifting under which the rich cared for the poor, and the healthy contributed to pay for the sick, has begun to crack under the strain of unequal payments and a burgeoning federal deficit.

PROBLEMS _____

1. {*economies of scale*} What major factors create economies of scale in hospitals? Diseconomies of scale? Are most hospitals of optimal size, too small, or too large?

2. {*case-mix, cost shifting*} Why do university teaching hospitals cost so much more per day of care than local community hospitals?

3. {*economies of scale*} Misericordia hospital had a 20 percent increase in admissions from 1990 to 1995. Total patient care costs went from $50 million to $61 million. Does Misericordia show evidence of economies of scale or diseconomies of scale? Might there be any other factors besides the number of admissions that would affect the costs of care?

4. {*economies of scale*} The number of patients at Harbordale Hospital's increased from 120 to 144 from Monday to Tuesday. The hospitals costs increased $720,000 to $722,000 as temp nurses were called in to deal with the heavy load. Does Harbordale Hospital show economies or diseconomies of scale? Which hospital is better managed for cost control, Harbordale or Misericordia (in problem 3)? Which is more costly, short-run adjustment between Monday and Tuesday, or long-run adjustment between 1990 and 1995?

5. {*marginal cost, accounting*} What is the cost of an extra admission to a hospital? Does it make a difference if it is an emergency service or scheduled in advance? Who bears the costs of an additional emergency admissions? Is there any difference in who bears the cost of a 50 percent increase in ER admission in the short-run and the long-run?

6. {*compensation*} Should hospital managers be rewarded for dealing with random fluctuations in demand, or for dealing with planned changes in demand?

7. {*efficiency, case-mix*} Costs per day are usually lower in community hospitals than in university hospitals. Does this mean that transferring patients from university hospitals to community hospitals would increase efficiency?

8. {*substitution*} Why do people spend so long waiting to be treated in the emergency room? Would it be more efficient if there were sufficient doctors available so that they could be treated right away?

9. {*economies of scale, discrimination*} Many rural counties have fewer hospital beds than urban and suburban counties, even when there are relatively more accidents and injuries for which immediate access to care is crucial. Does this disparity indicate systematic discrimination against rural counties?

10. {*transactions costs*} Why would a hospital that just expanded its home health care agency so as to service the patients of other hospitals in the region close down its clinical laboratory and purchase those services from a neighboring hospital?

11. {*quality*} Why have quality improvements in health care caused costs to rise while quality improvements in health care have caused costs to fall?

12. {*competition*} Wills Eye hospital in Philadelphia is a 114-bed hospital specializing in ophthalmologic surgery. Who do you think competes with Wills Eye?

13. {*competition*} Describe the factors that you would expect to be most important in competition for each of the following services. For which is price more important? location? quality? Would hospitals compete for patients or for doctors?

   a. heart transplants

   b. maternity

   c. immunization

   d. depression

   e. chemotherapy

   f. plastic surgery

   g. AIDS

14. {*technological change*} Automation has vastly increased the efficiency and accuracy of laboratory testing. The cost per test has fallen by more than 75 percent in many cases. Do you think that the cost of laboratory testing has fallen by more or less than 75 percent? Why?

15. {*price controls*} What would you expect to be the effect of a set of regulations limiting hospital revenues to an increase of 1 percent a year on the following?

   a. number of nurses hired

   b. number of doctors

   c. quality of care

   d. advertising budgets

   e. emergency room staffing

   f. new construction

   g. depreciation

   Would there be a difference if the regulation applied to just one hospital rather than all hospitals? Would there be a difference between short-run and long-run effects?

16. {*regulation*} CON regulations effectively limit the number of new hospital beds constructed in a region. Who would favor CON? Who would be against CON? When hospitals in a state with CON regulation renovate old buildings, would you expect the cost per bed to be more or less than in a state without CON regulation?

ENDNOTES _____

1. E. R. Becker and B. Steinwald, "The Determinants of Hospital Case-Mix Complexity," *Health Services Research* 16(4):439–458, 1981.
2. Frank Sloan, Roger Feldman, and Bruce Steinwald, "The Effects of Teaching on Hospital Costs," *Journal of Health Economics*, 2(1):1–28.
3. Howard Berman and Louis Weeks, *The Financial Management of Hospitals*, 5th edition, Ann Arbor, Mich.: Health Administration Press, 1990.
4. T. W. Granneman, R. S. Brown, and M. V. Pauly, "Estimating Hospital Costs: A Multiple-Output Analysis," *Journal of Health Economics*, 5(2):107–127, 1986; T. G. Cowing, A. G. Holtman, and S. Powers, "Hospital Cost Analysis: A Survey and Evaluation of Recent Studies," *Advances in Health Economics and Health Services Research*, 4:257–303, 1983.
5. Mark Pauly and Michael Redisch, "The Not-for-profit Hospital as a Physicians Cooperative," *American Economic Review*, 63:87–99, 1973.
6. Mark V. Pauly, *The Doctor's Workshop*, Philadelphia: University of Pennsylvania Press, 1980.
7. H. Luft, J. Robinson, D. Garnick, S. Maerki, and S. McPhee, "The Role of Specialized Clinical Services in the Competition Among Hospitals," *Inquiry*, 23(1):83–94, 1986.

8. Carson W. Bays, "The Determinants of Hospital Size: A Survivor Analysis," *Applied Economics*, 18:359–377, 1986.

9. Robert Sigmond and J. David Seay, "Community Benefit Standards for Hospitals: Perception and Performance," *Frontiers of Health Services Management*, Spring 1989.

10. American Hospital Association, *Hospital Statistics*, Chicago: American Hospital Association, various years.

11. CON, UR, PSROs, DRGs, and other regulations have all taken many different forms in different state or national programs over time. The brief discussion here refers to general conclusions about that type of regulation, rather than any particular specific program. The interested reader should consult one of the many comprehensive reviews that have been written, such as those in Paul Joskow, *Controlling Hospital Costs: The Role of Government Regulation*, Cambridge, Mass.: MIT Press, 1981; D. Abernathy and D. A. Pearson, *Regulating Hospital Costs: The Development of Public Policy*, Ann Arbor, Mich.: Health Administration Press, 1979; or the relevant chapters of Michael Rosko and Robert W. Broyles, *The Economics of Health Care: A Reference Handbook*, New York: Greenwood Press, 1988; or Sherman Folland, Allen Goodman and Miron Stano, *The Economics of Health and Health Care*, New York: Macmillan, 1993.

12. David Salkever and Thomas Bice, *Hospital Certificate-of-Need Controls: Impact on Investment, Costs and Use*, Washington, D.C.: American Enterprise Institute, 1979.

13. David Dranove and Kenneth Cone, "Do State Rate-Setting Regulations Really Lower Hospital Expenses?" *Journal of Health Economics*, 4:159–165, 1985; C. L. Eby and D. Cohodes, "What Do We Know About Rate-Setting?" *Journal of Health Politics, Policy and Law*, 10(2):299–327, 1985.

CHAPTER **10**

Managed Care

QUESTIONS

1. *What flaw in the U.S. health care system forced the development of managed care?*
2. *Does managed care reduce individual risks, or reduce system-wide average risks?*
3. *How do HMOs use financial contracts to align the interests of patients and doctors?*
4. *Did kickbacks and other fraud cause government to rely on capitation rather than fee-for-service?*
5. *Why do HMOs carve out or sub-capitate mental health and other special services?*
6. *Does capitation payment shift the risks of paying for ill health to hospitals?*
7. *Is a physician "gatekeeper" working for or against the patient?*
8. *How much profit can an HMO make? At whose expense?*

10.1 WHY *MANAGED* CARE? _____

Open or Closed Funding?

Funding for health care can be open-ended, dependent upon the separate decisions of many individuals and firms and expanding if demand increases, or closed, with a fixed total budget, usually set by the government. Most health care funding in the United States has traditionally been in the open-ended form of personal payments or indemnity insurance that paid fee-for-service bills (chapter 3). However, certain parts of the health care system have had closed-end budgets: immunization programs, city health clinics, Veterans Administration hospitals, and state mental hospitals, for example. When excess demands are placed on these closed-ended components with a fixed budget, the system cannot cope, and people are unhappy. In open-ended systems, if there are excess demands, either the insurance pool runs a deficit, or the individuals must reduce other consumption to pay medical bills.[1] For government insurance programs such as Medicare and Medicaid, excess demand means that money has to be obtained by raising taxes, diverting spending from other programs, or (temporarily) running a deficit.

It is possible to run the entire health sector as a closed-ended organization with a fixed budget. The National Health Service (NHS) in the United Kingdom is a notable example.[2] The different components common to all health care systems are shown in Figure 10.1: government, payers, insurers, providers and patients. In an indemnity fee-for-service system, all of these components are relatively distinct, as shown here. Government sets the rules, payers (usually employers) pick up the bills, providers (physicians, hospitals) decide what services to offer and how much to charge, and patients (along with their physicians) decide what service to use—and ultimately end up paying for the system through their wage contributions, taxes, copayments, and so on. Figure 10.2a shows that the National Health Service has the same components in a different configuration—government, payer, insurer, and providers are all one organization, the NHS. Other configurations are possible as well. Figure 10.2b shows an ASO self-insured employer, where the payer and insurer roles are combined. Figure 10.2c depicts Medicare, where the U.S. government takes on the roles of both payer and insurer. Figure 10.2d shows the role of HMOs. In each case, the same components are present, but the configuration differs.

Traditional corporate health insurance for employees, Medicare, and Medicaid, were all open-ended **entitlement** systems. The patient was entitled to some specified set of services and the payer had to cover the cost, regardless of how many services of each type were used. Insurance companies did not care about the size of the bill, since they were merely third-party intermediaries, raising premiums to match the rise in the cost of services. Patients had little incentive to moderate utilization, since services were being paid for with "other peoples' money" (taxes, insurance, employer's reserves). Providers had even less incentive to hold the line on costs, since larger total insurance reimbursements implied larger total payments to providers. Indemnity fee-for-service insurance has been the least restrictive form of payment, allowing providers to choose whatever expensive new technology they thought was appropriate, and then set charges at a level sufficient to cover the escalating cost. The end result was evident in Figure 9.6 of the previous

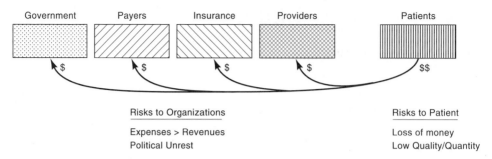

FIGURE 10.1   *Schematic Diagram of the Health Care System*

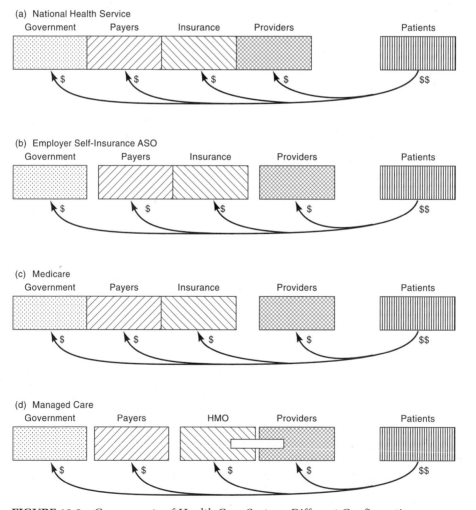

FIGURE 10.2   *Components of Health Care System: Different Configurations*

OPEN-ENDED ENTITLEMENT FUNDING

Patients	Providers	Insurance	Short-Run *Problems*	Long-Run *Problems*
Demand care	Produce services	Pays bills *(all risks are here and purely financial)*	Variability in costs	Costs escalate uncontrollably

CLOSED-END BUDGET FUNDING

Government	Providers	Patients	Short-Run *Problems*	Long-Run *Problems*
Allocates budget *(no financial risk—political unrest)*	Produce services *(consumer complaints)*	Receive care *(quality/ quantity risk)*	government blamed for everything	stagnant, unresponsive system since customers carry no $$

FIGURE 10.3   *Comparison of Open-Ended and Closed-Ended Health Care Financing*

chapter, which showed how hospital costs per day had soared out of control between 1945 and 1995 (see Figure 10.3).

Costs and Quality

In a system characterized by the lack of financial restraints, it is not surprising that by 1995 the United States was spending far more on health care than any other country in the world (chapter 19); the surprise was how little *health* the nation was able to buy with all the extra money. Despite years of insistence by politicians and physicians that the United States had the best medical care in the world, there is scant evidence that the additional expenditures led to improvements in longevity, infant mortality, morbidity, or days lost from work, relative to other countries spending less than half as much per person.[3] What has become apparent is that the real inflation-adjusted hourly wages of workers has stagnated, and even declined, while the implicit cost per hour of employer-provided health benefits has soared, and that the federal government has been dragged down by billions of dollars in deficits attributable to the soaring cost of Medicare benefits. The explosive increase in costs over the last twenty years has become the primary motivation for managing care. The nation has searched for an organizational format that would add the missing elements of planning, coordination, and control to the health care system in order to improve efficiency and limit total expenditures—and managed care is the evolving result of this search.

"Global budgeting" and other closed-ended financing systems used in the United Kingdom, Germany, Canada, and elsewhere are not without problems of their own, of course. A fixed level of funding eliminates the risk of financial loses, but the patients who are supposed to receive care may be turned away when the system is full, or accommodated only by overcrowding and the poor quality of services that is the inevitable result of stretching a budget thin to cover too many people with too many illnesses. There is an inherent trade-off between financial losses and service losses (Figure 10.3). Returning to the schematic diagrams of Figures 10.1 and 10.2a-d, it is easy to envision how deficits can be shuffled from one box to the other, but remain within the system, and so eventually shows up at one end or the other. The designer of a health care system can choose to have all the problems show up as financial deficits, or to have all the problems show up as service deficits, or try to obtain some balance—but the problems do not disappear. The wave of health care reforms that began in most countries during the 1980s appears certain to continue well past the year 2000, suggesting that neither escalating cost nor deteriorating service are satisfactory.[4] Success cannot be obtained by temporary measures that shuffle problems and unpaid bills from one pocket to another. Managed care is an attempt to solve some of the problems of the health care system by harnessing economic incentives to increase the efficiency of the system as a whole, thus providing better care for less money.

Individual and System Risks in Health Care

It is important to distinguish between the variation in individual costs, and variation in system costs. The variation between individuals with regard to medical costs is very large, more than a thousand to one. A fair number have minimal costs, while some unfortunate few would face bills of hundreds of thousands of dollars in the absence of health insurance. However, by placing everyone into a single insurance pool, individual risk is diversified away: each person can cover their expected losses by paying a modest premium in advance. A group of 10,000 people has reasonably predictable health care costs, and a group of 100,000 has negligible variation in average costs due to the random variation among the individuals that make up the group. To an individual even substantial differences in average costs mean very little. For two people worried about medical care bills, it is the one who gets most ill who will spend more, not the one who belongs to the more expensive health care system. On the other hand, at the aggregate level, random individual variation averages out and it is the systematic differences that dominate. Comparisons between small areas within the United States (see section 7.5) and between countries (chapter 19) reveal major differences in the average level of spending that are not explainable by differences in health status or random variation (Figure 10.4). Managed care seeks to capitalize on these systematic differences in the average level of health care costs between groups.[5] Whereas an insurer pools risks so that the individual can cover losses with an actuarially fair premium equal to the average, *the managed care organization seeks to reduce the average.* Since it deals in large groups, the **managed care organization (MCO)** must take on the function of an insurer as it tries to reduce costs, but those insurance

Cost Variability = Health Variability   +   Resource Use Variability
                          (individual 1,000 : 1)   5 : 1 between small areas
                          (group = diversified away)   (Wennberg)
                                                            4 : 1 between Countries
                                                            (OECD comparisons)

FIGURE 10.4   *Risks in Health Care*

functions are, in a sense, incidental to the central purpose of managing care: controlling costs while maintaining quality.

Management: The Distinctive Feature of Managed Care

The fundamental difference between traditional medical practice and managed care is that *a manager* intervenes to monitor and control the transaction between doctor and patient (Figure 10.5). An outside party, such as the plan medical director, a trained utilization review nurse, or a software program, will identify episodes of care that are potentially at variance with accepted clinical practice. This may be done through a statistical profile of each physician's practice, assessment of laboratory testing, or review of individual cases. The manager examines the process of care and controls the flow of funds, facilitating payments in some circumstances and holding back in others. Since the MCO takes financial responsibility for medical care, it has an incentive to provide care efficiently. In order to remain viable, it must compete on the basis of both quality and cost. A delicate balance must be maintained between expenditure control, administrative process, and medical uncertainty.

Managed care organizations are contractual intermediaries composed of contracts with the enrollees (or their employers or government programs) on one side, and contracts with providers to provide care on the other side. These linkages (and barriers) between the components of the health care system were depicted schematically in Figure 10.2d. The most prevalent and well-known form of MCO is an **HMO, or health maintenance organization.** HMOs receive a fixed payment in advance for all medical care received by a group and thus bear financial risk, but differ from traditional health insurance in the following ways. On the *demand side,* the contract between the managed care plan and the enrollees imposes some limits and responsibilities on enrollees: they can only receive care from specified hospitals and physicians, must use specified pharmacies and therapists, fill out forms, telephone for approval, and work with the system in many other ways in order to access their health care. In effect, patients do some of the work of management. The benefit to patients of all this effort and submission to administrative procedures comes from not having to pay any doctor or hospital bills or deal with any paperwork after treatment. Traditional health insurance pays bills with no questions asked, but costs more, often requires extensive recordkeeping, and may require months to finish settling claims. On the *supply*

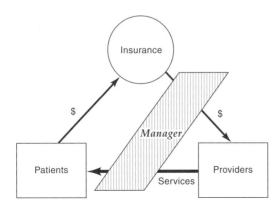

FIGURE 10.5 *Flow of Funds with Managed Care*

side, the managed care plan must contract with a sufficient number of physicians, hospitals, and so on to create a **provider network** that the patient can access for all necessary care. Often a single "gatekeeper" physician is in charge of the care provided by hospitals and other physicians, and bears some financial responsibility for controlling the total cost of care. When negotiating provider contracts, it is usual for an HMO to ask for discounts, projected or guaranteed expenditure limits, statistical utilization and quality reports, and guarantees of service (i.e., appointment within 3 days, full pharmacy line, etc.). None of this management supervision occurs in a traditional indemnity plan, where the insurer pays the bill but may have no other contact with the physician, and no rights of control, reporting, or approval.

10.2 THE RANGE OF MANAGED CARE PLANS

The variety and possible configurations of managed care are too diverse for any single definition. It is better to think in terms of a range from unmanaged fee-for-service to tightly managed, closed-staff health maintenance organizations, as diagrammed in Figure 10.6. The least constrained form of financing is **indemnity** fee-for-service (FFS) medicine. With pure indemnity insurance, the health plan plays a totally passive role. Whatever hospitalization, surgery, or drugs any physician decides to order are paid for by the insurance company without question. The only "control" comes from making the patient pay for some deductibles and coinsurance. Insurance can be made slightly more restrictive by **utilization review** (UR), evaluating the decisions made by the physician before the insurance company makes payment. Common UR procedures include:

- **Second opinion**—a second doctor must review the record and concur with the initial doctor's recommendation before surgery is performed.

- **Precertification**—obtaining approval in advance from the insurance company before elective surgery is performed.

- **Pre-admission testing**—a requirement that many tests be performed in advance on an outpatient basis so that the patient spends fewer days in the hospital.

- **Concurrent review**—regular evaluations by a case control nurse to authorize continued stay in the hospital or additional procedures.

- **Database profiling**—maintaining graphs and charts indicating the number of services used per 1,000 patients by each doctor or hospital to identify abnormally high or low patterns of utilization.

- **Intensive case management**—having a nurse in the insurance company individually follow and manage any case expected to cost more than $10,000.

Indemnity FFS — UR — PPO — Open HMO — Closed HMO
(no management controls) (tight management controls)

FIGURE 10.6 *The Range of Managed Care Plans*

- **Generic substitution**—a prescription for a brand-name drug is filled with a cheaper generic version if the two are biologically equivalent.
- **Discharge planning**—having a social worker meet with patient and family early on to facilitate rapid transfer back home or to a nursing home.
- **Retrospective review**—evaluation after discharge from the hospital to deny payment for any medically unnecessary services.
- **Audits**—making sure that all services billed for were actually performed.

A **Preferred Provider Organization (PPO)** limits the patient's choice of physicians and hospitals by paying in full only for care received from a **network**, an approved list of providers with whom the PPO has a contract. Patients obtaining care outside the network have to pay a significantly larger deductible and coinsurance rate (See Table 10.1). Often a health plan will establish a **pharmacy formulary**, a list of approved drugs that will be paid for, while drugs not on the list are not reimbursed. PPO plans also use UR to control utilization. The ability to steer patients to a specific group of hospitals, physicians, or pharmaceutical companies gives the PPO considerable buying power, and thus the ability to negotiate discounts. The providers are willing to accept a lower price in order to get a larger volume. Discounts and use of UR techniques allow PPOs to give patients a better benefit package at a lower premium than is possible with unmanaged FFS, while allowing more flexibility than in a fully managed HMO. In a PPO, patients can choose to see a specialist outside the plan, or to stay in a particular hospital that is not part of the preferred group, if they are willing to pay a larger portion of the bill out-of-pocket.

HMOs exert much tighter control over utilization. Since the less restrictive UR and PPO plans may be viewed as halfway steps, many commentators do not include them within their definition of "real" managed care. Two things mark the transition from partially managed care to HMOs: (1) mandatory authorization for hospitalization and (2) primary physicians who act as gatekeepers. Mandatory authorization means that the physician must get on the phone to the health plan and explain why the patient needs hospitalization and document the severity of illness to obtain approval before admitting any patient. Whereas UR precertification is usually applied only for elective surgery, in most HMOs every hospitalization or surgery must be precertified. Under a **gatekeeper** system, patients must receive all of their primary care from a single physician, and any specialty referrals, surgery, drug prescriptions, or hospitalizations must be approved in advance by that gate-

TABLE 10.1   Hypothetical PPO Payment

	Within Network	Outside Provider
Hospital	100%	80%
Physician	90%	75%
Therapist	90%	50%
Pharmacies	no copay	$10 copay
Drugs		
in formulary	covered	50%
not in formulary	not covered	not covered

keeper primary physician. The gatekeeper physician is commonly paid a **capitation rate**, a fixed amount per member per month (PMPM) (currently about $20–$40) for each person enrolled with them. They must provide all primary care for that person, and also act as a manager by coordinating and approving all other services. The gatekeeper primary physician will refer the patient needing additional treatment to a specialist physician, group practice, therapy center, or other provider who has a contract with the HMO. Referral services are usually paid for on a fee schedule using RBRVS relative values (see section 5.1), discounted FFS, or a negotiated rate for a service package (e.g., cesarean section or heart transplant). In this way the HMO is able to control the process of care and obtain price discounts. Only in unusual cases (e.g., emergency trauma, treatment of very rare diseases) will the HMO use noncontractual physicians or pay open market fee-for-service prices. Hospitals are most commonly paid per diem, but may have FFS or negotiated contracts as well.[6]

The health plan will often **withhold** some fraction of all payments, perhaps 20 percent, until the end of the year, and then distribute these held-back reserves only if utilization stays below the budgeted amount. This gives the primary and referral physicians some incentive to control utilization. The capitated primary physicians may also qualify for an end-of-year bonus tied to quality, patient satisfaction, and control over the cost of referral services (a more detailed description and analysis of withholds, capitation rates, and other payment mechanisms is given in sections 10.4 and 10.6).

In an **open HMO**, the physicians may have contracts with several other HMOs, and may see private fee-for-service patients as well. The physicians and hospitals are independent contractors, and such HMO plans are often termed *independent practice associations,* or **IPA HMOs.** In a **closed HMO** (often called a *group HMO* or *staff HMO*), the physicians do not see outside patients and in effect work as employees of the HMO. The premier example of a closed HMO is the Kaiser Permanente Health Plan, with its 6 million members (see chapter 11 for a more detailed description of the evolution of the Kaiser health plan). Kaiser owns its own hospitals, used exclusively by Kaiser patients. Closed HMOs provide the greatest degree of managerial control, because everything—physicians, hospitals, therapists, clinics—is all part of a single unified organization. The lack of exclusivity in open HMOs means weaker management control, but also allows a much wider choice of physicians for patients (since the physician do not see outside patients and in an IPA HMO can belong to several other HMOs and have FFS private practice, also). A closed HMO also has more difficulty accommodating growth, since it must hire and train new physicians to do so, while an open HMO must merely sign contracts or send more patients to those physicians with whom they have already contracted.

In order to create an HMO, the first thing an organization must do is negotiate contracts with doctors, hospitals, therapists, laboratories, and so on to build a **provider network** from which the enrollees will receive care. Then the HMO must meet certain regulatory obligations to assure financial solvency, provide quality control, and maintain records for reporting to the state so that it can obtain an HMO license to operate. Only after building a network and meeting state regulatory obligations can an HMO market its services, approaching various firms to try and have them include the new HMO among their employee benefit options. Occasionally the HMO can become the exclusive provider of medical care to the group, but in order to do so must usually include some out-of-plan coverage, so that it becomes a sort of a PPO/HMO hybrid. Some HMOs offer a **point-of-service** option (POS), where the patient is fully covered within the HMO network, and has lesser coverage from physicians and hospitals outside the network. In order to provide a full line of coverage to all employees, most large insurers now offer a **triple-option** in which the employee can choose an HMO, a PPO, or traditional unrestricted indemnity fee-for-service insurance. Since the HMO offers the most control over utilization, its premiums are the lowest; the PPO is intermediate, and the uncontrolled indemnity plan is most expensive.

10.3 SOURCES AND USES OF FUNDS _____

Managed care has been developed in the private sector, and primarily serves corporate employee benefit plans. Although two-thirds of hospital days, and two-fifths of all national health expenditures, are paid for through government programs, only about a tenth of HMO enrollees are publicly funded (see Table 10.2).[7] Around 60 million persons, approximately 20 percent of the employed work force and their dependents, received medical care through HMOs in 1995, paying total premiums of more than $60 billion. Of the 546 HMOs in operation, the nonprofit, closed-group Kaiser Health Plan, with 6 million enrollees, was the largest. But most enrollees were in commercial for-profit, open IPA HMOs. The largest of these firms in 1995 were United HealthCare, CIGNA Health Plan, and U.S. Healthcare, each with more than 2 million persons enrolled (see chapter 11).

Most HMOs take 15 to 20 percent of the premiums they receive for administration, marketing, and profit. The bulk of the funds are used to pay medical expenses (see Table 10.3 and Figure 10.7), and this fraction is known as the "medical loss ratio." The largest expense category is physician services. Although hospitals are the largest expenditure item in the National Health Expenditure accounts, HMOs' tight controls over hospitals, and coverage of a generally younger and healthier population, means that a less than a third of HMO premiums are used to pay for inpatient hospital services. Some of the HMOs' other expenses are reinsurance (to keep the plan solvent and ensure that patients' bills are paid even if the plan should have a catastrophic loss), taxes, emergency out-of-area services, and certain highly specialized treatments that must be paid for on a fee-for-service basis to noncontracted providers. Over time, the HMO business has become much more price-competitive. Administrative expenses and profit margins have been

TABLE 10.2   HMO Enrollment by Payer

Employee benefit plans	89%
Medicare	6%
Medicaid	5%

Source: Hoechst Marion Roussel *Managed Care Digest 1995*

(note: percentages are based on numbers of enrollees, not premiums).

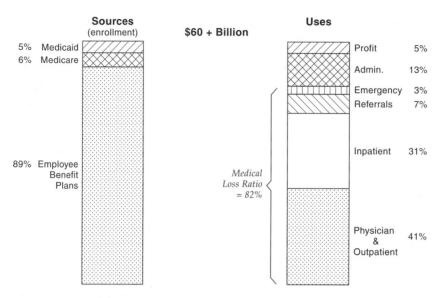

FIGURE 10.7   *HMO Sources & Uses of Funds, 1994*

TABLE 10.3   HMO Expenses as a % of Total Premiums

Physician and outpatient	41%	
Inpatient	31%	"Medical Loss
Outside referrals	7%	Ratio" = 82%
Emergency	3%	
Administrative	13%	
Profit	5%	

Source: Hoechst Marion Roussel *Managed Care Digest 1995*

cut as plans become more efficient, and so the percentage of total dollars going to treatment (the **medical loss ratio**) has risen. In earlier years, wide variations of ±25 percent were not uncommon. With more experience and better information, competitive standards have been set so that most HMOs will offer a similar price (perhaps ±10%) for most benefit packages (see Table 10.3).

10.4 CONTROLLING COSTS: CAPITATION, GATEKEEPERS, AND "WITHHOLDS" _____

Capitation

A distinctive feature of managed care is payment by **capitation**, a fixed dollar amount "per capita," usually specified as "per member per month" (PMPM). Paying for the number of persons enrolled rather than the number of services rendered changes the economic incentives from "doing more" (FFS) to "doing less" (capitation). With fixed payments per member made in advance, profits are greater when fewer services are used. What, then, keeps the HMO from doing less and less until it maximizes profits by providing no services at all? Quite simply, the need to attract new members and keep the old ones. Competition and the potential loss of enrollment makes HMOs strive to maintain quality and patient satisfaction. In FFS, profits increase as more is done. What keeps a surgeon from operating over and over again in order to make more money? Control over excessive surgery under FFS is largely a matter of professional ethics and disapproval by peers, since there is no external reporting or manager who intervenes to question the appropriateness of treatment.

Both FFS and capitation have incentives that are potentially harmful to the interests of patients. What differs is the locus of control. In an HMO, much of that control is placed with management and the development of information systems to track average recovery rates, readmission likelihood, number of complaints, average laboratory results, and so on. With FFS, control remains largely implicit, and in the hands of the individual physician. This difference in the way control is exercised explains why corporate benefit managers, public health advisors, and others used to dealing with medical care as a system and responsible for large numbers of people, are usually more comfortable with managed care. Conversely, physicians, who are used to taking individual responsibility for their own patients but not worrying about the system as a whole, are more comfortable with FFS. The reason that managed care has taken a rapidly increasing share of the market in the 1990s is that although most Americans are happy with their individual medical care, they are unhappy with the system, and overwhelmed by the uncontrolled increase in costs that indemnity FFS tends to foster.

The simplified discussions that take place in political arguments (or economics textbooks) tend to focus on the pros and cons of specific contract features taken separately. Yet in practice, it is how the system works as a whole that is relevant to the market. The informal understandings are often more important than the legal contract language. On paper, an FFS system with indemnity insurance is implausible, since it provides incentives for doctors to increase bills and utilization indefinitely; in practice, such a system worked fairly well for thirty years. On paper, capitation appears to make an HMO want to take the money and run; in practice, HMOs have been the most progressive organizations in trying to make sure that patients' rate of recovery matches or exceeds expectations (which must be defined statistically at the group level) and to create measures designed to improve patient satisfaction.[8] Economists have the expertise to analyze the incentives created by specific contract provisions. As social scientists, it is also necessary for them to examine the real world to see how those contract incentives work when they are used as part of a complex health care system.

Gatekeepers

A patient enrolled in an HMO plan must go through a single physician "gatekeeper" for all of their care. In this way, the plan is able to delegate responsibility for cost control and appropriateness to that primary care physician (PCP). Some PCPs are paid on a FFS basis, but it is more common to use capitation.[9] Payment of a fixed dollar amount per month, regardless of the number or length of visits, provides a mixed incentive with regard to the amount of care. On one hand, since PCPs are not paid more for extra visits, they will tend to encourage the patient to make fewer appointments. On the other hand, a fixed monthly payment encourages the PCP to send the patient to a specialist rather than taking a lot of their own time in treating complex cases. A withhold system may be used to limit the overuse of referral services with financial incentives, but most of the control is actually exercised by management through the information system. The HMO will print out a report each month showing the presenting complaints and symptoms of patients, the number and types of referrals, the number of hospitalizations and medicines prescribed, and so on. If a particular physician seems too far from the norm, then a clinical manager from the HMO will review selected patient charts and call the PCP to discuss appropriateness of care.

Education and understanding are usually much better motivational tools than monetary rewards. Although such a statement might seem a bit surprising for an economics textbook, it is consistent with what most people experience on the job, where they work on salary, with periodic performance reviews and promotions to reward good work. Direct cash bonus payments are a relatively minor and infrequent form of incentive compensation. HMOs prefer to use a more flexible and adaptive human resources approach to achieve system efficiencies, using cash penalties and rewards only in extreme cases or situations where managers lack the detailed information necessary to promote cost-effective care.

Once a patient is deeply involved in the system (e.g., chemotherapy for cancer, rehabilitation for spinal injury) the PCP may no longer be the best gatekeeper. The control function may shift to the specialist who is in charge, to an "intensive case manager" who works from the HMO central office, or to a contracted firm that specializes in that specific type of care. Mental health, obstetrics, and physical therapy are distinct services that may be separated from the bulk of acute care medicine for special reporting, management, and control procedures, with their own distinctive payment mechanisms.

The gatekeeper PCP model is used effectively by most open HMOs. Closed-staff HMOs often use a more diffuse "gatekeeper triage" system, where patients first see a nurse practitioner or discuss their problem over the phone with clinic staff before coming in. Since the closed-staff model limits the patient to using only specialists, laboratories, and hospitals exclusively designed for HMO patients, there is less need to force all requests for care to go through the PCP gatekeeper.

Withholds

All HMOs must use FFS payment for some types of care, especially for specialty services where use by enrollees is rare and unpredictable. Withholds are a way of incorporating part of the cost-control incentive of capitation into FFS payment. An HMO specialty referral withhold plan might work as follows. Each specialist receives 80 percent of the agreed amount at the time the patient is treated. The other 20 percent goes into the withhold pool. The HMO has projected a total dollar expenditure for specialty referral services for the year. If the total of referral bills from all specialists is at or below that amount at the end of the year, then the withhold pool is distributed in accordance with the amounts billed. In this case, the specialist receives 100 percent of the amount billed, but had to wait until the end of the year to receive 20 percent of it. However, if the total billings are more than 20 percent above the projected total, then the HMO keeps the withhold pool to help pay for the unanticipated extra volume. In this way, part of the risk of overutilization is shared with the specialists. If the total bills are more than 100 percent of the projected total, but less than 120 percent, then the specialists and the HMO split the withhold pool at the end of the year.

The withhold pool may cover all specialty services, just one type of specialty (e.g., thoracic surgery or allergy), or may sometimes be limited to a specific physician or medical group (in which case it becomes a modified FFS/capitation blend). It is also common to add or include other services, such as days in the hospital or laboratory tests, into the withhold pool. If the physicians contracting with the HMO hold down utilization of these services, then additional funds are available as a form of bonus payment.

Sub-Capitation and Carve-Outs

Whenever an HMO contracts with a separate organization to cover all of a certain type of care (laboratory testing, substance abuse, vision) for a fixed payment PMPM, it is said to have sub-capitated. A carve-out is a contract for a specific type of care, which is usually sub-capitated, but may be FFS or on some complex contractual blended payment formula. Since an HMO is in business to manage and accept the financial risks of providing care, why would it carve out or sub-capitate some portion of that care rather than doing the work itself? Carve-outs are done because separating out that distinctive type of care is more efficient than lumping it in with general medical services managed by the HMO. For example, mental health management requires special skills. Specialist firms become very adept at dealing with substance abuse, schizophrenia, and depression, and creating cost-effective specialty provider networks. The "make versus buy" decision for mental health and substance abuse so clearly favors external production that virtually all HMOs use outside contractors for such services. Indeed, some medical HMOs will buy a managed mental health firm, but continue to operate it as a separate entity, a "company within a company" to keep the distinctive practices of mental health management separate.

10.5 HOW CARE IS "MANAGED"—A MENTAL HEALTH EXAMPLE _____

The actual process of managing care to control costs and improve quality must always be tailored to the situation at hand, and is thus different for each type of medical care. It may be markedly different for different patients, even if they have the same diagnosis. Care management, although grounded in rules and guidelines, is done by and for individuals. Preauthorization, concurrent review, profiling, withholds, and other methods recur in a variety of contexts during specific interactions between physicians, health plans, case managers, hospitals, and patients. To illustrate how care is managed, some typical procedures in *managed behavioral health* (MBH) managed care plans for mental health and substance abuse, are presented here and contrasted with FFS indemnity practice.[10]

An insured person might seek help for a behavioral problem by calling a specialist (usually a psychiatrist or psychologist), or might have a behavioral problem noted during a medical visit ("Gee, Mr. X, as your doctor I would like to suggest that having five drinks after dinner every night may have something to do with your chronic fatigue and stomach pains"), but often the problem is not treated until it erupts and requires emergency attention (nervous breakdown, paranoid threats or abuse of family members, arrest for driving under the influence, etc.). Unfortunately, the closest hospital emergency room is usually not the best place for drug detoxification or treatment of a psychotic breakdown. Moral hazard and other difficulties in controlling the costs of mental health services led indemnity insurers to limit coverage, usually requiring patients to pay 50 percent coinsurance for outpatient (instead of the usual 10% to 20%) and placing separate limits on the number of inpatient days covered. Yet the costs for behavioral conditions continued to rise explosively throughout the 1980s. Payment limits alone still gave providers incentives to increase the number of treatments without limit, and did not create any mechanism for establishing overall fiscal responsibility.

Managed behavioral health (MBH) differs from FFS in the way that care is initiated when the patient first enters the health care system. Since behavioral health services are carved out from medical HMO benefits, MBH serves as the gatekeeper, not the primary care physician. Usually the MBH will establish an "employee assistance program" (EAP) to try and intervene before problems become emergencies. Workers with signs of depression or substance abuse may be referred to an EAP counselor, or they or their family members can call a confidential toll-free number to access services. If symptoms are first noted during a medical visit, the primary physician will refer the patient on to the MBH. After a call to the EAP or referral by a primary care physician, the patient will be scheduled for an evaluation to discuss his or her problem and treatment options with a trained counselor. An evaluation is conducted by trained counselors (CAC, MSW, PhD or MD) employed by the MBH, or a psych/substance abuse group practice doing evaluations under contract. Evaluations are usually done within 72 hours, with immediate arrangements made for placement in the appropriate form of therapy. Corporate employers benefit from EAPs, since earlier treatment helps to maintain the productivity of the work force. Sometimes people realize they have a drug problem, but are reluctant to enter treatment because of the stigma that alcoholism and drug addiction still carries, and out of worry regarding loss of wages. Waiting until the addicted worker acts out or has an accident means costly ($20,000 or more) inpatient drug rehabilitation under traditional indemnity insurance. The MBH evaluator can often place workers with addiction in less costly and confining intensive outpatient programs (four hours of therapy each night, close supervision, etc.) or halfway houses that allow people to continue to work while being rehabilitated, which are less disruptive to personal and family life, and tend to decrease the chance of relapse.

Many times an FFS physician with a patient displaying behavioral distress will suspect that substance abuse is a primary or contributing factor. Yet because the patient is in denial, or is afraid of stigmatization, the physician will continue treatment using some nondescriptive diagnosis (stomach pain, anxiety), or make a referral to a psychiatrist. This leads to costly and ineffective treatment. Talking with a psychiatrist while under the influence of drugs is just a way to waste $125 an hour. The trained MBH evaluator will recognize the symptoms and send the patient for cost-effective drug-abuse treatment (from a CAC-certified counselor at

$30 a visit) and rehabilitation first, and then on to psychological services once the patient is drug free and can benefit. In severe cases, the counselor will make a referral directly to residential programs that specialize in "dual-diagnosis" (i.e, mental illness with substance abuse) treatment. The coordinated treatment of mental health and substance abuse in MBH illustrates two principles: substitution (use the less expensive mode of treatment) and appropriateness (reduce length of treatment by more precise matching of services to patient's actual problems). Substitution and appropriateness are primary methods used by managed care to achieve cost reductions.

Negotiating for lower prices through selective contracting is another important way for managed care firms to reduce costs. Most working patients want to be seen at night or on weekends, while most therapists in private practice are overburdened during those hours. The MBH can contract with therapists who wish to work part-time (many of whom are employed during the day at salaried jobs in the mental health field) for $30 per session, while the FFS insurer would have to pay a therapist in private practice $60. Private-practice therapists have to charge more while netting less because they have to cover office overhead, secretarial services, and put up with erratic patient flow and missed appointments on an inefficient scale as solo practitioners. The MBH firm provides a suite of offices and guaranteed patient flow, so that their contractors can take home the full $30 paid. Hospitals, halfway houses, and other facilities are also willing to accept discounts from FFS rates in order to obtain a steady volume. Bulk contracting allows the MBH to insist on uniform reporting formats to better monitor the quality of care. Building a provider network by negotiating standard contractual agreements with hospitals, psych groups, and so on, is a crucial task for determining the efficiency of the managed care plan. With a network in place, the MBH can create statistical profiles to determine which therapists tend to take longer to complete treatment, or whose patients are most likely to be readmitted or suffer other problems. **Profiling** most clearly illustrates the difference between managed care and FFS approaches to quality. In managed care, quality is defined by the experience of the group, on how well most patients do relative to what can be expected. Only a large plan with a comprehensive and uniform information system can do the profiling necessary to measure quality in this way. While the individual examination of a single FFS case might appear more detailed, it is methodologically flawed because it lacks a standard and is subject to random variation. Consider how foolish it would be to assert that skydiving is safer than walking just because I survived 10 parachute jumps while my friend got killed the first time he went for a hike. Thinking in terms of the group and making comparisons to a standard based on large numbers of cases are the basic tools that make quality assurance under managed care more effective than individualistic efforts under FFS.

Managed care has made great strides in rationalizing the process of care, reducing the number of days spent in the hospital, and making better use of ambulatory services. In behavioral health, large and cost-effective improvements have been made in the treatment of emergency inpatient admissions. Under FFS, an emergency psychiatric patient will often be admitted for an inpatient stay at the receiving hospital. Since emergencies are often taken to inner-city hospitals, this may well be a research-oriented university facility geared to complex cases, costing more than $1,000 a day, and where the clinical professors have little interest in treating one more routine "crazy drunk." A Friday-night admission to a psychiatric teaching service may mean heavy sedation and nothing but passive observation over the weekend, so that a definitive diagnosis does not get made until Monday or Tuesday. In contrast, receiving an HMO patient obligates the emergency room staff to contact the managed care plan before admission. The patient may be transported to a more appropriate facility costing only one-half or one-third as much per day, and a treatment plan including provisions for discharge and community services must be filed within twenty-four hours in order for the bills to be paid. Once admitted, the case manager will authorize an expected number of days for treatment in consultation with the attending physician. Then, every day, a telephone call will be made by the case manager to conduct **concurrent review**, checking on the patient's progress, seeing if additional days are needed or if early discharge is possible, and arranging for post-hospital group services and community support.

A relatively large proportion of mental health care costs are accounted for by a small number of patients (less than 1%) who require repeated hospitalizations. Previously, most of these severely and chronically mentally ill persons would have been placed in state mental hospitals, or cared for in the community with public funds. Several MBH companies have established **risk-sharing contracts** that protect them from severe adverse selection by using the state funds as a form of reinsurance. The MBH firm will be responsible for care up to some limit (e.g., first 3 admissions, 30 days, or $30,000), at which point the state becomes responsible for 90 percent of all additional costs.

Although managed behavioral health care has sharply reduced inpatient hospital days, it is common for the number of people receiving treatment to increase. Additional outpatients and EAP counseling represent an improvement in quality that benefits patients by improving their mental health, even though it may currently cost extra. Employers may receive some financial benefit from greater worker productivity, but for the most part they gain from increases in employee satisfaction. Total savings come from contracting for services at lower prices through a provider network, reductions in inpatient days per thousand enrollees, and substitution of more appropriate but less costly forms of care. However, since mental health treatment needs were less able to be categorized by diagnoses, they were not subjected to the controls of the DRG prospective payment system (see chapter 8.2). Differences in payment mechanisms and supply conditions allowed managed care to reduce hospital utilization more for mental health and substance abuse than for most other types of medical care, on the order of 50 percent rather than the usual 10 percent to 25 percent.

Capitation gives the MBH firm an incentive to control costs, but direct financial incentives play a relatively minor role in the management of care. Most of the time, just knowing that costs are being monitored and that additional resource use must be justified and documented is sufficient to make providers work more efficiently. A therapist feels embarrassed being called to task for violating what he or she knows to be the principles of quality care, and that fear is enough to eliminate the biggest sources of waste—admissions made without any thought given to a treatment plan, heavy medications used to keep a patient in a holding pattern, weekend days in idle observation, and failure to consider discharge and community support services.

Since evaluators and case managers are paid on salary or a standard rate per case, they have no direct monetary incentives to authorize or deny more or fewer services. Most importantly, they lack the FFS incentive to increase revenues by admitting more patients, keeping patients for more days, or using more expensive hospitals. During the 1980s, admitting patients for inpatient psychiatric care had become so profitable that many hospitals aggressively sought to admit patients, and some stepped over the line by paying kickbacks to physicians for referrals or keeping patients longer than necessary—sometimes against their will and the wishes of family members. Abuses by one psychiatric hospital chain were so widespread that they were taken to court and fined $400 million.[11]

The most egregious problems of FFS mental health were typified by the "28th-day discharge." In some instances, patients were admitted and kept for a specified period with little regard to diagnosis, individual progress, or family situation, and then conveniently declared cured and ready for discharge just as their insurance benefits ran out (28 days). Indeed, it had become so common for all substance abuse cases to receive twenty-eight day inpatient treatment that it was considered a standard indicator of quality until questioned by managed care advocates—why does every addict need twenty-eight days, no more and no less? Why inpatient rather than outpatient, or continuing care in a halfway house? As managed care penetration increased in most markets, the "standard" twenty-eight day alcohol and substance abuse program was replaced by a variety of less-expensive programs more clearly matched to the needs of individual patients. Although the outright fraud and profiteering that characterized the worst part of the FFS psychiatric industry were relatively rare, they tainted the whole industry and indicated a lack of concern with the cost to the patient, the employer, and the government, that demanded a concerted response. The use of capitation rates structures profit incentives so that discipline is self-enforcing. Just as the quest for profit has reduced the cost of computers (and, in doing so, made sophisticated case management information available), so too, the quest for profit has lead to continual innovation and redesign in behavioral health care.

10.6 PAYMENT CONTRACTS AND INCENTIVE MODIFICATION _____

The success of an HMO is dependent on the structuring of the contracts that make up the plan and the capabilities of the management team. The incentives in the financial contracts must match the control mechanisms available to management. For instance, managed care plans communicate with their provider networks and authorize days of inpatient care. Since "days of care" is the unit of management reporting and control, it also becomes the best way of paying for care. Thus, a per diem rate is preferred to discounted FFS. On the other hand where management can authorize a package of services (a delivery, an organ transplant), paying a bundled price for the entire episode of care allows them to better predict and control expenditures than a per diem rate.

Capitation is preferred for gatekeepers because it pays for management services rendered (gatekeeping, patient education, marketing), is entirely under the control of and predictable to the plan, and provides none of the FFS incentives to overuse expensive services or raise charges. What about complaints that HMOs under-use or deny care? A capitated gatekeeper actually has mixed utilization incentives. With a fixed monthly payment for all care they do not wish to have any one patient taking up too much of their time, so that fixed monthly rates provides an incentive to refer the patient on to specialists in order to get them out of the office quicker, hence increasing utilization. At the same time, participation in a withhold pool for specialty services gives them some financial incentives not to refer. The incentive to withhold services becomes stronger as the percentage of the monthly cap placed in the withhold pool increases and the number of enrollees in the withhold pool decreases (since each action has a larger impact on the average cost).

An open HMO contracting with many primary care physicians who also have FFS practices and contracts with other HMOs has very little ability to exercise informal management control. The open HMO must depend on financial incentives and formal authorizations to limit inappropriate referral and hospitalization. In a closed-staff HMO like the Kaiser Health Plan where the doctors treat only plan enrollees, and usually spend their entire professional career with the HMO, the doctors are made part of the organization in a way that no open HMO can approach. These physicians carry on a corporate culture where control is embedded in a sense of "the way we do things here" so that direct financial rewards and penalties are less necessary.[12] Even though the Kaiser plan has a profit-sharing element, the pool is so large that a single physician making a decision to treat or not to treat, even for very expensive services, will see no impact on his or her own paycheck.

Capitation makes the primary care physician bear the financial consequences and risk for all primary care services (which they must provide for no extra charge), but not specialty services or hospitalization.* A 20 percent withhold implies a 80:20 sharing of risk between the health plan and the physicians up to 120 percent of expected costs, with the health plan bearing all risks above that. A health plan may reinsure in order to limit their exposure to catastrophic losses. For example, a typical reinsurance contract might call for the reinsurer to pay the health plan 90 percent of the amount by which any individual patient's bill exceeds $30,000 in a single year. Otherwise, just a few bad cases might swamp a

---

* Notice that the terms "risk" and "financial responsibility for" mean essentially the same thing in managed care discussions, and so the term "risk" *does not* carry the same connotation as it would in a finance textbook. In finance, risk is the deviation in actual asset returns around some expected mean. Bearing the risk due to such volatility is often implicitly or explicitly separated from business risk and systematic risk regarding changes in the expected average returns. In particular, finance experts talk about different portfolios as having different levels of risk even though on average, their returns are the same, or, more importantly, that an asset holder can obtain a higher average rate of return only by taking on a higher level of risk—a central proposition of the capital asset pricing model and arbitrage theory. In contrast, in managed care, "risk" simply means financial responsibility for paying the bills, and it is usually assumed that the holder of risk has some ability to change the expected loss. Indeed, a leading consultant writing in the journal of the Healthcare Financial Management Association admonished hospital financial officers "What cannot be controlled should not be assumed as risk" (Joseph Coyne, *Healthcare Financial Management* August 1994, p. 33)." This managerial control concept of risk and risk sharing is quite different from that used by currency and bond traders who daily take on exchange and interest rate risk outside of anyone's control.

small start-up HMO that did not have substantial reserves.[13] What about the physician who has several patients who are severely ill and justifiably require above average amounts of care? A contract in which the individual physician bears a large amount of risk gives physicians the greatest incentive to control costs, but also makes them most susceptible to adverse consequences from a few cases. At the extreme, it could lead to physicians who welcome only healthy people as new patients, and eschew serving the sick.

The business risks to an HMO should be distinguished from the risks to the participating physicians, hospitals, and patients (see Figure 10.8). The major risks to the individual, random variation in illness or health status, are diversified away for any HMO with a large number of members. The more relevant individual (client) risks to an HMO are related to marketing: selection and volume. An HMO attracting a larger proportion of seriously ill people will suffer financially from adverse selection much as any other insurer.[14] The more serious marketing risk is the inability to attract a sufficient number of clients. In order to break even, a certain volume must be attained, and growth is a primary determinant of profitability. In this, HMOs are similar to most other businesses. Indeed, the primary risks an investor must evaluate in considering HMO profitability are standard business risks: pricing (capitation rate); input prices (e.g., per diem hospital costs, cost of referrals); productivity (how much labor and capital does it take to run the HMO). The "core competency" of an HMO is identified in Figure 10.8 as allocative efficiency, the ability of an HMO to match patient needs to care providers so as to reduce costs while maintaining or increasing satisfaction.

The willingness to moderate and, when necessary, override the provisions in the financial contracts, is essential for managed care operations. Although most patients fall within the normal range, there are some exceptional cases, and the manager maintains the morale and motivation of the provider network by making appropriate exceptions. Just as government intervention is required to blunt

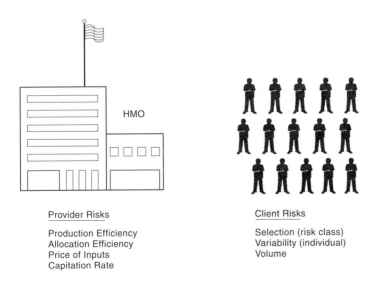

HMO

Provider Risks

Production Efficiency
Allocation Efficiency
Price of Inputs
Capitation Rate

Client Risks

Selection (risk class)
Variability (individual)
Volume

FIGURE 10.8 *Capitated Provider's Business Risks*

raw market forces to put a kind face on capitalism, the manager is required to judiciously consider medical realities and put a kind face on the HMO contract. If all contracts were perfectly self-enforcing, and there were no need for human intervention, then "managed care" would disappear and a legalistic software program could run the system. Rules are necessary, but analysts err when they identify managed care with the contracts that constitute the legal definition of the plan. In the real world, it takes people to deal with people, and often a physician to deal with other physicians. Two HMOs may have identical contracts and one could be very successful while the other fails, and the reason for the difference is *management*. There is good management and bad management, just as there are good surgeons and bad surgeons. Education and intelligence make a difference, but in the end there is some often-undefinable quality that that separates the winners from the losers. A major function of the market is to practice what Joseph Schumpeter called the "creative destruction" of capitalism,[15] rewarding those managers who come up with new ideas and organizations that meet consumers' needs, and allowing better organizations to grow by displacing those firms whose structure is out of date or whose management is bad.

SUGGESTIONS FOR FURTHER READING _____

Marsha Gold et al. "A National Survey of the Arrangements Managed-Care Plans Make With Physicians," *New England Journal of Medicine* 333:1678–83, 1995.
Interstudy, *The Interstudy Edge*, Excelsior, Minn. (annual).
Peter R. Kongstvedt, *The Managed Care Handbook*, Aspen: Gaithersburg, Md., 1996.
Managed Care Digest (annual), Hoechst Marion Roussel, Kansas City, Mo.
Charles W. Wrightson, *HMO Rate Setting and Financial Strategy*, Ann Arbor, Mich.: Health Administration Press, 1990.

SUMMARY _____

1. With **indemnity fee-for-service** health financing, **hospitals and physicians profit by seeing more patients** and the risk of excess utilization is borne by the insurance company, who passes it on to the employer or government in the form of higher premiums. **In managed care, the HMO forces the physicians and hospitals to bear some of the risks** for excess utilization, provides incentives to use fewer services by paying a fixed amount per month, and controls total premium expense by using withholds and other financial arrangements.

2. The **escalation in costs** under open-ended entitlement financing from Medicare, Medicaid, and employer-provided health insurance has been the primary force driving the development of managed care.

3. **Managed care** is a diverse set of contractual and management methods used to arrange the financing and delivery of medical services. Its distinctive feature is that *a manager* intervenes to monitor and control the transaction between doctor and patient. A primary physician usually serves as the **gate-**

keeper, coordinating and controlling most care, and bearing responsibility for clinical as well as financial outcomes.

4. Traditional insurance provides value through risk pooling so that medical expenses can be covered by an actuarially fair premium equal to the expected average loss. Managed care adds value by systematically **reducing the average** loss through utilization review, preauthorization, formularies, case management, statistical profiling, and other process controls.

5. In order to operate, an HMO (or other managed care firm such as a PPO) must first contract with doctors, hospitals, and pharmacies to create a **provider network**, and then **market to individuals and firms** who pay premiums based on the number of members who enroll.

6. HMOs **reduce costs by** saving money on both the demand and the supply side. They obtain **discounts** by contracting in volume with physicians and hospitals, **substitute** less expensive services (e.g., home care instead of hospital stays), and **control utilization** through the approval process. HMOs may use one-third to two-thirds fewer inpatient hospital days per thousand person than traditional fee-for-service insurance, although they often use more ambulatory services.

7. A **pharmacy formulary** limiting payment to those drugs listed, a **preferred provider network** that makes patients pay extra for using hospitals and physicians not on the list, and **utilization review** are some of the ways that managed care firms control costs.

8. The dominant mode of contracting in managed care is **capitation**, although discounted fees, negotiated per case and per diem payments, and budgeted costs are used as well. It is common for HMOs to **withhold** 20 percent or more of physician and hospital payments, which are only released to providers after the end of the year if overall utilization, quality, and budget goals are met.

9. About **80 percent of HMO premiums go to pay hospitals, physicians, and other providers**. This fraction is known as the "medical loss ratio." About 10 to 20 percent is used for administrative and marketing expenses, leaving up to 10 percent for profit.

10. Division of labor is practiced by HMOs that **carve out** and **sub-capitate** a particular service (such as mental health), letting another firm that specializes in that area bear the risk, contract with providers, and use its expertise in managing that aspect of the care process.

PROBLEMS _____

1. {*incentives*} What incentives does a capitated physician have to keep his patients happy? What incentive does an FFS physician have? If Mr. Jones is a cranky old man who smokes and drinks so much that his liver and other organs are going downhill, which payment system provides more incentive

to keep Mr. Jones satisfied? Which provides the most incentive to render extra care? Which provides the most incentive to make sure that the level of care is optimized?

2. {*costs*} What are the three main ways that HMOs act to reduce the cost of care?

3. {*marginal cost*} Suppose a family physician has HMO patients that are capitated for primary care, HMO patients that are capitated with a withhold for hospital care, and fee-for-service patients. For which patients is the marginal cost of doing additional laboratory services highest? For which is the marginal cost of admitting the patient to the hospital the highest?

4. {*distribution*} Why do "star" surgeons rarely work for HMOs, even the largest and wealthiest ones?

5. {*physician behavior*} What is the purpose of a "withhold" fund? Do HMOs have substitutes for financial incentives in controlling physician behavior? What factors will make these substitutes more or less effective?

6. {*incentives*} Which surgeons are more subject to financial incentives when deciding between alternative courses of therapy, fee-for-service physicians who own their own practice, or salaried physicians working for an HMO?

7. {*industrial organization*} If an HMO reduces the patient's marginal cost of surgery, hospitalization, chemotherapy and other expensive items to zero, how can it provide incentives for reduced utilization?

8. {*information systems*} In contracting for hip replacements, who would have an incentive to contract on a line-item basis, and who would have more incentive to contract on a bundled basis, an insurance company serving as a third-party administrator for a self-insured employer, or an HMO offering community rated plans to employers?

9. {*industrial organization*} Is an HMO able to obtain the biggest discounts where it has a large market share or where it has a smaller market share?

10. {*transactions costs*} Since managed care firms must hire managers and have all hospitalizations and surgeries reviewed by them, aren't they necessarily more expensive than unmanaged fee-for-service care due to this extra administrative cost?

11. {*selection*} Is a person who is chronically ill and has a long-term relationship with a physician more likely to choose an HMO, PPO, or indemnity plan? How will this affect the HMO capitation rates?

12. {*aggregation*} Which do HMOs reduce more, individual risks or system risks? (*Think* about this. Definitions are important, and relative risks are different than absolute risks.)

ENDNOTES

1. There was also some implicit insurance in the health care system. Providers acted as buffers by providing free care and absorbed losses to some degree.
2. Alan Maynard and Karen Bloor, "Introducing a Market to the United Kingdom's National Health Service," *New England Journal of Medicine*, 334(9):604–608, 1996.

3. Victor Fuchs, "The Best Health Care System in the World?" *Journal of the American Medical Association,* 268(7):916–917, 1992; Jack Hadley, *More Medical Care, Better Health?* Washington, D.C.: The Urban Institute Press, 1982; OECD, *OECD Health Data: Comparative Analysis of Health Systems,* Paris: Organization for Economic Cooperation and Development, 1995.

4. OECD, *The Reform of Health Care Systems,* Health Policy Studies No.5, Paris: OECD, 1994.

5. M. Chassin et al., "Does Inappropriate Use Explain Geographic Variations in the Use of Health Care Services? A Study of Three Procedures," *Journal of the American Medical Association* 256:2533–37, 1987.

6. Gerard Anderson et al.,"Setting Payment Rates for Capitated Systems: A Comparison of Various Alternatives" *Inquiry* 27(3):225–33, 1990.

7. *Managed Care Digest: HMO-PPO Digest,* Kansas City, Mo.: Hoechst Marion Roussel, 1995.

8. Paul Kenkel, "U.S. Healthcare 'Report Cards' Expanded to Primary-Care Docs," *Modern Healthcare,* April 11, 1994; Robert H. Miller and Harold Luft, "Managed Care Plan Performance Since 1980: A Literature Analysis, *Journal of the American Medical Association,* 271(19):1512–19, 1994; Maggie Mahar, "Time for A Checkup: HMOs Must Now Prove That They are Providing Quality Care," *Barron's* March 4, 1996, p. 29–35.

9. Marsha Gold et al., "A National Survey of the Arrangements Managed-Care Plans Make With Physicians," *New England Journal of Medicine* 333:1678–83, 1995.

10. Norman Winegar, *The Clinician's Guide to Managed Mental Health Care,* New York: Haworth Press, 1992. John K. Iglehart, "Managed Care and Mental Health," *New England Journal of Medicine* 334(2):131–135, 1996. The monthly publications *Open Minds* and *Behavioral Health Management* are also useful sources of current information on managed behavioral health care.

11. Sandy Lutz, "NME Totals Costs of Psych Woes" *Modern Healthcare* 23(43):20, October 25, 1993.

12. Robert H. Miller and Harold Luft, "Managed Care Plans: Characteristics, Growth and Premium Performance," *Annual Review of Public Health* 15:437–59, 1994.

13. Indeed, after several spectacular HMO bankruptcies that left the physician groups and hospitals that had rendered the services with millions of dollars in unpaid bills, most providers will not contract to join a network unless the HMO can demonstrate large financial reserves or a reinsurance policy that guarantees their solvency, and company benefits managers require the same assurance before enrolling their employees as subscribers in the HMO (see Richard Karp, "A Grade-A Battle" *Barron's,* October 30, 1995.)

14. Charles Wrightson, "Selection Bias and Premium Rate Setting," in *HMO Rate Setting and Financial Strategy,* Ann Arbor, Mich.: Health Administration Press, 1990, 245–92.

15. Joseph Schumpeter, *History of Economic Analysis,* New York: Oxford University Press, 1954. For a recent application of Schumpeter's ideas to health care, see L. D. Brown, "Policy Reform as Creative Destruction: Political and Administrative Challenges in Preserving the Public-Private Mix," *Inquiry* 29(2):188–202, 1992.

CHAPTER **11**

HMO Ownership and Growth: Risk, Capital, and Competition

QUESTIONS

1. *Who are the winners and losers from managed care? Do cost reductions mean that some doctors must take home lower incomes?*
2. *Does "financial innovation" improve productivity and consumer welfare like technological innovation does?*
3. *Does a surplus of doctors and hospitals foster or hinder the growth of HMOs?*
4. *What changed HMOs from social collectives into capital-driven enterprises?*
5. *How are HMO per-member-per-month capitation rates determined?*
6. *What made for-profit HMOs so attractive to investors in the 1990s?*
7. *University hospitals seek out the sickest and most demanding patients to practice and improve medical technology. Will HMOs support medical research? Will they seek out those most in need, or try to selectively enroll the healthy to keep costs down?*
8. *Are HMOs medical care organizations, or financial services companies in the insurance business?*

11.1 KAISER: THE EVOLUTION OF AN HMO —————————————————

Kaiser Health Plan, with more than 6 million members, is the largest HMO in the United States, and is one of the largest medical delivery systems in the world. Its origins lie in the efforts of a young surgeon, Sydney R. Garfield, to find a place to practice when he completed residency at Los Angeles County Hospital in 1933.[1] The disastrous economy of the depression made it impossible to open up a new solo fee-for-service practice in Los Angeles as he wished to do, so Dr. Garfield reluctantly began looking for a salaried job to tide him over until times improved. The Metropolitan Water District was building an aqueduct from the Colorado River to Los Angeles, and was looking for a physician to staff a small clinic to treat construction workers in the desert. Garfield thought the salary they offered, $125 a month, was too little for someone as well trained as himself. With the support of a local doctor as partner, he decided to open his own hospital at Desert Center. The construction companies were very anxious to have a doctor for their workers, and agreed to help Garfield and to send all of their industrial medicine cases insured under the new workers' compensation plan to his facility. Garfield opened a top-notch hospital, complete with modern operating facilities and air conditioning, an unheard of luxury for industrial workers at that time. The injured workers and the construction companies loved the facility, but two financial problems quickly arose. The workers' compensation insurance companies thought Dr. Garfield treated the workers too well, and argued over many of the bills submitted. Garfield also treated the men for nonindustrial illnesses, but few could afford to pay private practice fees for extended hospital stays or major surgery, even though Garfield felt obligated to treat them. Garfield threatened to close the hospital unless he could obtain a steady source of funding. The foundations of a major innovation in health care financing were laid when an executive of the major workers' compensation insurance companies suggested that they pre-pay Garfield by giving him an eighth of the worker's compensation insurance premium, which amounted to $1.50 per month for each of the 5,000 construction workers on the project, and for workers to voluntarily pre-pay an additional $1.50 per month to cover all nonindustrial accidents and illnesses.[2] Garfield's experiment in prepaid HMO medicine was very successful. He added two more hospitals; at the end of five years, as construction slowed and the hospitals began to close, Garfield had made a net profit of more than $250,000 (equivalent to $3 million after adjustment for inflation to 1995).

Although Garfield intended to take his profits and set up a private practice in Los Angeles, he was lured north to open another prepaid workers' clinic by one of the aqueduct contractors, Henry J. Kaiser, who had just been awarded a contract to complete the Grand Coulee Dam in Oregon. Kaiser had previously been impressed by the efficiency and high-class quality of Garfield's operation in the desert, and felt that establishing a similar facility would help him attract workers to another remote construction site. At Grand Coulee, SR Garfield & Associates provided twenty-four-hour medical coverage to 15,000 workers and family members in a modernized and, once again, air-conditioned hospital with a group of five physicians and six nurses. Garfield himself, however, remained in Los

Angeles undergoing more medical training and looking after business interests, flying to Grand Coulee and working in the clinic only once every six weeks. It was as a manager that Garfield made the health plan successful, albeit one whose status as a physician gave him a special connection with the professionals who worked under his direction. He was, in the words of one of the physicians who worked for him, "a genius at keeping salaries and expenses down."

With Grand Coulee nearing completion, and Garfield ordered up for service in the Army Medical Corps due to the war, it appeared that his days as an entrepreneur were over. However, Kaiser had just been given a new contract to construct sixty freighters at a hastily organized shipyard in Richmond, near San Francisco, and he wanted Garfield to provide the medical care for his wartime crew. Within a year, Garfield had built a hospital and was caring for 90,000 workers. His commitment to staying at the forefront of medical practice is evidenced by the establishment of a research program and a new journal, the *Permanente* (Kaiser) *Foundation Medical Bulletin*, in 1943. By 1944, Garfield had a hundred doctors working for him to care for more than 200,000 workers and dependents. Although his first recruits were outstanding doctors from Stanford, University of Southern California, and other leading schools who wished to join a prepaid group practice, others were signed only because they were unfit for military service and needed a job. From them, Garfield learned an important management lesson, which he later stated as, "No matter how the principles of our plan are meant, if you don't have the physician group who have it in their hearts and who believe in prepaid practice, it won't work," emphasizing that it is the culture and the people even more than the financial contracts that define a successful HMO.[3]

As fast as the war had created a need for the Kaiser medical plan, the end of the war took it away. The only clinic not to suffer major enrollment declines was the one at the new Kaiser steel mill in Fontana, in the desert outside of Los Angeles. The Alameda County and San Francisco medical societies, tolerant during the emergency, grew openly hostile. Kaiser doctors were denied membership, and hence could not join hospital medical staffs or participate in many forms of professional advancement. Yet Garfield, Kaiser, and many of their closest associates, including health economist Avram Yedidia, decided that the appropriate course of action was to regroup and expand their visionary health plan rather than shut it down. In the immediate postwar period, enrollment stabilized at fewer than 20,000. By 1948, it had rebounded to 60,000, with much of the growth coming from marketing to unions and firms whose employees would join as a group. Yet the pressures of fluctuating enrollment, requirements for capital, and a need for clearer lines of authority made the entrepreneurial organization with Sydney Garfield alone in charge of all the Kaiser health facilities untenable. The new structure had three entities, a charitable corporation for the hospitals, a nonprofit foundation for the health plan, and a private for-profit partnership for the physician group. Garfield was paid $257,000 for his interest in the hospitals, and subsequently gave up his interest in the partnership, so that by 1949 he was just an employee, albeit a very important one. By 1952, enrollment reached 250,000, but the organizational difficulties were not over, and financial disputes between the health plan and the physician groups had become serious. In 1955, Garfield resigned his post as executive director, and a new profit-sharing plan for the physician group was drafted. The medical group was to be paid on a capitation basis, to have a pension plan, and to get half of all revenues in excess of the funds needed for expenses, capital replacement, and reserves for distribution as bonuses. This financial agreement between Kaiser Health Plan and the Permanente Medical Group has continued essentially unchanged for the last forty years.

In 1962, enrollment exceeded 1 million subscribers and dependents, and by 1972, had surpassed 2.5 million. In 1992, more than 6 million persons were part of the Kaiser Health Plans nationwide. Thus over a forty-year span Kaiser had maintained a most enviable record of growth, more than doubling in most decades. Although Kaiser remains strongest in its initial market areas around San Francisco, Los Angeles, and Portland, it has expanded to Hawaii, Colorado, Connecticut, North Carolina, and Washington, D.C. Yet even as the forces of managed care began to revolutionize the U.S. health care system, Kaiser, the exemplar of prepaid organized medical practice, had begun to falter.[4] The Kaiser plan established in Hartford, Connecticut, was unable to grow past 30,000 members after ten years, below break-even size. To penetrate the competitive D.C. and North Carolina markets, Kaiser departed from its traditional closed-staff model and set up open, independent practice association (IPA) HMOs contracting with already-established local physicians. Despite these efforts, in 1994 Kaiser showed its first loss of enrollment in more than fifty years of operation. When the federal HMO Act of 1973 was passed, Kaiser accounted for over 2 million of the 3 million total HMO enrollees in the United States, a market share of 70 percent. By 1995, although still the largest, Kaiser's 6.6 million represented less than a 15 percent market share. As the remainder of this chapter will show, the times had clearly changed.

11.2   THE GROWTH OF HMOs _____

HMOs started during the 1930s, but most grew only slowly. Only a few—Kaiser, Group Health Cooperative of Puget Sound, and HIP (Health Insurance Plan of New York and New Jersey)—grew to a sustainable size, and Kaiser alone became large. As of 1970, there were just thirty-three HMO plans, and all but a few had less than 100,000 members.[5] Since then, growth has exceeded 10 percent a year, and as of 1995, more than 60 million Americans received their health care through HMOs.[6] Most of the growth that has occurred in the last ten years has come from the growth of existing commercial IPA HMOs, rather than new start-ups; closed staff group HMOs; or other nonprofit organizations. The number of HMOs actually peaked in 1987. Since then the industry has experienced some consolidation, as small HMOs merged or were acquired by larger plans (Table 11.1). The acceleration in enrollment growth after 1970 is probably attributable to several factors.

1. The industry matured, developing more efficient structures and administrative systems for managing care. Consumers became more accepting of the HMOs that had proven themselves over twenty years.

TABLE 11.1   Growth of HMOs from 1970 to 1994

	Number of HMOs	Enrollment (*thousands*)
1970	33	3,000
1975	148	5,600
1976	175	6,000
1977	165	6,300
1978	203	7,500
1979	215	8,200
1980	236	9,100
1981	243	10,200
1982	265	10,800
1983	280	12,500
1984	306	15,100
1985	393	18,900
1986	595	23,700
1987	700	29,000
1988	653	30,300
1989	591	34,500
1990	569	36,500
1991	550	40,400
1992	562	44,300
1993	541	49,100
1994	546	56,800

Source: Hoechst Marion Roussel, *Managed Care Digest 1995.*

2. The opposition by the medical establishment lessened as the post-Medicare boom increased the demand for all doctors and lessened worries about competitive pressures.
3. The Nixon administration, seeking to find a "market" solution to rising health care costs, supported the expansion of HMOs and passed the HMO Act of 1973, setting federal standards, providing planning and start-up grants, and mandating that corporations offer an HMO option to their employers wherever one was available.

The newer HMO organizations were mostly IPAs, and could expand much more rapidly than the older staff models. Physicians did not have to become employees of the HMO, but merely had to sign a contract, and physicians could sign with two, three, or more IPA HMOs if they wished and could still see private patients. This meant that many insured employees could switch to an HMO without having to switch physicians. By 1980, the commercial IPA HMOs had come to dominate the market, except in those areas where group and staff HMOs were already well entrenched. Even in California, the home of Kaiser, open HMOs now have more enrollees than group staff HMOs. Yet the tighter organizational structure and the more extensive ability to modify physician behavior through promotion of a corporate culture leads many analysts to suggest that the current situation is a transitory response to rapid growth, and that as managed care matures, more and more physicians will practice exclusively in one HMO, and follow the closed group model.

11.3   OWNERSHIP AND CAPITAL MARKETS: SIGNS OF FAILURE _____

Lack of Ownership Leads to Failure of Leadership

The Kaiser Health Plan operated as a nonprofit foundation; thus, there were no stockholders or individual owners who stood to gain by expanding into new markets. To some extent, it might seem as if the physicians were shareholders, but in one important way they clearly were not owners. When each new region got started, it took capital from the existing Kaiser foundation. However, once it was up and running, no "returns" were paid back. The physicians who had given up some current income to enable the new offshoot to grow gained nothing. Thus, it is not surprising that Kaiser plans grew robustly where they were already established (since that medical group stood to benefit), but had difficulty obtaining the resources to move into new areas. Garfield built Kaiser single-handedly, but after 1949, he held no legal ownership interest, and in 1955 he was forced out. Garfield was apparently willing to do it for the glory, but the fact is that someone of his talent and training would surely have ended up a wealthier man if he had stuck with his original plan to open an FFS surgical practice in Los Angeles. The incomplete and complex ownership structure was not able to protect his interest, nor was it able to maximize the potential of the Kaiser Health Plan.

GHA: A Consumer Co-Op Gets Bought Out by a Franchise Chain

The history of another of the first HMOs makes a similar point with regard to ownership. Group Health Association of Washington, D.C., was founded in 1937 as a consumer's cooperative to provide physician services to its members, largely federal employees. The physicians were employees, not partners. The AMA and the D.C. medical society sought to put GHA out of business, and the cooperative's victorious antitrust suit, which was affirmed by the U.S. Supreme Court in 1943, has been considered crucial to the survival and growth of all HMOs, including Kaiser. Yet ten years later, GHA still had less than 20,000 members. The cooperative structure legally makes every subscriber an owner. Some existing members were ambivalent about letting large unions join, since it would change the dynamics of control. A basic management function, marketing, was the subject of great ideological debates rather than concerted action. GHA did become more solidly established after becoming an option in the Federal Employees Health Benefits Program, reaching 50,000 members in 1962, and 100,000 in 1975. An attempt by the physicians to set up a medical group partnership similar to that at Kaiser met with resistance from the cooperative members and their elected board. As a chronicle of the cooperative observes, the physicians "failed to comprehend GHA's special environment, in which the members instinctively reacted against the notion of a profit motive."[7] Unable to form a corporate medical group, GHA's physicians formed a union in 1977 and went on strike in April, 1978. GHA continued to suffer financial reversals and labor disagreements. The nurses and physical therapists went on strike in 1982, and the physicians struck again in 1986. GHA weathered the storm, but continued to struggle. Enrollment reached 150,000 in 1986 and 200,000 in 1992. In 1994, unable to persevere in an increasingly competitive market, GHA was acquired by Humana. Thus, an organization that had begun as a consumer cooperative became part of a for-profit chain, one of whose founders had honed his business skills developing the Colonel Sanders Kentucky Fried Chicken franchise.

The rapid expansion of HMOs from 9 million enrollees in 1980 to 60 million in 1995 occurred mostly within the corporate for-profit structure. Many HMOs that started as nonprofits switched to for-profit to take better advantage of their market opportunities. Why have for-profit firms been more successful, and why didn't they emerge earlier? Sydney Garfield dreamed of "one organized integrality" that encompassed all of medicine as a business, including hospitals, laboratories, physicians, financing, and marketing under one roof. He was able to maintain unified control by force of personality during Kaiser's formative years, but lost control when confronted by these vital questions: Who can borrow enough money to build a hospital? How are wages to be set once profits start rolling in? How can one physician single-handedly manage a group of doctors too large for all of them to be personal friends? The common answer to all of these questions lay in the corporatization of health care organizations.[8]

Corporate Advantage

In a corporation, control is more clearly defined. The board of directors has the power to appoint senior management, who, in turn, has the power to hire and fire employees, purchase assets, and borrow money. The stockholders have a clear right to the profits. However, being numerous and diffuse, they usually have little control over the management of operations. Thus, the corporate structure is able to delegate authority and establish accountability reasonably well. Opponents of for-profit health care might argue that nonprofit organizations can be very well managed. In fact, nonprofit and for-profit hospitals both have boards of directors and suites full of administrators that seem to look and act quite similar in most ways. The difference is the nonprofit facility's lack of direct ownership. No one in a nonprofit organization has the incentive, or the power, to take a big risk in the hope of achieving a large capital gain. Furthermore, the lack of unified control makes it hard for any one person to make rapid and risky decisions on behalf of the whole organization in times of turbulent change and emerging opportunity. But these were precisely the conditions that characterized the managed care environment of the 1980s and 1990s. In a situation in which the leadership of an organization requires achieving a consensus among a large number of stakeholder groups, a nonprofit with diffuse ownership may actually be an advantage. Such a situation was characteristic for most community hospitals from 1950 to 1980. When profits and survival depend on hard bargaining, innovation, and making quick commitments to capture opportunities that expand and disappear in the moment, then the diffuse voluntary structure is overwhelmed. It is simply harder for an entrepreneur to work in a nonprofit structure, or to take the organization one has built and sell it for a large capital gain.

11.4   U.S. HEALTHCARE: A PROFITABLE GROWTH COMPANY _____

U.S. Healthcare, founded by Leonard Abramson in 1975, is a good example of the new for-profit HMO firms that are coming to dominate the market. Abramson was from a South Philadelphia family of modest means and had driven a taxi to put himself through pharmacy school. After working as a detailer calling on physicians for a pharmaceutical firm (see chapter 13), six years in retail pharmacy, and participation in equipment leasing and other health care businesses, Abramson was astounded by the freedom of doctors and hospitals to raise prices whenever they wanted. "It was a blank check," he said in a 1985 interview.[9] Abramson was much taken with the promise of HMOs to bring business methods to health care, and knew a number of physicians who shared his enthusiasm. Taking advantage of the government loans made available by the HMO Act of 1973, the "Health Maintenance Organization of Pennsylvania" was incorporated as a nonprofit prepaid health plan in January 1975, obtained a state HMO license in 1976, and designated as a federally qualified HMO in 1977.[10] Operations started in April 1977 by taking over the assets of an existing prepaid health plan, Family Medical Care. HMO/PA began enrolling members, and grew rapidly. In 1981, U.S. Healthcare went private, using venture capital from Warburg, Pincus and Company, paying back a $2.5 million loan to the federal government. Its initial public offering of stock came in 1983, as did its expansion into New Jersey.

The Philadelphia market of the 1980s was old-style traditional medicine: lots of specialists, lots of hospital beds, and fee-for-service indemnity insurance. With changing medical trends and the advent of Medicare's prospective payment by DRG (see chapter 8), it was becoming clear that there was a surplus of hospitals in the area, and that even good specialists were having some trouble attracting all the patients they wanted. There was room for an entrepreneur who could cut premiums by contracting in advance for surgery and beds at a discount. Abramson was a sharp negotiator. It often seemed that he came into a bargaining session knowing more about a hospital's operations and finances than its administrators knew. Discounts of 20 percent, 30 percent, or more were often won. Abramson made information a weapon in the fight for market share and low prices, and honed it to a fine edge in repeated competitive encounters.

Not everyone was enamored of U.S. Healthcare's tactics: some hospitals were terrified that they would lose so much revenue that they might go out of business, and the Philadelphia Blue Cross plan was furious that an upstart was trying to invade its market by cutting prices.[11] The acrimony spilled over into name calling, then full-page attack advertisements in the newspapers, and finally a series of lawsuits charging libel and unfair trading on both sides (most of which were settled or won by U.S. Healthcare, although bad feelings between the two companies continued to run high). By 1985 U.S. Healthcare, with over 500,000 enrollees, was the sixth-largest HMO in the nation, and probably the most profitable. Its medical loss ratio was only 75 percent, whereas the average was closer to 80 percent, and

Kaiser was above 95 percent.[12] The formula of aggressive contracting, meticulous claims review, and conscientious client service had made the company successful and financially sound, although with less than a 20 percent market share it was far from dominant and was not universally loved.

Abramson was not content to let the company rest on its laurels and pile up profits. He made a strategic decision to emphasize quality. Cost control was not neglected, but was now considered to have been built into routine operations and became less prominent. Whereas most of the incentive payments in the original HMO/PA primary care physician reimbursement plan had depended on reductions in the quantity of referrals and other services used, in the "Quality Care Compensation System" (QCCS) for primary physicians inaugurated in 1987, quality and consumer satisfaction were to account for 40 percent of practice bonuses. In 1992 the QCCS was amended so that 82 percent of incentives were determined by medical chart review, availability of evening hours, retention of existing patients, ability to attract new members, and ratings on questionnaires mailed to patients, and only 18 percent on reductions in utilization.[13] For hospitals, the "CapTainer™" payment system was introduced in 1992 paying a quality- and diagnosis-adjusted per diem rate. Quality incentive plans were introduced for OB/Gyns in 1994, and for other referral specialists in 1996.[14] However, the most important part of the new strategy was the development of a new corporate subsidiary in 1990, USQA, devoted solely to quality measurement. USQA created databanks based on millions of patient records, consumer surveys, pathology reports, and laboratory tests. The physician-information scientists working at USQA published significant studies on the cost-effectiveness of laparascopic cholecystectomy, asthma, influenza immunization, and autologous bone marrow transplantation for treatment of breast cancer. It used $2 million dollars to fund a fellowship in Managed Care and Quality Assessment at Jefferson Medical College. In 1993, U.S. Healthcare was the first HMO to release the full 1992 HEDIS (Health Employer Data and Information Set) report, and in 1994 the first to provide members with a detailed report card on each participating physician.[15] U.S. Healthcare had clearly gone far beyond compliance, and established a leading presence in the quality assurance and health care information field.[16]

Growth continued to climb, reaching 1 million members in 1989 and 2 million members in 1995. In the face of such rising demand, Abramson's announcement that he would cut premiums in order to build market share came as quite a surprise.[17] Publicly traded HMO stocks fell by as much as 16 percent on the following day. Yet the strategy of favoring long-term growth over short-term profitability was sound, and share prices soon recovered. U.S. Healthcare ended the year trading at 46½, with a total market capitalization of $7.1 billion. In April 1996, Aetna Life & Casualty declared that it would acquire Abramson's company, paying more than $8 billion.[18] The information and quality assurance systems of USQA would now be deployed to serve 14 million members, reaching roughly one out of every twelve persons with health insurance in the United States.

Why did Abramson decide to sell if U.S. Healthcare was such a successful company? Although any analysis of internal motivations and assessments must remain largely speculative, some plausible reasons do appear upon reflection. Although U.S. Healthcare had created start-ups and/or joint ventures in Florida, Illinois, Delaware and Maryland, as well as ten other states and even in Europe, by 1996 it was becoming harder and harder to maintain the 10 to 20 percent growth rates it had enjoyed. Every major market now had an established HMO, often several, and the indemnity insurers such as Blue Cross, CIGNA, and NY Life had developed their own HMO plans, so that signing up each additional employer group was a struggle. Merger with Aetna meant that their 11 million (mostly indemnity) members could be transferred over rather than fought for. Tremendous economies of scale in the use of USQA's software and statistical profiles could be immediately obtained. In 1992, heady with success, the management of U.S. Healthcare envisioned that USQA would attract other HMOs as clients, and that soon it would be spun off as a separate company, perhaps growing larger than its parent. Later, it became clear that such a strategy was not viable—monitoring quality and developing information systems is so intimately intertwined with the core business of an HMO that it would never allow a competing entity to participate in that task, or to access such sensitive data. Hence, USQA technology could only be used in-house or sold only in those regions (such as England) where U.S. Healthcare could never be a competitive threat.

In the end, it may have been Abramson himself who was the most compelling reason for selling the company. U.S. Healthcare never developed a faceless corporate style—it was always Leonard Abramson's company, where he personally made most of the important decisions. Although he had groomed several of his children for leadership roles, and brought in a number of senior executives, there was no clear successor in sight.[19] The genius and prime mover of the company was now sixty-three. Losing its CEO, or bringing in any conceivable replacement, would clearly have caused the company to decline, at least temporarily. With a merger, U.S. Healthcare's name may be absorbed and its chairman's seat vacated, but the contracting and information technology he created will live long and prosper.

11.5 WHY MANAGED CARE TODAY? _____

The primary impetus behind managed care has been the rise in health care costs, and in particular, the rise in the cost of employee health benefits. From 1970 to 1980, health care expenditures by businesses rose from 3.1 percent of employee compensation to 4.9 percent. Then, costs grew even more rapidly, and by 1990 reached 7.1 percent. Health benefits, equal to 36 percent of after-tax profits in 1970, and 43 percent in 1980, actually exceeded (108%) total corporate profits in 1990. Indemnity insurance premiums for Blue Cross and Blue Shield coverage rose by as much as 30 percent a year in many markets during the early 1980s. In the face of these large increases, prudence and survival demanded that something be done to reduce health care as a cost of business. The problems of businesses had actually been made worse by government cost-containment efforts in the 1980s, because reductions in Medicaid and Medicare rates forced hospitals to shift costs by charging more to insured patients (see section 8.4 for a discussion of cost shifting). Businesses became increasingly willing to turn to an outside contractor who could stabilize benefit costs, even if it meant having to accept some constraints and employee complaints. HMO contracts and membership exploded—from 3 million in 1970, to 9 million in 1980, 36 million in 1990, and 60 million in 1995, with employer group contracts accounting for 90 percent of the total membership.

Changes in **information technology** made management of care much more cost-effective. From the 1930s until 1970, utilization review (UR) meant manually retrieving a patient chart and reading it. Documentation had to be mailed from the hospital to UR reviewer, and read again. The rapid fall in the price of computing and telecommunications changed the way in which review was carried out. Software went through claims as they were submitted, checking for discrepancies and creating profiles for each physician, for each disease category, and for other variables of interest as needed. Documentation was either faxed or made available on-line for immediate retrieval. Patients called a toll-free number rather than traipsing downtown for a referral. Managed care as practiced in 1995 was neither technologically or financially feasible in 1960.

Changes in **medical technology** are also changing health care from a cottage industry in which skilled individuals do custom work to meet the specifications of individual clients into a corporate structure where teams engage in coordinated effort. Indemnity insurance was designed to pay bills as each separate general practitioner, laboratory, surgeon, neurologist, hospital, and physical therapist treated one patient at a time. A bundled payment for all services makes more sense now that quality is more a function of how well the organization works than the training or skill of each individual professional.

It has been suggested by some commentators that changes in medical technology were also responsible for the rapid rise in the cost of care, but this position is not entirely supported by the evidence.[20] Mental health, examined at length in chapter 10, section 5, had a higher than average rate of cost increase, but had no new expensive diagnostic machines or surgeries or artificial organs to which such costs could be attributed. The major technological advance in mental health treatment from 1960 to 1990 was the development of more powerful drugs to control symptoms, and this technology clearly reduced costs by allowing patients to be discharged earlier under medication. A comparison of the U.S. cost experience with that of other countries such as England, Germany, France and Japan (chapter 19), shows that these countries did not experience equally rapid rises in per capita health costs, even though all of the new technology that became available in the U.S. also became available overseas. Therefore, it is clear that something besides new technology must have been responsible for a large part of the rise in the cost of medical care in the United States during the last thirty years. Although all of the causes are not clear, some major factors were the rapid increases in hourly wages during the twenty post–WW II years, the *expectation* that wages and benefits would continue to increase and thus be able to support an expanded medical care system, a consensus that better post–WW II medical care had made life both better and longer, and expectations regarding continuous advances in medical practice (see chapters 15 and 18). These conditions favored the expansion of indemnity fee-for-service throughout the 1960s and 1970s. Its propensity for cost-shifting and the unrestrained growth inherent in an entitlement system were seen as positives, not negatives. As wages stagnated and the power of medicine was called into question, support for the continuous growth of medical technology and medical expenditures eroded.[21] Anxiety over the future of the economy and fears about the intrusiveness and futility of the most aggressive forms of medical practice made policies of moderation and cost-control more attractive.

Political and attitudinal changes since 1960 have shifted the climate of opinion and legal situation regarding HMOs from unfavorable to favorable in the 1990s. The relative importance of system versus individual interests has switched one way for physicians, and the other way for patients and payers. In the 1930s, physicians took a collective position in opposition to HMOs, with individual members willingly sacrificing hundreds of hours and millions of dollars in political contributions for what they perceived to be the good of the profession as a whole. At that time, employers and insurers did not speak out loudly for patients' collective interest in lowering costs. The rising price of medicine was "no problem," as long as you and your family could have insurance. These roles began to switch sometime during the 1980s. A surplus of physicians (created by the expansion of medical schools that started in 1970—see chapter 6) and a surplus of hospitals (created by overbuilding and changes in reimbursement and medical technology that shortened the length of time patients stayed in the hospital—see chapter 9) made providers scramble for business, putting individual concerns above common problems. Autonomy and a high income had previously come with the M.D. degree, but newer physicians were increasingly disillusioned by the years of sacrifice required to start a private practice, as well as the uncertain returns from doing so. More and more were willing to take an HMO job with steady hours, plenty of patients, and a guaranteed salary that had become significantly higher than they could expect to earn starting out in private practice. As physicians and hospitals in a down market became acutely aware that their colleagues were also their competitors, they became unwilling to sacrifice very much in the way of current income for the long-run good of the profession. Conversely, the patient's agents—government and corporate benefits managers—had acquired a much broader perspective, seeing that taking care of this or that person's illness would become ever more difficult to fund unless they could somehow change the big picture and reduce the overall cost of care. Medicare spending increases alone could account for most of the federal deficit, and Medicaid expenditures were the leading cause of state fiscal distress. Corporations simply choked on paying for an employee "benefit" that had become larger than their profits. Thus by 1990, HMOs were well positioned to take advantage of both sides: on the supply side, physician and hospital surpluses made them willing to provide these inputs at cut-rate prices in order to maintain patient volume; on the demand side, corporate benefit managers and government agencies were eager to find discounts for a total package and willing to turn the choice of provider over to the HMO.

The major legal barrier to HMOs had been the ban on the corporate practice of medicine. The AMA used a broad interpretation in its attack upon GHA in 1937—and lost. In 1965, the AMA fought Medicare as "socialized medicine"—and lost. By the time the HMO Act of 1973 guaranteeing employees the right to choose an HMO if one were operating in their area and providing small start-up grants to create new HMOs was proposed, most of the AMA opposition had faded. Years of coexistence with Kaiser, GHA, and other HMOs had led physicians to accept HMOs as a minor organizational variant that would not threaten the dominance of private practice and indemnity insurance—and indeed, for fifteen years it did not.

Legal restraints, as well as the supply and demand factors, go a long way toward explaining why none of the early HMOs were founded as corporations, and were thus so susceptible to the problems of ambiguous ownership and divided management. In a time when most doctors were still in private practice and people paid their bills in person, it would have been impossible to set up the kind of for-profit HMO that has come to dominate the managed care scene today.

11.6 MANAGED COMPETITION _____

The HMO Act of 1973 caused a flurry of activity, but only modest increases in enrollment took place. Although HMOs had become solidly established, they were only an "option," an alternative to the mainstream that remained FFS-financed through indemnity insurance. Despite the official endorsement implied by the HMO act, HMO enrollment of the patients whose care was directly funded by the government (Medicaid, Medicare, VA/DOD) stayed even lower than for the rest of the population, an almost negligible 2 percent. In 1978, Alain Enthoven published a provocative proposal in the *New England Journal of Medicine* calling for a "Consumer Choice Health Plan," envisioning a future in which managed care was the norm and FFS was the alternative.[22] Competition, but competition within a set of controls (i.e., "managed competition" to fit the special characteristics of health care as a human service) would be used to control costs while maintaining the technological dynamism of the market. The proposals have been through a number of iterations over the years, with the following points being among the most important.[23]

1. Competing HMOs would be created in each area.
2. Each plan would have a common set of basic benefits, but could add extra services to increase its market appeal.
3. Community rating, at least on a limited basis, would allow disabled individuals, companies with older workforces, and so on to obtain coverage at reasonable rates.
4. The tax subsidy of health insurance would be eliminated. Although employer payment sufficient to cover the basic services would be allowed, or perhaps even mandated, the employee would personally have to pay the full marginal cost of any additional premiums, and so would have an incentive to choose a more efficient or narrower plan.
5. FFS would be an option, but persons choosing FFS coverage would pay the full cost of the difference between indemnity and HMO premiums.

The managed competition strategy has become identified with an informal meeting of health policy experts led by Enthoven and Paul Ellwood (founder of Interstudy, a leading HMO consulting firm) called the "Jackson Hole Group." They became a major intellectual force, and strongly supported President Clinton's efforts to develop a new national health policy. In the end, however, disheartened by the number of compromises required to turn an idea into legislation, and perhaps sensitive to the polls predicting defeat, Enthoven declared that the Clinton Health Security plan of 1994 did not meet his criteria for a "Consumer Choice Health Plan" upholding the principles of managed competition, and publicly disavowed the final draft before a vote was taken.[24]

Critics claimed that the term *managed competition* was an oxymoron, two words that contradict each other. Indeed, on the surface it does appear confusing to argue that a plan eliminating consumers' out-of-pocket payments and limiting the choice of doctors promotes competition relative to the FFS alternative of increasing patient coinsurance and unrestricted choice. This confusion can be cleared by considering two premises:

1. In order to be socially beneficial, most competition must be highly organized and regulated (the "level playing field" with a referee that characterizes baseball, football, the stock market, commodities exchanges, etc.).
2. FFS indemnity insurance funded by employers and government had all but removed "price" as a factor relevant to consumer decision making: $50 in pharmaceutical copays had become more important than $50,000 hospital bills for heart surgery.

Enthoven's "consumer choice" health plan was based on the recognition that consumers, confronted with thousands of possible illnesses, millions of possible prices, and indemnity coverage that was (a) difficult to understand and (b) comprehensive enough to make the effort of comparing costs not worthwhile, actually made decisions that were very remote from the "market" in which suppliers operated. Consumers looked for plans with low copayments, or coverage of eyeglasses and orthodontics, or benefit maximums set at reassuringly astronomical amounts—factors that had nothing to do with the cost of health care overall, or the rising premiums that employers had to pay each year that were reducing profits and wages. In contrast, "consumer choice" as envisioned by Enthoven was between two or three competing plans. Each plan was to have a price that was known in advance, and the consumer was to pay the full difference between the low-cost plan and the high-cost plan if they preferred to obtain greater choice, more coverage, or higher quality. Far from being an intellectual abstraction, Enthoven's proposal was based on the Federal Employee's Health Benefits Plan (FEHBP), which had worked that way for years, offering federal employees a choice from a menu of HMO and indemnity plans in each area.[25] Since the FEHBP has been in operation for more than thirty years, it is easy to verify that consumers do make choices, that they are satisfied with the choices they are given, that such a system is administratively feasible on a large scale, that price differences do matter, and that some efficiencies can be gained. What is not so clear is whether or not such "consumer-choice" managed competition will revolutionize the health care system and solve the problem of ever-rising costs that hobble economic growth nationwide and drive the federal budget into deficit each year.

11.7   IS MANAGED CARE THE SOLUTION TO RISING COSTS? _____

Evidence on Cost Reductions

A large number of studies in many markets over many years have consistently shown that medical care managed and financed through an HMO costs 10 to 20 percent less than under indemnity insurance.[26] Most of the savings comes from two factors: A substantial reduction in the number of hospital days per 1,000 enrollees, and the ability to obtain lower prices by contracting for large volumes of hospital, physician, laboratory, and pharmacy services. The reduction in hospital days is somewhat offset by a greater use of ambulatory physician services and outpatient surgery among HMOs, but since these substitutes are less expensive than inpatient services, overall dollar savings are realized even when the quantity of services used stays the same or increases. The following questions have arisen regarding this record of HMO cost reductions, and will be discussed at length.

1. Are some of the apparent savings overstated because HMOs enroll people who are at lower risk to begin with?
2. Is the quality of care as good when costs are lowered?
3. Can newer forms of managed care (IPAs, PPOs) reduce costs as much as closed HMOs?
4. Will cost reductions be offset by higher administrative costs and profits?
5. Does the switch to managed care give just a one-time 20 percent reduction in health care costs, or can it slow the rate of price increases?
6. If most patients and payers are winners, are there also some people who stand to lose from the spread of managed care?

Risk Selection

Some companies that added an HMO option found that although the cost per person was significantly lower for those employees who chose the HMO plan rather than the indemnity plan, the company's overall health care cost for all employees (HMO and indemnity) rose just as rapidly as before. The reason was that there had been positive risk selection into the HMO option, which attracted the younger and relatively healthy people, and adverse selection into the indemnity plan, which kept the older and sicker people (see chapter 3, section 3 to review adverse selection).[27] Sicker people are more likely to opt for a less-restrictive FFS plan rather than the HMO, since they are more likely to have become attached to a particular physician whom they visit often, and are thus unwilling to accept an HMO that limits their choice of doctors; and people with serious illness are more likely to want "the best" care at famous (and expensive) academic research hospitals rather than be limited to the providers within the HMO network. Young, healthy couples are often attracted to HMOs because they provide more extensive preventive services, and cover many prenatal and baby visits at no charge. (There are, however, also some reasons that sicker people might prefer the HMO: better coverage of pharmaceuticals, lower copayments and no deductible.)

Evaluation studies have shown that on average, HMOs tend to have a more favorable risk selection, attracting healthier enrollees. Yet even after adjusting for differences in age, sex, prior hospitalizations and other factors, the costs per person in an HMO are still 10 to 20 percent lower than for comparable groups under FFS. The differential cost savings have been maintained over time as HMO enrollees aged and began to use more care. HMO cost savings have also been shown to occur in companies that switched to 100 percent HMO coverage where there was no possibility for positive selection. The one area for which the ability of HMOs to generate savings has not been consistently demonstrated is among those chronically ill elderly and disabled persons who are not covered by employer insurance in the first place (which may be a very significant exclusion for purposes of public policy; see later discussion).

Quality of Care

From the time prepaid medical plans were first developed, they have been attacked for providing incentives to reduce services, and hence to reduce quality. However, decades of research shows that on average, the quality of care in HMOs is comparable to or better than that provided under indemnity insurance.[28] In particular, HMO patients are more likely to receive preventive services, to see physicians more often, receive coordinated care from a variety of providers, appropriately use primary physicians rather than the emergency rooms for acute illnesses, and be subjected to less unnecessary surgery. On the other hand, HMO patients are less likely to receive treatment for some disorders such as depression and back pain. Also, HMOs use less aggressive therapy and thus more frequently err on the side of doing too little surgery rather than too much. Surveys of consumer satisfaction show mixed results. Patients are usually more satisfied with the financial aspects of an HMO than an indemnity insurance plan (no paperwork and billing hassles, no deductibles). However, patients may be less satisfied with service and amenities, particularly when they feel forced to accept an HMO option, even though extensive research has shown little difference in morbidity, mortality or extent of functional recovery from accidents and chronic illness.[29] The net effect is that quality is roughly comparable in the two sectors, a little better in the HMO for some things, a little better under FFS for others.

Since care in an HMO is not rationed by price, administrative barriers are used to sort those who need, or want, or can get, immediate care from those who are willing to wait or do without. HMOs thus tend to favor those people and families who can manage their own care. Although it might seem that not charging to see a doctor would favor poor people, in practice it is the middle- and upper-class patients (i.e., those who are most successful at working within the system) who are likely to receive more and better care in HMOs. Managed care requires active involvement that people who have been disenfranchised and have low expectations for service sometimes find difficult to achieve.

An early experiment with Medicaid managed care contracting ended disastrously when many shoddy clinics (often termed "Medicaid mills" because they treated hundreds of patients per hour with little personal attention, or medical care, like an assembly line) signed up as providers and made millions in the California Medi-Cal program—and subsequently were sued for malpractice, and frequently went bankrupt. In order to keep Medicaid patients from getting second-class service, regulations were written requiring federally qualified HMOs that wanted to accept Medicaid patients to be able to attract 75 percent of their enrollees from private employer-funded groups. While well meaning, this legislation had the effect of forcing indigent people into managed care systems designed for the employed. Yet in order to provide effective care for a traditionally underserved and disenfranchised population, it is often necessary to use aggressive outreach and health promotion, to design clinics, appointment systems, and paperwork that is user-friendly to indigent patients. Maintaining the quality of care provided to Medicaid enrollees has been a constant challenge for HMOs. These quality problems in Medicaid HMO enrollment would be more troublesome were it not for the fact that in comparison, most FFS care available to Medicaid patients is much worse, or simply unaffordable. Although Medicaid indemnity insurance has paid for thousands of heart transplants, MRI scans, and other high-tech medical interventions, it has not done a good job of providing prenatal care, treatment for drug abuse, or control of blood pressure among the indigent population. Although the quality of care provided to Medicaid HMO enrollees may not be quite as high as that received by employed HMO enrollees, the cost is significantly lower than with FFS Medicaid, and the overall quality has usually been equal or better.[30]

Costs Reductions in IPA-HMOs, PPOs, and POS Plans

The more open and less restrictive a managed care plan has been, the more acceptable it has been to new enrollees who were accustomed to FFS care. That is why the great expansion of HMO membership in the 1980s occurred in IPA HMOs, and more recently, the new preferred provider organization (PPO) and point-of-service (POS) plans (see chapter 10). Can these less-tightly managed plans control costs as well as the more-tightly managed closed-group HMO? They can, but only to the extent that they adopt stringent UR procedures, careful assessment of each day of hospitalization, aggressive substitution of less costly drugs and therapies, and in general, tighten up the management of care to an equivalent degree as the traditional closed HMO.[31] When HMO enrollment accounts for less than a quarter of a physician's practice, that physician's behavior shows little change. When most of a physician's patients are in a single HMO, that physician begins to act much more like a physician in a closed HMO, with lower rates of hospitalization, more careful attention to administrative procedures, awareness of drug and laboratory reimbursement limits, and so on. PPOs are able to obtain volume discounts, but since they do not have primary care physician gatekeepers, and cannot use administrative procedures or financial withholds (chapter 10, section 4) to control physicians' referral and admitting patterns, they usually do not have much effect on utilization. In short, to get something (cost control), something must be given up (freedom of choice and clinical autonomy).

Administrative Costs and Profits

Some commentators have worried that reductions in the cost of medical care do not benefit consumers, but are taken up by the higher administrative costs required to manage care, and by the profits that for-profit HMO companies pay to shareholders as dividends. Since 20 percent of the premiums HMOs receive go toward administrative costs and profit, the reason for concern is evident. However, management is a cost of doing business, and a cost that has increased over time as business has become more complex *and more efficient.* Douglass North, who received the 1994 Nobel Prize for his work in cliometrics (the use of statistical measures to study economic history), estimated that in 1800 less than 10 percent of the GDP of a largely rural U.S. economy went to transaction costs, but that by 1970, more than 50 percent of economic activity was accounted for by managers, salespeople, consultants, accountants, telecommunications, and other administrative costs.[32] The production of high-technology equipment or services requires more of the "management" input than it does of raw materials, unskilled labor, or other inputs. It was sensible for the solo physician of the 1950s to do his own billing, office maintenance, and recordkeeping; it is not very efficient in the 1990s when the treatment of any serious illness will usually require the services of a dozen doctors and hundreds of ancillary personnel. All this is not to say that some HMOs do not have excessive levels of administrative costs. There are well-managed HMOs that can do a better job of quality control and negotiation with 11 percent of premiums than others can do with 15 or 20 percent—and that is one reason that some HMOs are more profitable than others. Profits are a cost of doing business; they are a means of rewarding entrepreneurial effort, insightful planning, and correct anticipation of market demands.

Profits tend to follow the flow of business. Without profits, there is no clear signal of which firms are most efficient, or produce services of greatest value to consumers. As HMOs became more able to control where patients received care, they not only reduced utilization to improve efficiency, but were also able to obtain some of the profits that had previously been received by hospitals and physicians. This made shareholders happy, but not the hospitals and physicians, who quite rightly resented being managed and having some of "their" producer's surplus taken away. Over time, competition between HMOs will transfer that surplus to employers (who pay lower premiums), and ultimately to workers (who receive higher wages as health benefit costs decline).

One-time Savings?

Will the search by HMOs for market share and greater profits revolutionize U.S. health care, just enrich a few owners and shareholders? This question lies at the heart of speculation about whether the switch to managed care will yield a one-time-only savings of 10 to 20 percent, or cause a permanent reduction in the rate of growth in health care costs (Figure 11.1). In most evaluations so far, only one-time savings have been demonstrated.[33] Kaiser premiums, for example, although

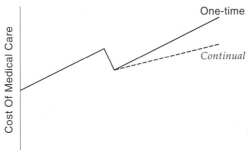

FIGURE 11.1 *Do HMOs provide one-time or continued cost reductions?*

consistently lower than Blue Cross premiums, have grown at about the same annual percentage rate over the last fifty years. However, HMOs have become a significant market force only in recent years. Therefore these results, based on HMOs
as a minor optional alternative, may not be indicative of what will happen if
HMOs come to dominate the market. Just as physicians with few HMO patients
have been shown to still treat them almost the same as FFS patients, markets with
little HMO penetration may mostly continue with traditional patterns of treatment and so would not reveal the changes that might occur if most corporations
and government agencies were constantly shopping for value in health care benefits on the basis of price and quality information. The advent of managed care on
a large scale is so recent, and adaptive change to societal structures takes so long,
that any conclusions about what will happen to the trajectory of health care costs
over the next fifty years must be considered fairly speculative at this point in time.
Managed care may prove to be the revolution that brought price sensitivity and
continuous quality improvement to health care, or just another management fad
that caught the attention of the politicians for a few years.

Are There Losers as Well as Winners?

Most of the opposition to managed care has come from the traditional powers on
the supply side of medicine, licensed professionals and nonprofit hospitals, who
clearly stand to lose money as costs are cut.[34] Yet it is on the demand side that the
weakness of managed care as a strategy for controlling cost is revealed. The problem is that the rather small groups of people who need a lot of care (the chronically ill, children with AIDS, the frail elderly, etc.) are quite separate from those
who can afford to pay for care (the employed). Managed care has been developed
to serve groups that are mostly healthy and have resources, not the dependent
sick. Yet the healthy three-fourths of the population that has money, family support, and skills in dealing with management, accounts for less than one-fourth of
the costs. This split between the sick and the well, between those who pay taxes
and those who receive subsidized benefits, will get wider and wider as life expectancy lengthens. At the same time, the curable, randomly-occurring illnesses
that still affect employees and their children will increasingly be reduced in importance relative to chronic conditions and social disorders. It may be difficult to
get the majority to agree to forgo fancy medical advances in order to continue to
improve care for the minority that is most in need.

Managed care techniques can be applied to reduce the costs of AIDS, of diabetes
and genetic defects, just as it already has (sometimes) reduced the cost of heart
disease and cancer. Yet even with the most effective management possible, people
with AIDS or diabetes or birth defects will still have treatment costs much greater
than the average, and so inevitably raise the question of who should pay. Surely
employees will take care of each other, from president to parking lot attendant.
But will working people willingly pay for treatment of AIDS in intravenous drug
abusers, or the years of therapy for a child born with Down's syndrome to a single unemployed mother, or the final years of decline in an Alzheimer's patient?
For a hundred years, the U.S. health care system has funded care of the indigent,
chronic disease treatment, and medical research through cost shifting (see chapter

8, section 4, for a review). Managed care seeks lower costs for the group of patients being managed, and roots out costs that belong to others. When an intoxicated patient is shifted from an academic hospital psychiatric unit costing $1,200 a day to a community hospital costing $400 a day, and then on to a halfway house costing $80 per day, the health plan is not only saving money by using more appropriate services, it is also avoiding the costs of teaching residents, uncompensated care, and medical research. Shifting coronary-artery bypass grafts to efficient high-volume providers means that those fees can no longer be used to subsidize organ transplants. The profit margins in HMOs are around 5 percent. Managers are constantly searching for an extra 0.5 percent. Avoiding enrollment of the seriously ill, or even reducing the number slightly, will usually reduce costs by more than that. Managed care gives an incentive for efficiency, but it gives an even bigger incentive for exclusion of expensive cases. In this way it may act to further separate those who are well off from those who are needy.

The principle that all citizens should have equal access to health care has been put under increasing pressure.[35] A federal deficit that could be entirely attributed to the unanticipated cost increases in the Medicare program, and state budgetary problems largely due to Medicaid cost increases, make it harder and harder to maintain the hidden transfer tax implicit in cost-shifting. The advance of managed care to more employer groups will make this problem much worse, revealing ever more starkly that the group picking up most of the cost through wage and income taxes is not the same as the group of needy persons who take most of the health care resources. Although managed care techniques are likely to reduce the cost of treating AIDS, diabetes, drug addiction and manic depression, managed care pricing will make the differential between the average cost of caring for worker and nonworker more and more apparent. Most people would agree that those who need medical care should receive it, and that those who can afford to do so should pay to support the system that cares for us all. Managed care forces the question: How much? In managed care, employees pay premiums that cover only themselves and their dependents. Will these workers take their savings and vote to use them to raise taxes and pay more for Medicaid, for medical research? $100 billion a year? Managed care will force the public to confront these questions. It will not solve the problems.

SUGGESTIONS FOR FURTHER READING _____

Alain Enthoven, *Theory and Practice of Managed Competition in Health Care Finance,* Amsterdam: North-Holland, 1988.

E. Hoy, R. Curtis and T. Rice, "Change and Growth in Managed Care," *Health Affairs* 10(4):18–36, 1991.

Association of American Health Plans, *HMO Performance Report* (annual).

Robert H. Miller and Harold Luft, "Managed Care Plans: Characteristics, Growth and Premium Performance," *Annual Review of Public Health* 15:437–459, 1994, and "Managed Care Plan Performance Since 1980: A Literature Analysis, *Journal of the American Medical Association,* 271(19):1512–1519, 1994.

John G. Smillie, M.D. *Can Physicians Manage the Quality and Costs of Health Care: The Story of the Permanente Medical Group,* New York, McGraw–Hill, 1991.

SUMMARY _____

1. Contractual medical practice has existed in different forms for centuries, but the HMO only took shape over the last sixty years. **Payment systems and capitation rates have evolved through trial and error** and are usually based more on prior experience and practice patterns than on actuarial science or economic theory.

2. **Kaiser,** founded just after World War II, is **the largest HMO** with over 6 million members. However, the lack of a clearly defined ownership structure, limited access to capital, and a resistance to capital mobility between regions have been major impediments to further growth.

3. Most HMOs started as nonprofit organizations. Some were explicitly collectivist and anti-capitalist in origin, but have become increasingly businesslike. Over time, the more rapid **growth of for-profit firms** has led them to dominate the industry, and now even many nonprofit HMOs have for-profit subsidiaries.

4. **Excess capacity** in the health care industry allowed HMOs to obtain **discounts** from providers in the 1980s. A burgeoning surplus of hospital beds, and a rapid expansion in the number of physicians graduating from medical schools and residencies made it easy for the hard bargaining HMOs to trade volume for lower prices.

5. Managed care has begun to force a much greater degree of **vertical and horizontal integration** upon a medical system that had resisted organizational change. Changes in telecommunications and **information technology** make it possible for management to practice utilization review and monitor quality of care at dispersed sites around the country.

6. **"Managed competition"** is based on the premise that consumers will become more price sensitive as they are able to take home the difference between more and less expensive health plans in their paychecks, while competing HMOs strive to offer the best value for money, and not just "the best."

7. Managed care has been shown to **reduce costs**, but may not be the answer to all of America's health care problems. Some HMOs have made money by **risk selection**, accepting mostly healthier patients. Other HMOs **may find it hard to maintain quality of care** once the easy savings from discounting and substitution have been taken, and thus may be tempted to reduce services in precisely those areas where patients, hampered by information asymmetry, depend most on professionals for monitoring quality. Extending coverage to the homeless, those born with birth defects, the disenfranchised, and the chronically ill will provide the true test of managed care as a strategy for universal cost control.

8. On the whole, it appears that most patients, employers, and the government are clear winners and are well **satisfied with the expansion of managed care**. However, at least some of their gains come from the **doctors and hospitals**, who are clearly **losers in the short run** as increased competition, discounting

and tight management control over utilization reduces professional autonomy and incomes.

PROBLEMS _____

1. {*incidence*} If ABC corporation shifts from an indemnity plan to an HMO plan that lowers its cost of employee benefits by 35 percent over three years, who benefits? Who loses?

2. {*dynamics*} Does a surplus of hospital beds in an area make it easier or harder to start an HMO? A surplus of doctors? A surplus of insurance companies?

3. {*pricing*} How did Sydney Garfield set the monthly premiums for his first pre-paid health plan? How are premiums set for Kaiser today?

4. {*property rights*} Who owns Kaiser Permanente? Is there stock? Have ownership rights ever been sold?

5. {*regulation*} Did the HMO Act of 1973 have affects on competition and capital expenditure similar to the CON acts passed during the same period?

6. {*dynamics*} What technological change has been most important in fostering the growth of managed care?

7. {*selection bias*} If a company offers both an HMO and indemnity plan, which employees will choose which?

8. {*property rights*} Why is it that HMOs formed in the 1930s were often collectives attracting physicians with liberal or socialist leanings, while today HMOs are most often formed by entrepreneurs with capitalist ideals?

9. {*property rights*} What are the advantages and disadvantages of (a) nonprofit status and (b) publicly traded stock that provides incentives to physicians?

10. {*selection*} Would an HMO entering the Medicare market expect to experience favorable or adverse selection? Would the magnitude of the selection bias be larger or smaller for an HMO entering the commercial employee benefit market? The Medicaid market?

11. {*dynamics*} Will a contract that lowers the amount an HMO pays providers be more important with regard to short-run or long-run profitability? Why?

12. {*information*} In what ways can an HMO use information to increase profits? As information technology has become more efficient and cheaper to use, have health care firms invested more or less in computers?

13. {*competition*} Since HMOs limit choice of doctors relative to indemnity fee for service, why are they considered to be the centerpiece of managed competition as described by Alan Enthoven in his "Consumer Choice Health Plan"?

14. {*incidence*} Which groups are favored by a general move toward capitated managed care? Which groups tend to lose?

15. {*incidence*} If an HMO provides inadequate maternity coverage, who gets hurt? Is it likely to cause an employer to look for a different insurance plan? How would your answer be different for treatment of psoriasis? For treatment of drug addiction? Suppose that it is an indemnity insurer who provides the inadequate treatment; would this change your answers? Would your answers

change if it were the doctor who was providing inadequate care, and not a limitation due to coverage?

ENDNOTES _____

1. Much of the information in this section comes from John G. Smillie, M.D. *Can Physicians Manage the Quality and Costs of Health Care: The Story of the Permanente Medical Group,* New York, McGraw-Hill, 1991; and Paul de Kruif, *Kaiser Wakes the Doctors,* New York: Harcourt, Brace & Co, 1943.

2. Prepaid medical group practice had existed in America since at least 1790, when such a plan was used at the Boston Dispensary. The innovative prepayment contract between The City of Los Angeles Department of Water and Power and Drs. Ross and Loos to provide all medical services to 12,000 employees and 25,000 dependents for $2 per month (excluding hospitalization) was a more proximate example that probably influenced Garfield.

3. Quoted on page 55 of John G. Smillie, M.D. *Can Physicians Manage the Quality and Costs of Health Care: The Story of the Permanente Medical Group,* New York, McGraw-Hill, 1991.

4. Louise Kertesz, "Kaiser Retools to Fight for Lost Ground," *Modern Healthcare,* July 17, 1995, pp: 34–40.

5. E. Hoy, R. Curtis, and T. Rice, "Change and Growth in Managed Care," *Health Affairs* 10(4):18–36, 1991.

6. Hoechst, Marion, Roussel, *HMO-PPO Digest 1995,* Kansas City, Mo.: Hoechst, Marion, Roussel, 1995.

7. Edward D. Berkowitz and Wendy Wolff, *Group Health Association: A Portrait of a Health Maintenance Organization,* Philadelphia: Temple University Press, 1988, p. 144.

8. Paul Starr, *The Social Transformation of American Medicine,* New York: Basic Books, 1982.

9. As quoted in Gilbert Gaul, "U.S. Healthcare's Abramson: Dedicated, Perhaps Ruthless," *The Philadelphia Inquirer,* April 2, 1996, page A5.

10. Much of the information in this case study comes from interviews with Sandra Harmon-Weiss, M.D., Medical Director of U.S. Healthcare, and other executives, "A Brief Overview: U.S. Healthcare" by Hyman R. Kahn, M.D. (mimeo, November 28, 1994), and annual financial reports of U.S. Healthcare.

11. In the words of Pulitzer-Prize-winning journalist Gilbert Gaul, "For years, some of the most prestigious hospitals in Philadelphia refused to sign contracts with U.S. Healthcare. Those that did often complained bitterly about the hard-line negotiating style of Abramson and his colleagues, which resulted in lower reimbursement rates for the hospitals." in "U.S. Healthcare's Abramson: Dedicated, Perhaps Ruthless," *The Philadelphia Inquirer,* April 2, 1996, page A5.

12. Accounting practices are significantly different in the nonprofit Kaiser plan, so the figures are not entirely comparable. It is, however, generally accepted that of the major HMOs, Kaiser probably has the highest percentage of premiums going to medical costs, while U.S. Healthcare is among the lowest.

13. Neil Schlackman, "Evolution of a Quality-Based Compensation Model: The Third Generation," *American Journal of Medical Quality* 8(2):103–110, 1993.

14. Nicholas Hanchak, Neil Schlackman, Sandra Harmon-Weiss, U.S. *Healthcare's Quality-Based Compensation Model* 32 pages (mimeo), Blue Bell, Pa.: U.S. Healthcare, 1996.

15. Paul Kenkel, "U.S. Healthcare 'Report Cards' Expanded to Primary-Care Docs," *Modern Healthcare,* April 11, 1994.

16. Eleanor H. Kerns, health care analyst for Alex Brown & Sons, a leading investment banking firm, has opined publicly that U.S. Healthcare's information systems are su-

perior to those of its competitors: see Marian Uhlman and Andrea Knox, "Aetna, U.S. Healthcare Plan Merger," *The Philadelphia Inquirer,* April 2, 1996, pages A1,A5.

17. George Anders and Ron Winslow, "HMO Stocks Skid on U.S. Healthcare Announcement," *The Wall Street Journal,* April 20, 1995.

18. Leslie Scism and Steven Lipin, "Aetna Near $8 Billion Deal to Acquire U.S. Healthcare," *The Wall Street Journal,* April 1, 1996, page A3.

19. Gilbert Gaul, "U.S. Healthcare's Abramson: Dedicated, Perhaps Ruthless," *The Philadelphia Inquirer,* April 2, 1996, page A5.

20. S. Altman and S. Wallack, "Technology on Trial—Is It the Culprit Behind Rising Health Costs? The Case For and Against," in *Medical Technology: The Culprit Behind Health Care Costs?* S. Altman and R. Blendon, eds., Washington, D.C.: U.S. Department of Health, Education and Welfare, 1979.

21. Victor Fuchs, "The Best Health Care System in the World?" *Journal of the American Medical Association,* 268(7):916–917, 1992; Jack Hadley, *More Medical Care, Better Health?* Washington, D.C.: The Urban Institute Press, 1982; Institute of Medicine, *Innovation at the Crossroads,* Vol. 3, *Technology and Health Care in an Era of Limits,* A. Gelijns, ed., Washington, D.C.: National Academy Press, 1992; Ivan Illich, *Medical Nemesis: The Expropriation of Health,* New York: Pantheon Books, 1976.

22. Alain Enthoven, " Consumer Choice Health Plan," *New England Journal of Medicine,* 298:650–658 and 709–720, 1978.

23. Alain Enthoven, *Theory and Practice of Managed Competition in Health Care Finance,* Amsterdam: North-Holland, 1988.

24. Paul M. Ellwood and Alain C. Enthoven, " 'Responsible Choices:' The Jackson Hole Plan," *Health Affairs* 14(2):24–39, 1995.

25. Alain Enthoven, "Management of Competition in the FEHPB," *Health Affairs,* 8(3):33–50, 1989.

26. Harold Luft, *Health Maintenance Organizations: Dimensions of Performance,* New York: John Wiley & Sons, 1981; Robert H. Miller and Harold Luft, "Managed Care Plan Performance Since 1980: A Literature Analysis, *Journal of the American Medical Association,* 271(19):1512–1519, 1994; J. Hill et al. *The Impact of the Medicare Risk Program on the Use of Services and Costs to Medicare,* (Princeton, N.J.: Mathematica Policy Research, 1992); D. K. Freeborn and C. R. Pope, *Promise and Performance in Managed Care: The Prepaid Group Practice Model,* Baltimore: Johns Hopkins University Press, 1994.

27. Gail Wilensky and Louis Rossiter, "Patient Self-Selection in HMOs," *Health Affairs* 5(4):66–80, 1986; S. E. Berki and M. L. Ashcraft, "HMO Enrollment: Who Joins and Why: A Review of the Literature," *Milbank Memorial Fund Quarterly,* 58:588–632, 1980; Kyle Grazier, William Richardson, Diane Martin, et al; "Factors Affecting Choice of Health Care Plans," *Health Services Research* 20(6):659–682, 1986.

28. S. M. Retchin and B. Brown, "The Quality of Ambulatory Care in Medicare Health Maintenance Organizations," *American Journal of Public Health,* 80:411–415, 1990; I. S. Udvarhely et al., "Comparison of the Quality of Ambulatory Care for Fee-For-Service and Prepaid Patients," *Annals of Internal Medicine* 327:424–429, 1991; J. E. Ware et al., "Comparison of Health Outcomes at a Health Maintenance Organization With Those of Fee-For-Service Care," *Lancet* 1986, I:130–136.

29. Karen Davis, Karen Scott Collins, Cathy Schoen, and Cynthia Morris, "Choice Matters: Enrollees' Views of Their Health Plans," *Health Affairs,* 14(2):99–112, 1995; H. R. Rubin et al., "Patients Ratings of Outpatient Visits in Different Practice Settings: Results from the Medical Outcomes Study," *Journal of the American Medical Association,* 262:57–63, 1989.

30. Robert Hurley, Deborah Freund, and John Paul, *Managed Care in Medicaid: Lessons for Policy and Program Design,* Ann Arbor, Mich.: Health Administration Press, 1993.

31. Robert H. Miller and Harold Luft, "Managed Care Plans: Characteristics, Growth and Premium Performance," *Annual Review of Public Health* 15:437–459, 1994.
32. John J. Wallis and Douglass C. North. "Measuring the Transaction Sector in the American Economy, 1870–1970," pp: 95–161 in Stanley L. Engerman and Robert E. Gallman, *Long Term Factors in American Economic Growth,* NBER Studies in Income and Wealth, #51, Chicago: University of Chicago Press, 1986.
33. Robert H. Miller and Harold Luft, "Managed Care Plan Performance Since 1980: A Literature Analysis, *Journal of the American Medical Association,* 271(19):1512–1519, 1994.
34. Council on Ethical and Judicial Affairs, American Medical Association, "Ethical Issues in Managed Care," *Journal of the American Medical Association,* 273(4):330–335, 1995; Ezekiel Emanuel and Nancy Dubler, "Preserving the Physician-Patient Relationship in the Era of Managed Care," *Journal of the American Medical Association,* 273(4):323–329, 1995; Marc Rodwin, "Conflicts in Managed Care," *New England Journal of Medicine,* 332(9):605–607, 1995.
35. See Julie Rovner, "The Safety Net: What's Happening to Health Care of Last Resort?" and Howard Larkin, "Employed but Uninsured: Why Business is Cutting Back on Health Insurance," in *Advances,* quarterly newsletter of the Robert Wood Johnson Foundation, Princeton, N.J., Issue 1, 1996.

CHAPTER 12

LONG-TERM CARE

QUESTIONS

1. *Do the elderly pay to be cured or to be cared for?*
2. *Who provides most long-term care for the disabled elderly? Who is the largest insurer?*
3. *What do nursing home owners compete for? Do they want patients who are sicker?*
4. *How can substituting nursing homes for hospitals increase costs if the cost per day is lower?*
5. *Have government payments and regulations raised or lowered the quality of care?*
6. *How can Medicaid payments create an "excess" and a "shortage" of patients at the same time?*
7. *Do Certificate of Need (CON) rules reduce costs or reduce access?*
8. *Are retirement communities "managed care" for aging? Is there "managed death?"*

Of the $100 billion paid for long-term care, most is spent for institutional services in nursing homes. Yet for every person in a nursing home, there are two equally disabled people living in the community who are cared for by family and friends. Hence, more of the actual care comes from unpaid labor, acts of obligation and love, rather than patient fees or third-party payments. **Long-term care (LTC)** revolves around *care* rather than cure, around quality of life rather than treatment of disease. LTC needs are defined by functional status, the ability to carry out activities of daily life. Most patients will continue to require assistance for the rest of their lives. Food, housing, comfort, and social relations are more important than diagnostic tests or surgical procedures. Although doctors, hospitals, nurses, drugs, and all the other elements of modern medicine are employed, they are actively involved in only a small portion of the care that patients receive, and long-term care is not "medical" in the same way that most acute care is. These differences—long-term chronic disabilities that continue rather than short-term diseases capable of being cured; predominantly human caring rather than medical science; and a reliance on unpaid acts of love and obligation rather than services purchased in the market—all tend to make the long-term care transactions quite different from acute medical care transactions, and from the ordinary two-party transactions for most economic goods and services.

The challenge of meeting both medical and social needs has also left public policy in a confused state, with legislators uncertain as to which aspects of care are to be funded through social welfare programs, and which are to be financed as part of the health care system. The response to people with chronic illness and disability is a long-term care "system" in which boundaries are often unclear and many fundamental issues still unresolved. This chapter can present only a few aspects of the many and multifaceted economic entities that make up the fragmented long-term care sector.

12.1 DEVELOPMENT OF THE LTC MARKET

The original hospitals were long-term care facilities. They served destitute patients who could not work and could no longer live at home. Most people had family members who took care of them at home when they became sick, old or infirm, and the wealthy could also call upon the services of paid home nurses, so that only a small group of disabled and indigent paupers were forced to reside in hospitals. However, after the scientific revolutions of the nineteenth century, curative medicine was increasingly separated from caring for the disabled. By the start of World War II, the distinction between acute medical care and chronic long-term care was clearly demarcated in the mind of the public, and in the flow of funds. It was hoped that the poorhouses and "almshouse hospitality" would disappear as infectious diseases were cured and the desperately poor were elevated by a rising economy. To a large extent, sanitation and Social Security did cause the old system to fade, but some problems were troublingly persistent. No cure was found for mental illness, and ever more people were confined to state hospitals. These institutions made limited attempts at cure, and often served more to relieve the community of a burden rather than to improve the patients' quality of life.

Rising incomes meant that fewer and fewer old people were left truly destitute, but there were always some who had no friends, no family, and no place to go except a county "home" once they could no longer work. Although people with severe mental illness and homeless elders had persistent needs, they were small in number and almost ignored in planning for the overall health care system. In 1940, nursing home expenditures constituted less than 1 percent of the nation's total health spending.

The number of elderly people rose rapidly in the postwar era, from 10 million in 1940 to 17 million in 1965 and 32 million in 1995. This burgeoning group of elderly Americans was relatively healthy, thanks to years of good nutrition and sanitation, and relatively wealthy, thanks to pensions and years of saving. For the first time, there was a sizable population that could look forward to living for many years after working with no need to depend on their children to support them. This emerging group of retirees constituted a distinct market. They wanted to enjoy their "golden years," and often looked to each other for social activity. "Retirement communities" sprang up in Florida, California, and Arizona that catered to this growing group of middle-class elderly. Retirement communities were specially designed to appeal to the elderly, featuring single-story dwellings without steps; limited traffic; a social center for bridge games, dancing and crafts; and often discouraging or excluding families with children. This market response to the special needs of the elderly occurred without any reference to medicine or long-term care.

"Nursing home patients" were another small group within the elderly population that was also destined to grow rapidly during the postwar era. The fraction of total health expenditures devoted to nursing homes, which had been less than 1 percent in 1940, more than doubled by 1950, doubled again by 1960, and nearly doubled again by 1970, but was increasingly constrained after that (see Table 12.1). The fraction of total health spending devoted to nursing homes peaked at 8 percent around 1980 and has held steady since then, while the number of active retirees living in segregated housing with special amenities continues to soar. Distinguishing the active senior citizens from the institutionalized patients is easy at the extremes, but there is a range in between for which neat separation is impossible. The simple dichotomy of "at home" versus "in a nursing home" has been replaced by a range of organizational settings, from high-intensity facilities that are almost like hospitals, through a variety of intermediate care and assisted living facilities, to houses identical to those occupied by young families. The picture is further clouded by the provision of visiting nurse services, Meals on Wheels, home IV and physical therapy, and other supplemental services that make it possible to provide a wide range of care in the same place the person lived before they became disabled.

Although there are a limited number of disabled younger persons who receive long-term care, the vast majority are above age 65, and the rate of institutionalization increases with advancing age (Table 12.2). Residents in nursing homes are disproportionately female (74%) and poor. Older males who are disabled are more likely to be married, and hence receive assistance from a spouse or adult child. Traditionally, care of disabled elders has been provided by adult daughters who were expected to take on the task of caring for one or more parents or parents-in-law after their own children were raised. This informal system was adequate in

TABLE 12.1 Changes in the LTC Market

	1940	1950	1960	1970	1980	1990
Persons aged 65+	9,540,000	12,400,000	16,600,000	20,100,000	25,710,000	30,390,000
% of population	7.2%	8.1%	9.2%	9.8%	11.3%	12.2%
Nursing Home $ (*millions*)	$28	$178	$980	$4,867	$19,989	$54,810
% of Total Health $$	0.7%	1.5%	3.6%	6.5%	8.0%	7.9%
Home Health $ (*millions*)	—	—	$37	$143	$1,347	$11,056
% of Total Health $$			0.1%	0.2%	0.5%	1.2%

TABLE 12.2 Percentage of Population in a Nursing Home by Age

under 65	0.1%
65-74	1.3%
75-84	5.8%
85+	22.1%

Source: National Center for Health Statistics, *Health, United States, 1990.* Hyattsville, MD: USPHS, 1991.

the 1950s, when most women married and had children early, and did not have careers. In the 1990s, with the vast majority of adult women in the labor force, and births frequently delayed so that children do not leave home until the mother is in her fifties, finding time to care for a 78-year-old parent is much more difficult. The "shadow price" (forgone wage opportunity) of unpaid middle-aged females has become much greater. At the same time, demand has risen. In the immediate post-war 1950s era, families were larger, fewer parents lived past age 70, and so each middle-aged woman was likely to have several sisters to help share the burden. As family size shrank and longevity increased, there were more elderly disabled parents per potential care-giving daughter. The stress and family complications became greater. As the supply of unpaid labor fell and demand rose, what had formerly been care provided within the household became care purchased in the marketplace.[1]

The services provided by family members are invisible in the national income accounts: no one is billed, no one is paid, and from one point of view, no "transaction" has taken place. Yet from another point of view, one that pre-dates the existence of money, the obligations of parents to care for children, for neighbors to care for the sick, and for any person present to ease the pain of dying, are fundamental transactions that define society. In long-term care, the boundary between market and nonmarket activities is quite blurred. The mere fact that nursing home admissions or expenditures double does not mean that twice as many disabled persons are getting care, or that they are getting more or better services. Some of that increase is simply the movement from the realm of household production and family obligation into monetarized commerce.

12.2 DEFINING LTC: TYPES OF CARE _____

A person's potential need for long-term care can be analyzed as occurring in three dimensions: physical illness (medical diagnoses), functional disability (ADLs and IADLs, see section 12.5) and psycho/socio/economic deficits (family support, see Table 12.3). That care can then be provided either at home or in an institutional setting. Institutional settings can be ranked by the intensity of medical intervention: acute hospitals, long-term hospitals (rehabilitation, psychiatric), nursing homes (skilled and intermediate), and assisted living/board and care homes. Placement depends on the interaction between medical, social, and functional needs rather than any single dimension. A post-operative patient who only needs regular

TABLE 12.3   Dimensions of Long-Term Care Need

	Medical Need	*Functional Need*	*Social Need*
Acute Hospital	********	– – –	– – –
Rehab Hospital	***	***	– – –
Nursing Home	*	********	********
CCRC	– – –	– – –	*
Skilled Home Care	********	***	*
Personal Home Care	*	***	***
Family/Community	*	*	*

******** high

*** medium

* low

– – – varies or not applicable

bathing and hourly medication could be cared for at home if there were sufficient support from the family. A patient without actively involved family members may be a candidate for nursing home placement, and if there were no available nursing home beds, might continue to stay in the hospital for hundreds of days.[2] To some extent, the boundaries between different types of care are ambiguous, and the flow of funds somewhat arbitrary.

Home health care is growing rapidly in two different directions.[3] On the one hand, medical treatments that used to be performed in the hospital are being pushed out into the patient's home, paralleling the trend away from the hospital evidenced in shorter lengths of stay, the growth of ambulatory surgery, and the development of outpatient rehabilitation. In order for home medical care to be effective, the physician and nurse must be able to count on a high degree of family support to assist in monitoring the patient, administering medication, and carrying out basic nursing functions of feeding, bathing, and changing clothes. In contrast, personal home care is provided to otherwise healthy but homebound individuals whose lack of relatives at home is compensated for by having unskilled aides do ordinary cleaning, cooking, and other household tasks. Meals on Wheels, a publicly funded program that delivers hot meals to the homebound, provides a good example. Even though the services are quite different, the terminology and provision can become confusing, since a single provider may do both. A visiting nurse could stop at one house to change an IV antibiotic, and proceed to a next visit where the only service provided was to help someone into a wheelchair.

A person who has good friends, good health, and no functional limitations, can have an active life in the community. As elderly people begin to need more care and protection, their likelihood of being placed in a nursing home depends most of all on the presence of social support. For example, most married people with Alzheimer's can continue to live at home and be cared for by their spouse at least through the early phases of their decline. Those who have children, but no spouse, are less likely to be able to remain at home, and those with no family nearby are apt to be institutionalized. The extent of disability is the second most important factor. Eventually, almost every family who cares for a parent with Alzheimer's becomes overwhelmed by the necessity for constant attention, as well as by the pain and alienation of caring for someone who may not know or appreciate any of the things being done. Mental dysfunction is a significant cause in more than half of all LTC institutionalization. Medical needs, while often critical in precipitating a crisis, are relatively less important than social, housing, and functional needs as determinants of long-term care.

The goal of acute care is to increase the level of functioning and reduce the risk of dying. In contrast, most LTC is supportive. Attempts are made to slow the decline and stabilize functioning, but only rarely is an attempt made to achieve a definitive cure, and it is expected that the person will remain in a state of dependence. Since acute medical care is focused on cure, the quality of the meals, the room, and social functions are incidentals, and contribute only a little toward the total cost of a hospital stay. Most of the cost of LTC, on the other hand, is for helping people with their daily lives, not treatment. A physician may show up at a nursing home only once a month, drugs are supposed to help the patient get through the day, not to get better, and curative procedures account for a relatively minor fraction of total expenditures. In studies of nursing costs, physician services account for only 1 percent, as do drugs, while wages, salaries, and benefits, mostly for unskilled labor, accounts for 69 percent. A breakdown of nursing home inputs by category (Table 12.4) shows that most LTC expenses are for the costs of supported living rather than of medical care.

12.3 MEDICAID: NURSING HOMES AS A TWO-PART MARKET _____

The nursing home market was radically transformed, almost created anew, by the passage of "Medicare," Title XVII, and "Medicaid," Title XIX, of the Social Security Amendments of 1965. When Medicare was drafted to provide health insurance for the elderly, Medicaid was somewhat of an afterthought. Medicare explicitly did not pay for the kind of supportive care provided by most nursing homes.[5] It was presumed that housing, nutrition, and personal assistance were

TABLE 12.4   Breakdown of Nursing Home Costs

Physician services	1%
RNs (estimated)	9%
Other wages & salaries	53%
Employee benefits	7%
Food	10%
Fuel	4%
Drugs	1%
Other supplies	3%
Insurance	2%
Taxes	2%
Rent, debt, service, profit, etc.	8%

Source: HCFA detailed breakdown of Nursing Home Input Price Index Weightings, BLS Employment Statistics Survey.

individual or family responsibilities. Inability to provide for oneself indicated a need for charity or welfare assistance, not medical insurance.[6] Medicaid was originally intended mostly to expand and consolidate insurance coverage of medical services for indigent women and children who received AFDC welfare payments. Since it was directed toward a dependent indigent population, Medicaid did pay for social support of the kind given in nursing homes. Therefore, elderly people who were poor, or who could become indigent after spending down or giving away their savings, could obtain government insurance payments for institutional long-term care. Soon Medicaid was funneling billions of dollars each year into nursing homes; it now accounts for 52 percent of total nursing home funding, with Medicare paying 8 percent (mostly for the skilled medical nursing care and therapy), as illustrated in Figure 12.1. Medicaid is actually a joint state/federal program, with poor states getting as much as 80 percent of their total medicaid funding from the federal government, while wealthy states get only 50 percent. States are required to cover basic medical services for all people who are on welfare and/or who meet federal poverty definitions, but have discretion to increase benefits and eligibility above that limit. (Please note that any brief description must necessarily be qualified, because there are more than fifty different Medicaid payment systems with numerous clauses, exceptions, and special programs.)

Although nursing homes had been only a minor consideration in the creation of the Medicaid program, cost quickly rose over a billion dollars and soared out of control, more than doubling in cost every five years. State governors and budgetary officials discovered that Medicaid, even with federal matching funds, was an onerous financial burden. In most years since 1965, Medicaid has been the most rapidly growing category of state spending. The surge of Medicaid money into what had been a tiny market caused a rapid increase in prices and a shortage of spaces for the millions of new patients. As prices rose, state financial burdens increased. Any new homes built were quickly filled with more of the waiting Medicaid eligibles, adding millions to state budget outlays. States responded to

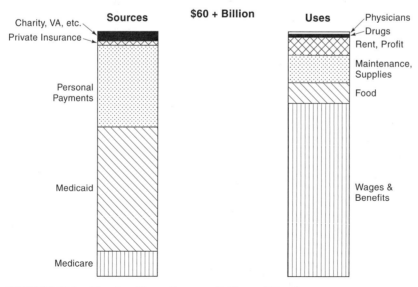

FIGURE 12.1 *Nursing Home Sources & Uses of Funds*

this financial drain in two ways: capping the price that they would pay for each day of nursing home care, and halting the construction of new homes. The methods of price control varied, but usually regulations were based on costs incurred, or on a set percentage increase over prior years (see section 12.5). Control over the number of beds was established by requiring that owners obtain a "Certificate of Need" (CON) before building or expanding any facilities (see section 12.4 and hospital CON in chapter 9.7).

With these two moves, price controls and capacity constraints, government created a unique market for nursing home beds. Its distinctive feature is a constant excess demand, but an excess only of below-market-price Medicaid patients. Consider Figure 12.2. On the left side is the private market demand, with a normal, downward-sloping demand schedule. The middle panel shows the Medicaid demand. Since price is fixed by government regulation, there is no change in price as quantity increases, so the demand "curve" is a right angle. Nursing homes can get as many patients as they want at the state regulated price, until there are no more Medicaid-eligible patients in the area. The right panel shows the combined "private and Medicaid" demand. Only private-pay patients can be served above the fixed Medicaid price, so the initial portion of the demand curve is composed solely of private patients, and is downward sloping. Once the Medicaid price is reached, the demand curve flattens out, since the nursing home can get more patients without reducing price. If a nursing home got too large, it would eventually exhaust the excess Medicaid demand and have to attract additional private patients with even

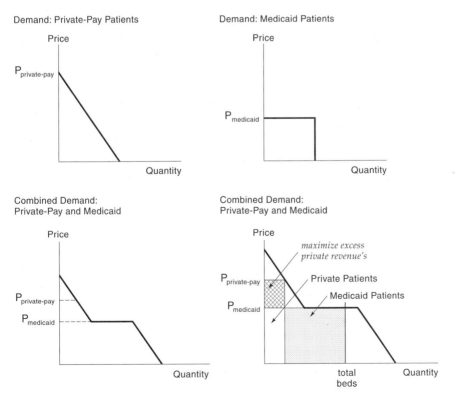

FIGURE 12.2   *Two-Part Nursing Home Market*

lower prices, as shown by the bottom third, downward-sloping, segment. Increasing the number of beds sufficient to force nursing home owners to dip into the demand of those only willing to pay an amount less than Medicaid pays is usually unintentional, since expansion typically ceases before all Medicaid patients are served. The two-part market faced by the nursing home owner is described in more detail in the bottom center panel of Figure 12.2. The vertical line represents the total bed capacity of the nursing home, the maximum number of patients that can be cared for. In order to maximize profits, the owner first sets a price for private pay patients P_{pp} that maximizes the total amount of excess revenues above the Medicaid rate (i.e., maximize the dotted rectangle $Q_{pp} \times [P_{pp} - P_{medicaid}]$), and then fills the remaining beds from the waiting list of Medicaid patients who pay the state regulated price $P_{medicaid}$ (shaded rectangle $[Q_{max} - Q_{pp}] \times P_{medicaid}$).[7]

The two-part market structure causes nursing home utilization to have an unusual "U-shaped" relationship to income. Although most normal goods show demand steadily rising as income rises, in this market utilization is high at low incomes (where patients readily qualify for Medicaid), drops for middle incomes (where lack of coverage reduces demand), and then rises at high incomes (where wealthy people can afford $30,000 or more per year for care).

The real world is, of course, more complicated than the straight lines drawn in Figure 12.2. Often a nursing home will only admit private paying patients. Many patients come into a nursing home with considerable assets, but over the years **spend down** all their savings by paying for care, and only then become poor enough to be eligible for Medicaid.[8] There are stories of couples becoming divorced solely to allow the spouse who is disabled to qualify for Medicaid so that the one who is still living at home can keep the savings accounts. Elderly couples are protected to some extent by federal guidelines that allow the spouse at home to keep the house, car, and some additional assets. Elderly single people may give their assets to their children in anticipation of entering a nursing home. This must be planned with care, since most states include recently transferred assets as part of personal funds to be used before Medicaid reimbursement is allowed. Families that would never consider "going on welfare" use asset transfers to make aging parents dependent upon state funds as indigents. With 52 percent of all nursing home bills being paid for by Medicaid, the conclusion that many middle-class and wealthy people are benefiting from a program designed for the poor is inescapable.[9] The fact that a certain amount of subterfuge is required (fake divorces, paper transfer of ownership of cars and land, "giving" money to children that the parent still controls) only makes this process more distasteful and morally undermining.[10] Medicaid is an entrenched part of the nursing home market, but it is not well liked by taxpayers or beneficiaries, and is hard to justify as being either equitable or ethical.

12.4 CON (CERTIFICATE OF NEED): WHOSE NEEDS? _____

It is important to understand the implications of regulatory constraints upon the long-term care market, and to examine whose interests are served by creating a situation of chronic excess demand in which frail and sick patients must wait months for a bed. For example, the surge of Medicaid money into nursing home care after 1965 meant that there would be a shortage of beds for the years it would take until the market could catch up. In addition, imposing a construction moratorium through the **Certificate of Need (CON)** process increased the shortage and made it permanent.

Money and Quality

It would seem that pushing more money into nursing homes during the late 1960s would have improved the quality of care provided. However, for perfectly reasonable economic reasons, conditions actually became worse in most nursing homes. For instance, a nursing home owner does not choose furniture or service based on what can be afforded, but on what will maximize profits. With a long line of Medicaid patients waiting to get in, it was not necessary to keep up the appearance of the nursing home to attract new clients, nor was it necessary to provide good nursing service or good food to keep them there. Since every bed was always filled from the waiting list, profits were maximized by reducing costs (fewer hours of nursing, less-skilled nurses, less repairs and maintenance, etc.). The flood of Medicaid money washed away any incentive to provide high quality in order to attract more patients.

The perverse dynamics of a two-part market are such that sometimes an increase in rates can cause a *reduction* in quality.[11] Consider the simplified scenario illustrated in Figure 12.3. The upper-left panel shows the two-part market, with the nursing home owner able to fill all of the extra beds with Medicaid patients (i.e., there is chronic excess Medicaid demand). Additional profits can be obtained for each bed that is filled by a higher paying private patient. The amount of excess revenue (shaded rectangle) is a function of the number of private pay patients attracted to the home, and the differential between the private pay and Medicaid rates, $P_{private\ pay} - P_{Medicaid}$. In the upper-right panel, it is shown that the owner who raises quality is able to obtain additional revenues (dotted rectangle, less notch for excess private pay revenues that could have been obtained even without any quality increase) by attracting more private pay patients who are willing to pay extra for better service, but in order to do so the owner must incur additional costs (striped narrow rectangle at base of diagram) for better food, new paint, more nurses, and so on. Note that for purpose of profit maximization, higher quality and the attendant costs are "wasted" on Medicaid patients, since, with chronic excess Medicaid demand, the owner does not need to do anything special to attract them. The choice of whether or not to improve quality depends on whether the additional extra private-pay revenues exceeds the additional costs or not. Raising $P_{Medicaid}$ has two effects: it makes it easier to pay for high quality, but it also reduces the incentive to use quality as a means of attracting private-pay patients as the revenue differential ($P_{private\ pay} - P_{Medicaid}$) becomes smaller. In the bottom left panel, Medicaid rates are very low, and the owner chooses to bear the additional costs of high quality to fill most of the beds with private-pay patients. In the bottom right panel, Medicaid rates are much higher, so high that the nursing home owner would get very little additional revenue from increased quality. Therefore, the owner maximizes profits

Demand with low quality

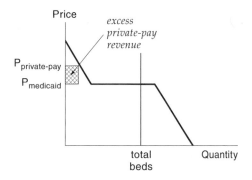

Higher quality increases private pay demand, but also incurrs additional costs

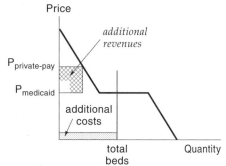

Medicaid price low: additional revenues from high quality are larger than additional costs–increase profits by raising quality

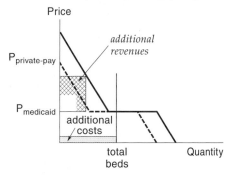

Medicaid price high: potential additional revenues too small to justify added costs—leave quality at low level

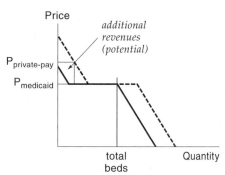

FIGURE 12.3   *Results of Raising Medicaid Payment Rates May Actually Cause Nursing Homes to Provide Lower Quality Since the Extra Profits From Attracting Private Pay Patients Become Smaller.*

by minimizing costs, filling most beds with the highly reimbursed Medicaid patients.

Whether or not a particular rate increase would actually create incentives for a profit-maximizing owner to reduce quality depends on the specifics of the private demand curve and the cost/quality function. Certainly, the decline of quality in the face of billions of dollars in extra government spending was very disappointing to nursing home advocates during the decade following the passage of Medicaid. The fact that a two-part quasi-regulated market can occasionally show such a backward response indicates how government intervention can distort the normal flow of information through prices and have unintended adverse effects. The particular conditions necessary for inverse price/quality response are less likely to occur today, because state budget pressures have reduced the level of reimbursement. Some Medicaid rates are so low that only inadequate and understaffed homes are economically viable. In these instances, any further reductions in payment can threaten the lives and health of the patients.

Competing for CONs (but not for patients)

With chronic excess demand guaranteeing full occupancy from the first day, new nursing homes were sure money-makers. If placed in nice locations to attract a sizable share of private-pay patients, even more money could be made. CON slowed, but did not entirely stop, the construction of new nursing homes. Since a certificate was now required, how was it to be determined who got to build these facilities, and where they were to be placed? State officials faced a dilemma. If the beds were built in a nice area, they would generate higher profits, and would not cost the state as much money, since only a few places would be taken by Medicaid patients. On the other hand, placing a nursing home in a poorer area of high need would do more to relieve the shortage of Medicaid beds, but cost the state more money. The conflict between patient needs and state budget pressures made it necessary to compromise. It is unlikely that CON regulation actually did much to change or improve the location of new nursing home beds.

Who gets to build?   Certainly the state might favor church groups that had donated money to help care for patients, but, being political, might also favor owners who donated money to help elect a congressman or senator. With chronic excess demand, the CON itself became valuable property. In effect, one could "buy" patients by obtaining a CON from the government. Once an owner had a CON, the supply of (Medicaid) patients was assured, and so the owner would not have to do any marketing or quality improvements to attract them. Competition was thus shifted away from the market into the political regulatory arena.

Windfall profits accrued to anyone who was able to obtain a CON for new construction, or who already owned a nursing home. This does not mean that the next owner would make excess profits. When the facility was sold, the new owner had to pay for the building and also implicitly for the CON permit—a piece of paper whose value would be roughly equal to the expected future profits of the facility. The new owner having paid $10 million for a $5 million building in order to get the CON, would have high fixed costs and find it hard to make a profit unless they reduced operating costs, and hence often reduced quality.

Who Pays?   CON restrictions succeeded in reducing state Medicaid budgets and providing excess profits to nursing home owners. So the question then becomes, if both owners and regulators benefited, who got hurt? The answer is that patients and their families paid, directly or indirectly, to generate those financial gains. Without competition, patients were often forced to take whatever bed they could get. Instead of market research to meet patient needs, nursing home operators sensibly devoted their dollars to lobbying for continued regulation. Restrictions on supply also meant higher prices for private pay patients. The biggest cost of CON regulation is all of the hours of unpaid labor and disruption imposed on families who could not get their loved ones into a needed nursing home bed, or who had to wait months to do so. In the highest need category (mentally confused, multiple impairments in activities of daily living), over 90 percent are in nursing homes in states where there is no shortage of beds, but only 50 percent of similarly impaired patients are in nursing homes in states that continue to impose tight limits on bed supply.[12] What happens to the other 40 percent? Who cares for them? At what personal sacrifice? Just because family labor and unnecessary declines in quality of life are not charged for in the market does not make them any less costly.

The Effects of CON: Evidence from Recent Years

The primary purpose of CON from the beginning has been to limit the growth of states' Medicaid expenditures. The crisis atmosphere generated after Medicaid suddenly flooded the market has eased over time, and with it, the reflexive need to use regulations to impose order on a market out of control faded. The shortage of beds created by restricting supply became more of an issue. Long waiting lists and the protests of families whose lives were disrupted by unpaid caregiving put pressure on states to relax or eliminate their CON rules. The differences between states that have continued to use CON and those that have stopped illustrate some of the effects of artificial controls on supply. The length of time a patient has to wait for a bed has fallen in those states where CON has been repealed. Also, the large disparity in waiting time between private-pay and Medicaid patients has been reduced or eliminated as shortages have disappeared. It has often been assumed that nursing homes with a high percentage of Medicaid patients were less successful in attracting private pay patients, and were thus of lower-than-average quality. A study comparing states with and without CON showed that higher percentages of Medicaid reimbursement were indeed associated with lower quality in those states where CON caused a chronic shortage of beds.[13] However, this was not the case in the deregulated states without CON. As free entry made more beds available, even Medicaid patients had to be competed for with better quality. Since 1990, the supply situation has continued to ease, so that more and more states show declines in occupancy. With empty beds, competition for all types of patients has intensified.

12.5 CASE-MIX REIMBURSEMENT _____

Even with an adequate supply of beds, the fact that the state pays only a single fixed rate per day for nursing home care means that some patients may be denied care. A patient who is very sick, or whose disruptive mental condition requires frequent attention, will cost more than a patient who is not a problem. With revenue per day fixed, a nursing home can increase profits by selectively accepting only those less costly patients who need very little care. In order to provide nursing homes with incentives to admit more severely ill patients, some states have developed **case-mix reimbursement** systems that increase payments based on some index of need. Whereas the starting point for acute medical case-mix reimbursement is the diagnosis (see chapter 8, section 2 for a discussion of diagnosis-based DRG reimbursement in hospitals), in LTC it is the level of functioning. Most frequently, this is measured in terms of **ADLs**, the number of "Activities of Daily Living" for which the individual needs assistance (dressing, grooming, bathing, eating, bed mobility, transferring, walking, and toileting—see Table 12.5) as well as the level of assistance required.[14] In New York state, the association between number of ADLs and cost of care was used to create a number of "resource utilization groups," referred to by the acronym RUGS.

TABLE 12.5   Activities of Daily Living (ADL) Evaluation Form

For each area of functioning listed below, check description that applies. (The word *assistance* means supervision, direction or personal assistance.)

BATHING—either sponge bath, tub bath, or shower

☐	☐	☐
Receives no assistance (gets in and out of tub by self if tub is usual means of bathing)	Receives assistance in bathing only one part of body (such as back or a leg)	Receives assistance in bathing more than one part of body (or not bathed)

DRESSING—gets clothes from closets and drawers—including underclothes, outer garments and using fasteners (including braces, if worn)

☐	☐	☐
Gets clothes and gets completely dressed without assistance	Gets clothes and gets dressed without assistance except for assistance in tying shoes	Receives assistance in getting clothes or in getting dressed, or stays partly or completely undressed

TOILETING—going to the "toilet room" for bowel and urine elimination; cleaning self after elimination and arranging clothes

☐	☐	☐
Goes to "toilet room," cleans self, and arranges clothes without assistance (may use object for support such as cane, walker, or wheelchair)	Receives assistance in going to "toilet room" or in cleansing self or in arranging clothes after elimination or in use of night bed pan or commode	Doesn't go to room termed "toilet" for the elimination process

TRANSFER—

☐	☐	☐
Moves in and out of bed as well as in and out of chair without assistance	Moves in and out of bed or chair with assistance	Doesn't get out of bed

CONTINENCE—

☐	☐	☐
Controls urination and bowel movement completely by self	Has occasional "accidents"	Supervision helps keep urine or bowel control; catheter is used or is incontinent

FEEDING—

☐	☐	☐
Feeds self without assistance	Feeds self except for getting assistance in cutting meat or buttering bread	Receives assistance in feeding or is fed partly or completely by using tubes or intravenous fluids

Adapted from Katz et al., "Studies of Illness in the Aged. The Index of ADL: A Standardized Measure of Biological and Psychosocial Function" *Journal of the American Medical Association,* 185:94ff. 1963.

The U.S. General Accounting Office has issued a report showing that the problem of "heavy care" patients having greater difficulty in obtaining a nursing home bed is substantially reduced in those states with systems that adjust reimbursement according to case-mix. However, the adjustment is always imperfect, and even with differential payment rates, nursing homes may find it profitable to accept some patients while turning others away.[15] In Minnesota, the state created a system with eleven levels of reimbursement running from A (0 to 3 ADLs with no problems) to K (7 to 8 ADLs and special nursing). To the extent that differences in payment rate correctly adjusted for differences in cost, a nursing home would have no reason to selectively admit one group rather than another. However, researchers at the University of Minnesota estimated that categories H and J were significantly overcompensated, while categories C and F were significantly undercompensated.[16] The total number of days of care remained basically the same from 1986 (the first year of the case-mix reimbursement system) to 1990, but nursing homes admitted more patients in the over-compensated categories over time, and admitted fewer patients in the under-compensated categories (Table 12.6). Even though some of the change may have been due to "gaming" of the regulatory system by reclassifying patients into more profitable categories, at least some appears to have been a result of selective admissions policies. The lesson of this study is that nursing homes, even non-profit nursing homes, will respond to any remaining inaccuracies in case-mix reimbursement.

12.6 SUBSTITUTION _____

The lack of extra payment for those patients needing extra care may mean that they cannot be transferred to a nursing home, and hence must remain in a high-cost acute hospital bed for additional "administratively necessary days" (ANDs). Some hospitals have even purchased nursing homes primarily to make it easier to discharge their post-acute patients. Yet opportunities for system-wide savings are often passed up because different parties are paying different bills. For instance, Medicare (federal) pays most hospital bills, while Medicaid (state) pays most nursing home bills. A state may be unwilling to pay for additional nursing home days even though each additional hospital day is much more expensive—because the cost of hospital days is born by the federal government, not the state.

A larger and more general problem in trying to use service substitution as a means for reducing costs is controlling who gets the additional days of nursing home care. Increased bed supply and changes in reimbursement that make it easier to transfer patients from the hospital will also make it easier for new patients to obtain care. The cost of providing care to these new patients tends to outweigh the savings obtained by switching some patients from hospitals to nursing homes. A large experiment was run trying to demonstrate cost savings by "channeling" patients at high risk of repeat hospitalization into less expensive nursing homes, home health, and social services.[17] The channeling project was not able to generate savings because only a few hospitalizations could be avoided, counseling patients was itself expensive, and mostly resulted in the utilization of additional services rather than substituting for hospitalization.

It was once thought that expanded home health and ambulatory surgery would

TABLE 12.6 Nursing Homes Admit More of the Patients that are Relatively More Profitable

	(care level)	Case Index	Revenue	Estimated Cost	Profit	Days of care 1986	Days of care 1990	change %
A	(0-3 ADLs)	1.00	$47.50	$43.64	9%	3,008,098	2,781,037	-8%
B	(0-3 ADLs with behavior problem)	1.30	$51.40	$55.31	-7%	1,236,058	1,066,884	-14%
C	(0-3 ADLs and special nursing)	1.64	$55.83	$68.09	-18%	193,084	76,229	-61%
D	(4-6 ADLs)	1.95	$59.86	$66.96	-11%	1,466,417	1,457,940	-1%
E	(4-6 ADLs and behavior problem)	2.27	$64.01	$61.40	4%	1,252,917	1,071,265	-14%
F	(4-6 ADLs and special nursing)	2.29	$64.28	$89.53	-28%	249,083	105,049	-58%
G	(7-8 ADLs and heavy feeding)	2.56	$67.79	$66.00	3%	1,791,836	2,471,990	38%
H	(7-8 ADLs, heavy feeding & behavior)	3.07	$74.42	$60.66	23%	1,225,666	1,370,201	12%
I	(7-8 ADLs and very heavy feeding)	3.25	$76.76	$79.85	-4%	1,182,752	954,488	-19%
J	(7-8 ADLs, feeding & severe neurology)	3.53	$80.39	$62.79	28%	1,688,881	2,345,085	39%
K	(7-8 ADLs and special nursing)	4.12	$88.06	$89.86	-2%	1,364,042	835,112	-39%
average			$66.39	$67.64	-0.3%	14,658,834	14,535,280	-0.8%

Source: J. A. Nyman and R. A. Connor, "Do Case-Mix Adjusted Nursing Home Reimbursements Actually Reflect Costs? Minnesota's Experience," Journal of Health Economics 13(2):145–62, 1994.

save money for Medicare by reducing hospitalization. Part A (hospital) expenses have indeed declined in recent years, but Part B (professional services) have increased by a much greater amount. For example, cataract surgery, intravenous antibiotics, and physical therapy are all cheaper when performed on an outpatient basis, but once the need for a hospital admission was eliminated, so many new patients utilized these services that the total cost of treatment more than doubled.

12.7 LONG-TERM CARE INSURANCE_____

Although most medical care is paid for through third-party insurance, private long-term care insurance did not even come into existence until the 1980s, and still pays for less than 3 percent of nursing home and home health bills. There are several major reasons why LTC insurance is not as attractive to consumers as insurance for acute medical care, summarized in Table 12.7. The incidence of disability requiring long-term care is not so much random, as delayed. If we live long enough, almost all of us will need some form of long-term care. Yet if we wait until age 70 to purchase LTC insurance, the premiums must be very high, since the likelihood of loss is so great. A more prudent course would be to plan in advance. However, someone who purchases LTC insurance at age 40 will have to wait many years to obtain benefits. Financially, they may do almost as well if they put aside savings to be used for LTC if the need should arise, letting interest accrue over the intervening years. At age 70, one may already have died without entering a nursing home, and hence the money could be passed on to one's heirs. If one did end up needing a lot of LTC and ran out of savings, there would always be Medicaid to fall back on. Why should people pay premiums for thirty years when the government would pay if they really needed help?

A final barrier to LTC insurance is the nature of the benefit: payment for a nursing home stay. Unlike payment for acute medical treatment, which is expected to improve health or reduce the risk of premature death, payment for nursing home care just makes it easier to be taken from home and be placed in an institution. Although there may be some improvement, for the most part the health "benefits" of nursing home care are a slowing of the rate of decline so as to extend the number of years spent in a mode of assisted living with limited function. Many people find it hard to get excited about paying thousands of dollars for that. Upon reflection, it becomes clear that the greatest beneficiaries of LTC insurance are not

TABLE 12.7 Reasons Long-Term Care Insurance is Not Popular

1. Incidence of LTC is less random than acute illness.
2. Insurance must be purchased so far in advance of anticipated need that savings become a good alternative to insurance.
3. Medicaid is always there, providing a stop-loss against large expenditures.
4. To get benefits paid, purchaser must be admitted to nursing home. Unlike treatment for acute illness, the person would usually rather make treatment more rather than less difficult to obtain.
5. Benefits mostly reduce expenditures by heirs and Medicaid, rather than helping the patients who pay the premiums.

the patients, but their children and the Medicaid program. Children benefit because they may find it easier to send a disabled parent to a nursing home if the charges are paid for by insurance, and also protect their inheritance by having this risk insured. Medicaid benefits because the nursing home charges are being paid for by premiums rather than state and federal tax monies. Expansion of private LTC insurance will be quite limited until (a) the benefits are modified so that they help patients to continue living at home rather than making it easier to be admitted to a nursing home; (b) payments are made in advance with favorable tax treatment by employers like most group medical insurance; and (c) policies are coordinated with Medicaid so that they yield financial benefits to patients, their spouses and heirs, instead of offsetting government expenditures.

12.8 CCRCs AND THE WEALTHY ELDERLY _____

Elderly people with enough money to afford long-term care insurance have not been particularly interested in purchasing it. However, the wealthy elderly have flocked to retirement communities and other market alternatives. Among the most successful have been Life Care or Continuing Care Retirement Communities (CCRCs). In essence, these residential developments combine an LTC insurance HMO with a retirement community, guaranteeing the person a pleasant place to live and nursing care for the remainder of their life.[18] In most retirement communities, new entrants (usually married couples in their 70s) pay a substantial fixed-up-front fee ($75,000 to $250,000) for their apartment, and then a monthly fee ($500 to $1500 a month) that includes maintenance, housekeeping, social services, and some or all meals. Home health nurses are provided when needed. As a person becomes more disabled, they can enter a nursing home located on the premises. Residents do not own their apartment, but do have the right to live in it until they die or are admitted to the nursing facility. Major advantages of CCRCs are the controlled environment geared toward elders, the possibilities of creating a new circle of friends even as health declines, and the ability to continue seeing them daily even after entering the nursing facility. CCRC communities range from modestly nice to quite luxurious. The nursing facilities tend to be less institutional than most nursing homes. Even severely impaired people may still have table linens, candles with dinner, and a homelike atmosphere.

The large up-front fee and sizable monthly payments generate two problems: fraud/bankruptcy and affordability. The first life-care communities depended almost entirely on the entry fees, with very low monthly rates. Many of these were "sponsored" but not financially supported by religious denominations. After taking the up-front fee (sometimes, the entire savings and estate of the couple), the CCRC was obligated to provide care for life—and should have invested the money wisely so that interest income could be used to pay for maintenance and nursing home care. Unfortunately, the actuarial estimates were often quite far from the mark. Financial projections assumed that apartments could be turned over and resold every ten years or so, but the people who chose to enter lived much longer than usual for their ages (a form of adverse selection). In many cases the husband began to need nursing care (which cost extra) while the wife continued to live for many years (occupying a large apartment that could not be resold). Some religious leaders were uncomfortable about raising monthly fees when millions of dollars in investments were in the bank, even though the future obligations for nursing home care and maintenance were greater than could be covered by the interest. Necessary financial reserves were depleted over time when monthly rates were not raised promptly. These factors alone would have been sufficient to cause problems, but were compounded in case after case when unscrupulous CCRC operators paid themselves excessive sales fees or salaries, or simply embezzled funds. Immediately after a facility opened there would be millions of dollars of entry fees in the bank. The loss or mismanagement of those funds would not become evident until years later, when buildings needed repair or residents needed nursing care. By then, the money was sometimes quite literally out of the country. Numerous reforms have been instituted to maintain the financial integrity of CCRCs. Now, if a religious denomination agrees to sponsor a facility, it must legally guarantee future expenses. Reserves must be routinely reported and financial viability, including coverage of medical and nursing expenses, must be demonstrated. The risky "pay everything up front" financing has been supplanted so that more of the costs are covered by monthly fees, and often the nursing-care component is paid for separately, and subjected to standard underwriting practices (e.g., waiting periods, extra fees, or exclusions for those entering with preexisting conditions such as cancer or Alzheimer's).

More and more elderly can afford the cost of entering a CCRC. Definitions of *wealthy* are to some extent always subjective, but by any measure the wealth of the elderly has risen dramatically in both absolute terms and relative to the younger population. In the 1950s, many elderly were poor, still struggling with the aftermath of the Depression. In contrast, young families faced bright economic prospects and relatively few children lived in poverty. By 1990, Social Security, marital patterns, and other factors had reversed the incidence of poverty. The elderly were much better off than children. Favorable tax and transfer treatment, along with years of savings, have made the elderly aged 55–64 the wealthiest group in America with a net worth of $371,000 in 1992, and the elderly aged 65–74 almost equal at $369,800 (see Table 12.8).[19] This does not mean that there are not sub-groups of the elderly with high poverty rates (the single black elderly are notably poor, as are the oldest old, above age 85), but it does mean that many can afford to buy care and protection in the market using their own substantial assets rather than depending on government programs. Married couples reaching age 65 have higher average incomes than the rest of the population, and twice as many financial assets. At least half of them can readily afford a CCRC or other market-based LTC financing mechanism. Public protection for the poor will always be necessary. What is important to change now is the perception that all or even most of the elderly are "poor."

Medicare Catastrophic Coverage Act of 1988 and the Taxpayer Revolt

Policies designed without regard to the diversity in wealth among the elderly may be seriously flawed, and are apt to be rejected in the marketplace. A prime

TABLE 12.8 Average Income and Wealth for Different Age Categories, 1992

	Income	Net Worth
All Households Surveyed	$44,900	$220,300
Head of Household Aged		
less than 35	$33,800	$60,200
35–44	$52,300	$157,000
45–54	$62,100	$304,500
55–64	$55,200	$371,000
65–74	$34,600	$369,800
75 and more	$27,300	$257,600

Source: Survey of Consumer Finances, 1992, *Federal Reserve Bulletin,* October 1994.

example is the Medicare Catastrophic Coverage Act (MCCA) passed by Congress in 1988—and repealed in 1989. The act was intended to extend Medicare coverage by reducing copays, deductibles, and limits, add a pharmaceutical benefit, and make several other benefit increases. It appeared that the MCCA would be quite popular, since many of the elderly had been buying Medigap insurance at far greater cost, since pharmaceuticals were a major source of out-of-pocket expenditures, and since the largest lobbying group for the elderly, the AARP (American Association of Retired Persons) strongly supported passage of the bill. The problem came in designing a payment mechanism. MCCA was intended to be "budget neutral," in that additional premiums and taxes would pay for the cost of the new benefits. Unlike Medicare Part B premiums, which are the same for all participants, MCCA premiums increased with income. The poor elderly would not have to pay anything. In order to subsidize the poor elderly, the higher income elderly would have to pay as much as $800 per year, more than the expected value of the additional benefits. Although perhaps willing to vote for higher taxes (which mostly fell on working people), the wealthy elderly were outraged at being forced to personally pay extra to cover the poor. Congressmen visiting their local districts expecting accolades were pelted with questions and complaints. Angry older people blocked cars, wrote letters, and swore revenge. In short order, the biggest extension of Medicare since 1965 had been repealed. Although it benefited most elderly, MCCA was not financially beneficial to the upper-income elderly, and it is this group that is most politically active.[20]

12.9 DEFINING BOUNDARIES: IS LONG-TERM CARE "MEDICAL"? _____

The Medicare program is immensely popular (and immensely expensive) because it serves every elderly person without regard to need or indigency, and therefore provides an upper-middle-class standard of care to all by using taxpayers' money. Attempts to forge an equally popular long-term care program have failed. While numerous cultural and political factors are involved, a major reason is that most of the features that characterize medical care (randomly occurring illness, reliance on physicians when quality can be a life and death issue, rapid technological innovation) are missing in long-term care. Instead, much of the cost of LTC is for housing, food, social amenities; things that would normally be identified as personal responsibilities or lifestyle rather than medical care. The boundary between medical care, social services, and living expenses often becomes quite ambiguous. Distinctions between professional services and unpaid family help are often similarly unclear. The divergence between medical and long-term care suggests that the types of health insurance financing developed for medical care may not be very appropriate for supporting the costs of assisted daily living characteristic of most long-term care.

What difference does it make if long-term care is called *medical* or not? In a word, money. Distinguishing services as *medical* makes it more likely that they will be insured, more likely that the people providing services will be licensed, and more likely that quality will be regulated and that choices by consumers in the marketplace will be supplanted by professional standards. Long-term care has more in common with social insurance programs such as disability, workers' compensation, pensions, and Social Security. Yet the tremendous cost of expanding entitlements and the lack of taxpayer support has caused many advocates to try to find ways to "medicalize" long-term care so as to increase the flow of funds to professionals and institutions.

SUGGESTIONS FOR FURTHER READING _____

Connie J. Evashwick, ed. *The Continuum of Long-Term Care*, Albany, N.Y.: Delmar Publishers, 1996.

John Nyman and Robert Connor, "Do Case-Mix Adjusted Nursing Home Reimbursements Actually Reflect Costs? Minnesota's Experience," *Journal of Health Economics* 13(2):145–162, 1994.

William Scanlon, "A Theory of the Nursing Home Market," *Inquiry* 17(1):25–41, 1980.

P. Short, S. Feinleib and P. Cunningham, "Expenditures and Sources of Payment for Persons in Nursing and Personal Care Homes," AHCPR Pub.94-0032, Agency for Health Care Policy & Research, PHS; Rockville, Md., April 1994.

US General Accounting Office, *Nursing Homes: Admission Problems for Medicaid Recipients and Attempts to Solve Them*, GAO report #GAO/HRD-90-135, September 1990.

SUMMARY _____

1. Most LTC **expenditures are for nursing home care**, but **most care** of the disabled elderly **is actually provided by family members and friends without pay.**

2. As the **number of elderly** rose, and the **shadow price of labor** by adult daughters increased, more and more long-term care was **shifted from unpaid household production to commercial market purchases** of care.

3. Nursing home economics is dominated by a **split two-part market**. Private-pay patients tend to pay more and sometimes receive better care. Medicaid patients must demonstrate to the state that they qualify by being poor. The state pays their bills, but will not pay as much, and so there is a chronic excess of Medicaid patients trying to get into beds that nursing home owners would prefer to fill with private-pay patients.

4. There is a great **range of LTC** arrangements. Much care, both professional and unskilled, is now provided at the patient's home. Institutions range from intensive rehabilitation hospitals to simple board and care homes that provide little more than a room with meals.

5. CON (certificate of need) **regulations** were intended to halt the construction of new nursing homes after the passage of Medicaid in 1965 greatly increased demand, and hence the tax burden on the states. CON has exacerbated the **shortage** of nursing homes and caused patients to wait months for a bed.

6. **Competing for CONs** has helped regulators and nursing home owners, but has not the patients who are forced to wait months for a bed or accept substandard care.

7. In a shortage situation, those patients most in need of care are more likely to be denied a space, since they also tend to be more costly. To alleviate this problem, some states have replaced the flat rate per diem with a rate that is **case-mix adjusted** for differences in need. Such systems help to match reimbursement with cost, but can never be perfect.

8. **Substituting** lower-cost LTC for hospital care (or home health for nursing home care) sounds good, but usually actually increases total system costs because so many new patients are brought in.

9. Long-term care is mostly assistance to the disabled for activities of daily living, and financing should properly be made by social insurance. **"Medicalizing"** LTC enables providers to tap new sources of funding, allows workers to justify licensure, probably increases quality, and clearly increases total costs.

PROBLEMS _____

1. How much is the average cost per day of a nursing home day? On a typical day in the United States, are there more patients in hospitals or nursing homes? Which type of care is growing more rapidly? What is the most rapidly growing form of LTC?

2. {*incidence, social insurance*} Who provides most of the care for elderly people who need assistance with the daily tasks of life? How do these helpers get paid?

3. {*case-mix selection*} Does the administrator of a hospital want to admit patients that are sicker than average, or less sick than average? Doe the administrator of an LTC facility wish to admit patients that are sicker than average or healthier than average? Why do LTC administrators face different financial incentives than hospital administrators?

4. {*competition*} Hospitals compete for doctors, and for the newest technology. How do nursing homes compete? Does price play more or less of a role? Technology?

5. {*supply controls*} Draw a set of supply and demand diagrams illustrating how a CON law could cause waiting lists and increase the price of care.

6. {*labor markets*} Several major trends have characterized labor markets in the U.S. over the last 80 years; wages have increased, life expectancy has increased, and female (but not male) labor force participation has increased. Discuss how each of these has affected the market for LTC services. Which has been more important in determining the shape of LTC markets, changes in labor market factors, or changes in medical technology?

7. {*substitution*} Use supply and demand diagrams to show what would happen if additional LTC insurance allows more substitution of nursing home care for hospital care. According to your diagram, do LTC expenditures increase or decrease? Do hospital expenditures increase or decrease? Do total expenditures (LTC + hospital) increase or decrease?

8. {*rent seeking*} If there is competition for CONs, what is the price? Who gets paid? Is the CON worth more than is paid for it? If so, who obtains those gains from trade?

9. {*shortages, discrimination*} Would a shortage of beds created by regulation make it easier or more difficult for a nursing home administrator to racially discriminate among patients for admission? Draw supply and demand graphs to illustrate.

10. {*risk*} Are the risks born in long-term care insurance different than the risks in hospital insurance?

11. {*substitution*} Does the federal/state-funded Medicaid program expand or contract the market for private long-term care insurance? Who would benefit from a federal subsidy of private LTC insurance plans?

12. {*productivity, outcomes*} In order to measure the productivity of medical care, economists attempt to measure outcomes of treatment: increases in longevity, fewer sick days, increased earnings. What measures would you use to compare the productivity of two nursing homes?

13. {*Medicaid, two-part market, tax incidence*} If you were elderly, would you be in favor of or against a proposal to increase the amount paid per day under Medicaid? What factors would your response depend upon?

14. {*management, vertical integration*} In what ways is a CCRC like an HMO? In what ways is it different? Are payments made on similar or different bases? Which is more subject to adverse selection? To moral hazard? Which relies most on gatekeepers? On financial incentives to physicians?

15. {*incidence*} What socioeconomic groups in the United States benefit most from extensive government funding of long-term care? Is the flow of funds progressive or regressive?

16. {*risk aversion, Medigap insurance*} Virtually all elderly persons in the United States qualify for Medicare. Almost 70 percent also purchase "Medigap" insurance, which covers copayments, deductibles, and often some additional services for home health care, pharmaceuticals, etc. Which insurance, Medicare or Medigap, provides the largest "welfare gain from risk pooling" (see chapters 3 and 4). Does Medigap insurance increase or decrease the cost of Medicare?

ENDNOTES _____

1. A. E. Benjamin, "An Historical Perspective on Home Care," *Milbank Quarterly* 71(1):129–166, 1993.
2. Robert L. Kane, Joseph G. Ouslander and Itamar B. Abras, *Essentials of Clinical Geriatrics,* New York: McGraw-Hill, 1989, pages 30–44.
3. Susan Hughes, "Home Health Care" in Connie J. Evashwick (ed.), *The Continuum of Long-Term Care,* Albany, N.Y.: Delmar Publishers, 1966, pp:61–81.
4. Detailed breakdown of cost categories used by the Health Care Financing Administration in their study of actual expenditures are used to construct the Nursing Home Input Price Index. *Source*: Office of the Actuary, HCFA.
5. Brian Burwell, William H. Crown, Carol O'Shaunessy and Richard Price, "Financing Long-Term Care," Chapter 13 in Connie Evashwick (ed.), *The Continuum of Long-Term Care,* Albany, N.Y.: Delmar Publishers, 1996, page 199.
6. William Aaronson, "Financing the Continuum of Care: A Disintegrating Past and an Integrating Future," Chapter 14 in Connie Evashwick (ed.), *The Continuum of Long-Term Care,* Albany, N.Y.: Delmar Publishers, 1996, page 225.
7. William P. Scanlon, "A Theory of the Nursing Home Market," *Inquiry* 17(1):25–41, 1980.
8. Korbin Liu, Pamela Doty, and Kenneth Manton, "Medicaid Spenddown in Nursing Homes," *The Gerontologist* 30(10):7, 1990; H. Temkin-Greener, M. Meiner, E. Petty, and J. Szydlowski, "Spending Down to Medicaid in the Nursing Home and in the Community," *Medical Care* 31(8):663–679, 1993.
9. Brian Burwell, *Middle-Class Welfare: Medicaid Estate Planning for Long-Term Care Coverage,* Lexington, Mass.: Systemetrics, 1991.
10. S. Moses, "The Fallacy of Impoverishment," *The Gerontologist* 30(1):21–25, 1990.
11. John A. Nyman, "Prospective and 'Cost-Plus' Medicaid Reimbursement, Excess Medicaid Demand, and the Quality of Nursing Home Care," *Journal of Health Economics,* 4(3):237–60, 1985; and "Excess Demand, the Percentage of nursing Home Patients, and the Quality of Nursing Home Care," *Journal of Human Resources,* 23(1):76–92, 1988.
12. U.S. General Accounting Office, *Nursing Homes: Admission Problems for Medicaid Recipients and Attempts to Solve Them,* GAO Report #GAO/HRD-90-135, September 1990.
13. John Nyman, "The Demand for nursing Home Care," *Journal of Health Economics* 8(2), 1989; *Journal of Human Resources* 23(1), 1988. *JHE* 4(3), Sept. 1985.
14. S. Katz, A. B. Ford, R. W. Moskowitz, B. A. Jackson and M. W. Jaffee, "Studies of Illness in the Aged. The Index of ADL: A Standardized Measure of Biological and Psychosocial Function," *Journal of the American Medical Association,* 185:94ff, 1963.

15. U.S. General Accounting Office, *op. cit.*
16. J. A. Nyman and R. A. Connor, "Do Case-Mix Adjusted Nursing Home Reimbursements Actually Reflect Costs? Minnesota's Experience." *Journal of Health Economics* 13(2):145–162, 1994.
17. P. Kemper, "The Evaluation of the National Long-Term Care Demonstration," *Health Services Research* 23(1)(special issue), 1988.
18. H. S. Ruchlin, "Continuing Care Retirement Communities: An Analysis of Financial Viability and Health Care Coverage," *The Gerontologist* 28(2):156–162, 1988.
19. Arthur Kennickell and Martha Starr-McCluer, "Changes in Family Finances from 1989 to 1992: Evidence from the Survey of Consumer Finances," *Federal Reserve Bulletin,* 80(10):1–18, October 1994.
20. William Aaronson, Jacqueline Zinn, and Michael Rosko, "The Success and Repeal of the Medicare Catastrophic Coverage Act: A Paradoxical Lesson for Health Care Reform," *Journal of Health Politics, Policy & Law* 19(4):753–771, 1994.

CHAPTER 13

The Pharmaceutical Industry

QUESTIONS

1. *What three things occurred in the 1940s that gave rise to the modern pharmaceutical industry?*
2. *What governmental agency regulates the marketing and promotion of pharmaceutical products? How did it come about?*
3. *Why are patents important to the pharmaceutical industry?*
4. *What is the difference between a branded and a generic product?*
5. *What are the major market segments for pharmaceutical products and how/why are they different?*
6. *What is a drug formulary?*
7. *How have drug formularies changed the market for pharmaceutical products?*

The pharmaceutical industry has existed in its current form only since the 1940s. Before then, local pharmacists (or chemists) mixed potions and elixirs from bulk chemicals using either standardized formulas or their own concoctions. Today, the modern U.S. pharmaceutical industry is comprised of more than 1,200 firms that produce a wide range of products used to treat disease and injury. The total expenditures on pharmaceutical products are likely to exceed $98 billion in 1997, or about 8 percent of all health care expenditures. Recently, the pharmaceutical industry has drawn considerable attention for its pricing and promotional policies. Some politicians have alleged that the industry charges excessive prices and spends too much money promoting products to physicians. These allegations have resulted in calls to regulate prices in this industry.

The pharmaceutical industry consists of many small companies, each producing only one or two products, and approximately thirty large global corporations that have broader product lines. Even in the largest corporations, however, only one or two "block-buster" drugs are responsible for most of the revenues at any point in time. Competition for the development of these key products, through research and development (R&D) activities, is fierce. The success or failure of even a single product could mean the success or failure of the corporation. As a result, R&D activities drive competition in the pharmaceutical industry. The average cost of developing a new drug is $230 million and the process can take up to ten years. Once developed, patents protect the new product from competition. Patents give the innovator the exclusive right to manufacture and sell that product, once approved, for up to twenty-two years from the time of discovery.

Since the early 1980s, several smaller generic manufacturers have entered the pharmaceutical industry. These companies do not conduct large-scale research and development programs, but compete with the larger pharmaceutical houses by producing identical, **generic** products after the patent has expired. Competition from the generic manufacturers has created incentives for the research-based companies to introduce and subsequently patent minor changes in their most important products. These changes might include introducing a sustained release or once-a-day formulation, or changing the route of administration from injection to inhaler or pill.

Managed care has also had a major impact on the way the pharmaceutical industry conducts business. To control the budget spent on pharmaceutical products, many managed care organizations have established **formularies**, lists of drugs for preferential reimbursement. To have its drug included on the formulary, the pharmaceutical manufacturer must agree to provide large discounts to the managed care organization. Today, discounts to managed care companies average about 15 percent. The extent that doctors are permitted to prescribe off-formulary varies across managed care groups and is one distinguishing feature of these plans.

Independent Pharmaceutical Benefits Management (PBM) companies have also arisen in recent years. These companies manage the prescription drug benefits of large self-insured employers. They help the employer by administering claims

This chapter was prepared by Thomas Abbott, Ph.D., Department of Economics and Center for Research in Regulated Industries, Rutgers University and Senior Economist, Outcomes Research Management, Merck & Co.

and by developing benefit plans that often include a formulary of preferred drugs. These PBMs consolidate the purchasing power of individual patients and employers and negotiate with the pharmaceutical manufacturers to obtain price discounts. Unlike managed care plans, PBMs do not have any direct control over physician prescribing behavior. However, by placing restrictions on which drugs are covered by the plan, they indirectly influence the physicians' choices through the patient's pocketbook.

As a result of pressure from managed care and pharmaceutical benefits companies, many research-based pharmaceutical firms are conducting economic research on the impact of their products. This research is used to establish the "economic value" of their products and is the basis of the emerging disciplines of outcomes research, pharmacoeconomics, and disease management. The overall objectives of these disciplines are to understand how and when pharmaceutical products can be most economically used to treat patients.

13.1 HOW THE FUNDS FLOW IN ————————————

As with health care services, funding for pharmaceutical products comes from a variety of sources, including: patients, employers and private insurance, and federal and state governments (see Table 13.1). 61 percent of the cost of pharmaceuticals is paid out-of-pocket. This is much higher than the out-of-pocket costs of other health care services. For people over age 65, out-of-pocket costs are even higher (64%) because Medicare does not cover the cost of outpatient pharmaceuticals, although drug coverage is frequently included in the supplemental "Medigap" policies, which most elderly persons purchase on their own. The large fraction that must be paid from personal funds is particularly burdensome for the elderly, because they consume a disproportionate amount of all pharmaceuticals.

Outpatient Pharmaceuticals

The process of obtaining a drug begins with the patient visiting a physician. After making a diagnosis, the physician may give the patient a prescription for a specific drug and directions for its use. Although all drugs are approved for sale by the Food and Drug Administration (FDA) based on specific indications, physicians can prescribe drugs as they think appropriate. Moreover, when writing a prescription, physicians do not have to provide a specific indication for the medication, although some exceptions occur in managed care plans.

TABLE 13.1 **Sources of Funds for Pharmaceutical Products**

Out of pocket	61%
Private insurance	26%
Medicare	0%
Medicaid	11%
Other public programs	2%

Source: Health Care Financing Administration, Office of the Actuary.

In most outpatient situations, the patient takes the prescription to the local pharmacy, where the pharmacist fills the prescription. Pharmacists often provide additional information about how to take the drug and its potential side-effects. Patients often pay the full cost of the drug when they receive it and later get reimbursed by their insurance provider or employer. In some cases, patients may present a pharmaceutical benefits card and pay the pharmacist only their portion of the cost (either a percentage of the drug cost or fixed amount). In the latter case, the pharmacist bills the insurance provider, employer, or third-party administrator the balance due on the drug, less any agreed-upon discounts.

The local pharmacy purchases inventories from a drug wholesaler, who in turn buys it from the manufacturer. Because of the many drugs available, most local pharmacies do not carry a large inventory of each drug but rely on computerized inventory systems to get deliveries from the wholesaler daily. Wholesalers and pharmacists usually cannot switch patients from one product to another (except for generic products). As a result, they are unable to exert market power against the pharmaceutical manufacturer, but instead must pay the full, list price of the drug.

If the patient belongs to a managed care plan, the process of obtaining a drug is a little different. In some cases the managed care plan has its own pharmacy and the patient may pick up the drug at the managed care facility. In other cases, particularly for chronic treatment, the managed care plan may use a mail-order pharmacy. In this case, the physician will often phone in the prescription and the product will be sent directly to the patient. In still other cases, the managed care plan has an arrangement with specific local pharmacies and the patient must fill a prescription at one of these. The primary difference between a managed care plan and traditional fee-for-service (FFS) medicine is that a managed care plan will often have a restrictive formulary, or list of drugs from which the physician may prescribe. That is, the managed care plan will intentionally restrict the physician's choice of drugs. In exchange for being included on the formulary, the pharmaceutical company gives the managed care plan a significant discount. The tighter the control of the managed care plan, the higher the discount. On average, the discounts to managed care are about 15 percent.

Pharmaceutical Benefits Management companies essentially operate as a managed care plan for self-insured employers. Although PBMs have less direct control over the prescribing patterns of physicians, they are becoming increasingly more sophisticated about designing benefit plans to cut out the higher-priced drugs and only provide coverage for the generics or cheaper products. Often, the PBM will use a co-payment structure that favors the generic products. For example, a patient may pay ten dollars for a branded product but only a dollar for the generic drug. This is an attempt to have the patient influence the physician's writing behavior. In addition, PBMs have become sophisticated about calling physicians and suggesting product substitutions.

Medicaid is the primary government program providing pharmaceutical coverage. Under the Medicaid program, a qualified beneficiary is able to receive prescription drugs at little or no cost. To receive a drug, the patient must first obtain a prescription from a participating physician, and then take it to a participating pharmacy. At the pharmacy, the patient presents the Medicaid benefits card and receives the drug. The pharmacy bills the Medicaid program directly for the cost of the drug, plus a dispensing charge, which averaged \$4.10 in 1990. The state Medicaid agencies keep track of the drugs purchased through their program and obtain rebates from the manufactures of the single source drugs. These rebates are the maximum of 15.2 percent or the highest discount given by the manufacturer to a single buyer. In 1994, an estimated \$1.56 billion was refunded to Medicaid programs under the Medicaid Rebate law.

Inpatient Pharmaceuticals

The process of receiving a drug as an inpatient differs significantly from that used for outpatients. Again, the process begins with a physician writing a prescription, but the prescription goes directly to the hospital pharmacy. The prescription is filled by the staff pharmacist and administered to the patient by the nursing staff. All medications are carefully noted on the patient's hospital chart.

Payment for the drug depends on how the hospital is reimbursed for its services. Under Medicare, the hospital receives a flat, fixed payment based on the patient diagnosis and the average cost of treating a patient of that type. A component of that payment is based on average drug utilization, but the hospital receives no payment that is linked directly to drug utilization. A number of states have adopted all-payer diagnostically related group (DRG) payment systems (i.e., a pre-set payment per case as described in chapter 8, section 2) that extend this form of payment to all patients. If the hospital is being paid on a per diem rate, average drug utilization is generally incorporated into the daily rate. Again, the hospital does not receive any payment directly associated with drug utilization. It is only in cases where the hospitals are paid on a "charges" basis that the drug utilization is itemized and billed directly to the patient or their third-party payer. Thus, in many cases, the hospital bears the full marginal cost of the drug.

Because the hospital often bears the marginal cost of the drugs it administers to its patients, it has a strong financial incentive to try to minimize the overall pharmaceutical departmental budget. In pursuit of this objective, hospitals often establish their own formulary of drugs that they keep in stock and from which physicians may prescribe. By negotiating with the pharmaceutical companies over inclusion in the formulary, hospitals are able to utilize their market power to obtain discounts on drugs that have close competitors. At the same time, the hospital must balance these economic decisions against antagonizing the physicians on the medical staff on whom the hospital must rely on for admissions.

13.2   HOW THE FUNDS FLOW OUT _____

The funds that flow into the pharmaceutical industry are used in a variety of ways. For example, they are used to support the research and development efforts of the firm as it seeks to develop newer and better drugs before its competitors. These funds are also used to support the marketing and promotional efforts needed to get physicians to prescribe their drug rather than a competitor's drug. In addition, some of these funds are used to cover the costs of manufacturing, distribution, and administration that go along with any production process. And a

TABLE 13.2   Where the U.S. Prescription Dollar Goes

Cost of goods	30.1%
Distribution and administration	10.0%
Research and development	16.0%
Marketing and advertising	22.5%
Taxes	8.4%
Profits	13.0%

Source: U.S. Senate, Special Committee on Aging, 1993.

portion of these funds are profits, which are either given to stockholders in the form of dividends or reinvested in the company in the form of retained earnings. A breakout of the uses of funds is shown in Table 13.2.

From Table 13.2 we see that more than 30 percent of the funds go to cover the cost of manufacturing the drugs. Most studies have shown that there are constant returns to scale in the manufacturing of pharmaceutical products; that is, the average manufacturing cost is independent of the amount produced. This is, in part, due to the fact that most drugs are manufactured in small batches rather than in a continual process. Production in small batches is a result of the need to maintain high quality standards. Although large batches are generally more economical to manufacture, there is also a greater variance in the quality of the product and a greater chance that some of the units will have either too much or too little of the active ingredients. With pharmaceutical products, such deviations could be deadly; hence, small manufacturing batches are the norm.

Advertising and promotional activities account for another 22.5 percent of the pharmaceutical dollar. These activities primarily consist of detailing, sampling, and journal advertising. Of these, detailing and sampling are the most important. Detailing involves a representative of the pharmaceutical firm calling on an individual physician. During this meeting, the representative will discuss one or two products with the physician. For each drug discussed, the representative will give the physician the results of recent tests, explain how the drug works and what the potential side-effects are, and discuss the advantages of this drug over some of the competitors. The representative may leave the physician with some literature on the drug, as well as some free samples to pass on to patients. In addition, the detailer can answer many of the questions the physician might have about the drug or its use. The information presented and literature given to the physician must meet with strict guidelines developed by the Food and Drug Administration. Empirical studies have shown that detailing can have a large impact on a physician's prescribing behavior and on the elasticity of demand for individual products. As a result of these studies, a number of politicians have charged that the promotional activities of the industry are wasteful and excessive and have called for increased regulation of the industry. Whether such actions are justified, and what the overall social impact of such actions would be, are the subject of ongoing research and debate.

Research and development also accounts for another 16 percent of the total pharmaceutical dollar. Viewing R&D in this manner is, however, unfortunate. It gives one the impression that R&D activities are "funded" by current sales, a notion perpetuated by current accounting practices and the industry itself. It is more appropriate to view R&D expenditures as investments in intangible capital, rather than a current period expense. In this manner, it is clearly seen that current cash flows are the result of past R&D expenditures and that the primary incentive for current R&D efforts are the future cash flows that are expected to result from these investments in the future. When viewed this way, it is also clear that policies or environmental changes that jeopardize future cash flows adversely affect the incentives on the current R&D.

Profits account for about 13 percent of the pharmaceutical dollar. Looking at the profits per dollar sales may not be the correct way to examine the issue. It is necessary to examine the implied rate of return on the capital invested in the pharmaceutical industry to determine if the returns are excessive. Doing so requires a complicated set of adjustments, in part because of the need to capitalize the R&D expenditures as just discussed. Depending on how R&D is treated, on the cost of capital used for the industry, and on the time period examined, researchers have arrived at opposite conclusions.

13.3 BACKGROUND HISTORY AND REGULATION OF PHARMACEUTICALS_____

The regulation of the pharmaceutical industry and its products has evolved during the twentieth century in response to increased potency, effectiveness, and toxicity of these products. Until the late 1800s, most "pharmaceutical preparations" had an immediate effect of making the patient feel better, although in most instances they did little to cure the underlying disease. This meant that patients could directly evaluate the benefits of the drug and did not need extensive guidance from health care professionals in choosing which products to use.

The first "modern" pharmaceutical product, the diphtheria antitoxin, was developed the mid-1890s and dramatically reduced the incidence of diphtheria. However, because this new drug did not have an immediate effect on the patient (it prevented the person from becoming sick), it was much more difficult for the patient to evaluate the drug's benefit. (Would they have gotten sick without the drug?) And, although the benefits were not readily apparent to the patient, some of the dangerous side-effects were all too obvious. Thus, health care professionals with specialized knowledge about drugs became involved in helping patients decide which products to use.

The first regulation of pharmaceutical products was the Biologics Control Act of 1902. This legislation was a direct response to contaminated diphtheria antitoxin that fatally infected thirteen children. This incident contributed to overall concerns about the safety of the food and drug supply, which were being raised in the popular press and in books, such as Upton Sinclair's *The Jungle*. These events were quickly followed by the passage of the Pure Food and Drug Act of 1906. Although it focused primarily on the food supply, it required drug manufacturers to provide adequate labeling. The manufacturer either had to use a standardized formula for making their product or provide a complete list of the product's contents. In addition, the Food and Drug Act expanded the Agriculture Department's Bureau of Chemistry, and gave it authority to oversee testing and compliance of food and drug manufacturers. In 1931, the regulatory aspects of the Bureau of Chemistry

TABLE 13.3   Major Legislation Affecting the
Pharmaceutical Industry

1902	Biologics Control Act
1906	Pure Food and Drug Act
1938	Food, Drugs, and Cosmetics Act
1962	Harris–Kefauver Drug Act Amendments
1984	Drug Price Competition and Patent Restoration Act

became known as the Food and Drug Administration (FDA), which today is responsible for evaluating new products and overseeing their manufacture (see Table 13.3).

Despite a few notable breakthroughs, during the first part of the nineteenth century the pharmaceutical industry produced primarily bulk commodities for sale to packaging firms and local pharmacies. Thus, pharmaceutical firms were not manufacturing drugs in the sense of today's integrated firms. Moreover, despite producing many "drugs," there were few diseases that could actually be cured or controlled by drugs. A poster for a 1931 symposium on fighting diseases, for example, indicated only seven diseases that could be controlled using drugs, and another seven that could be partially controlled.

Against this backdrop of many ineffective products, the Federal Food, Drug, and Cosmetics Act was introduced in 1933 and eventually passed in 1938. Final passage was, in part, due to the Elixir Sulfanilamide incident, where more than one hundred people died painfully because the solvent used to make the drug in liquid form had not been adequately tested for toxicity in humans. Before this legislation, manufacturers could market any product as soon as they wished, and the burden of proof fell on the FDA to show that the product was unsafe.

The Food, Drug, and Cosmetics Act established several important provisions. First, it required preregistration of all new drugs with the FDA, giving them the opportunity to test the drug before marketing. It also gave the FDA the mandate of preventing unsafe drugs from *entering* the market. The new law, however, specifically excluded drugs that were administered by "trained professionals" for testing purposes. Second, it increased the amount of information that had to be included on the label of any drug sold without a prescription. This information included statements of recommended uses and potential dangers. Drugs sold by "prescription only" were not held to these same labeling standards.

Through these labeling provisions, the Food, Drug, and Cosmetics Act created the first real distinction between prescription and over-the-counter (OTC) drugs. Although previously any non-narcotic could be sold as either prescription or OTC, after 1938 nearly all new drugs were classified as prescription only. This was an unintended impact of the law; the original intent was not to restrict self-medication, but simply to restrict the use of the most dangerous drugs to professional supervision. Manufacturers, however, soon realized that *restricting sales of a product to prescription only had the effect of reducing the elasticity of demand,* since the physicians writing the prescription were not directly paying for the drug, and the patients paying for the drug rarely challenged the physicians authority. The lower price elasticity, in turn, allowed the firm to charge a higher price, since the patient and pharmacist could not substitute cheaper products once the prescription was written. Moreover, requiring a prescription gave the appearance that the drug was more potent or effective. Finally, the medical profession strongly supported these moves, in part, because they directly benefited from forcing patients to see a physician before receiving treatment.

During the 1940s, three key changes built on these regulatory changes that dramatically altered the pharmaceutical industry. First, new techniques for discovering and isolating potentially beneficial substances were developed in the process of discovering streptomycin. Second, the U.S. Patent Office ruled that the chemical modifications made to streptomycin, which enable it to be isolated and purified, created a new product. Moreover, the process that developed this product and the product itself were patentable. Third, instead of licensing patents to competitors, as had been done in the past, pharmaceutical firms began to exercise their patent rights to control the production, distribution, and price of the product. Together, these changes ushered in the era of the modern pharmaceutical firm. These firms are R&D driven and use patents to maintain prices above short-run marginal cost and reap the rewards of the research and development activities.

The 1950s and early 1960s represented a heyday of drug development, as one firm after another introduced "wonder drugs." Many states also passed "anti-substitution" laws, which further reduced the elasticity of demand by requiring pharmacists to fill the prescriptions as written rather than substituting cheaper generic products. However, questions began to arise about the effectiveness of some of these new drugs and whether the prices were too high.

In 1959, Senator Kefauver's Antitrust and Monopoly Subcommittee began hearings on the question of whether too many drugs that were minor variations of existing drugs were being introduced to extend the patent life of a product line—something that has a familiar ring today. However, it was the Thalidomide incident in 1961–62 that triggered passage of the 1962 Harris–Kefauver Drug Amendments and brought this heyday of drug development to a screeching halt.

Thalidomide was a drug used to treat nausea during pregnancy. Although it had not yet received FDA approval, it was being widely distributed to physicians for "experimental purposes" when it was discovered that it caused major birth defects in some babies of women who had taken the drug. This inflamed the fears that drug companies, in their rush to market new drugs and earn large profits, were "egregiously exposing humans to potentially harmful drugs during clinical trials."[1] As a result of this fear, Congress passed legislation that greatly increased the burden on pharmaceutical firms to not only show that their products were safe, but that they were also effective when used in the manner directed. In addition, the testing procedures used to establish these results were put under the oversight of the FDA. The 1962 amendments also required pharmaceutical firms to follow "good manufacturing and laboratory practices," as defined by the FDA, and gave the FDA the authority to inspect the manufacturing plants. Finally, the 1962 amendments extended these testing requirements to both generic (identical) and similar (me-too) drugs. Previously, these drugs could avoid pre-market testing through certification from the FDA that they were in effect the same as the original drug.

These amendments had the effect of dramatically increasing the costs and time of new drug development and, as a result, slowed the rate of new drug introductions. The average number of new drug introductions fell from fifty-one a year between 1956 and 1961, to only twenty a year between 1962 and 1967. Although these restrictions increased the cost of drug development to the pioneering firms, it also reduced competition once the patent had expired, by creating larger barriers to entry for the producers of generic products. Thus, over the years, considerable debate erupted over whether these restriction were excessive, whether they increased or decreased consumer welfare, and whether they have increased or decreased the profitability of pharmaceutical firms. What is clear, however, is that after the passage of the 1962 amendments, the length of time between the discovery or synthesis of a new drug and its market introduction increased dramatically. In 1960 the average development time was 35 months; by 1980 this had increased to 145 months. It is also clear that these amendments had a chilling effect on the introduction of generic products, since generic manufacturers had to duplicate all of the research conducted by the pioneering firm to gain approval for their own new drug application.

In 1984, Congress passed the Drug Price Competition and Patent Term Restoration Act, which attempted to remedy some of the problems created by the 1962 amendments. First, it established the Abbreviated New Drug Application (ANDA), which allowed a generic manufacturer to show that its drug was "bioequivalent" to the pioneer's product, rather than repeat all of the safety and efficacy studies. Since 1984, hundreds of products have been introduced under the ANDA provisions. Second, the act established a formula for increasing the patent life of a new product to restore some of the time (up to five years) lost due to the pre-market regulatory process.

As we have seen, the regulation of the pharmaceutical industry has evolved since the turn of the century by responding to the perceived needs for consumer protection and industry development; attempting to balance the benefits and costs of regulation. What began as a requirement for adequate labeling, ensuring that the public was protected from adulterated or misrepresented products, grew into a system where consumers no longer make choices about the drugs they receive, but rely on their physicians (and sometimes even third party payers) to make these choices for them. Along the way, the entire industry was transformed from simply manufacturing bulk products to one that spent over $12.6 billion of dollars actively searching for new products in 1993.

13.4 PRODUCT RESEARCH AND DEVELOPMENT _____

New product research and development plays a critical role in the pharmaceutical industry as firms compete to provide the most effective drug for treating specific diseases and as patent expiration opens the market to competition from generic manufacturers. To understand competition in this industry, one must be familiar with the R&D process and its role in the industry.

The research and development of a new product takes place in several distinct steps, with the pharmaceutical company making decisions of whether to continue the project or abandon it at each step. The first step is either the discovery stage or the synthesis stage—reflecting two very different approaches to new drug development. In the discovery stage, natural chemical compounds having desired properties are isolated from biological samples. Alternatively, in the synthesis stage, a new synthetic compound is created in the laboratory based on the results of previous research or computer models. Once the new compound has been isolated, regardless of its source, it is generally immediately patented and is then screened for pharmacological activity and toxicity, first *in vitro* (i.e., test-tubes with tissue cultures) and then in animals. This preclinical phase can take up to three years and literally thousands of compounds are examined and rejected for each one that moves on to the next stage of testing. Once a promising compound has been found, the firm files an **Investigational New Drug (IND)** application with the FDA and, unless rejected, the firm can begin testing in humans within thirty days of making the application.

Clinical trials (i.e., human testing) is generally conducted in three distinct phases. Phase I testing is generally performed on a small number of healthy patients, although cancer drugs are typically tested on terminal patients because a high level of toxicity is generally necessary to kill the cancer cells. The objective of these studies is to obtain some preliminary information on the toxicity and tolerable dosage range in humans. Generally, the drug is given sequentially to sets of three patients at each dosage level, until a preset toxicity threshold is crossed (the acceptable toxicity level depends greatly on the nature of the disease that the drug is intended to treat and the availability of alternative therapies, or until some predetermined dose is reached.) During the phase I trials, data are also collected on the drug's absorption, metabolic effects, and the way in which the body eliminates the drug. These trials generally last slightly more than a year. Although signs of efficacy are always encouraging, they are not necessary for moving on to the phase II trials because of the small size of the sample.

In the second phase of testing, the drug is administered to a limited number of patients whom the drug is intended to benefit (generally 30–300 patients). In phase II, the first evidence of efficacy is obtained, even though the general focus of the trial is still on safety. The trial also begins to examine the cumulative effects of the drug. On average, these trials last about two years. If the safety profile continues to look good, and there are signs of beneficial effects, the drug is moved into the final stage of human testing.

The final stage of clinical testing, the phase III trials, are intended to establish the efficacy claims of the manufacturer. Large samples, frequently thousands of patients, are exposed to the new drug. Often, these trials are double blind, where neither the patient nor the treating physician know whether the individual patient is on the experimental drug or the control drug (perhaps a placebo). In addition to looking for evidence of efficacy, researchers continue to look at the safety profile of the drug as well as beginning to look for potential adverse reactions to the drug.[2] In order to obtain information on the long-term effects of the drug, these phase III clinical trials can go on for several years and on average last nearly three years.

At the same time as the clinical trials are underway, pharmaceutical firms typically continue their long-term animal testing, looking for possible adverse genetic and/or reproductive effects. Once the firm believes that it has sufficient information to show that the product is both safe and effective, it files a New Drug Application (NDA) with the FDA. On average, only one of five drugs that enter the IND phase reach the point of an NDA. Once the NDA has been filed, the FDA has sixty days to determine if there is sufficient information in the NDA for the agency to conduct a substantive review. Although the FDA is supposed to render a decision within six months, the Office of Technology Assessment has estimated that for drugs approved during 1990, the average approval time took nearly thirty months. Part of this delay was the result of additional testing required by the FDA before granting approval.

As a result of the lengthy testing and approval process, from the time the firm first began spending money on researching a new product, a total of more than ten years has generally elapsed before a successful product is ready for the market. Because of this lengthy period of time, it is very important to take into account the opportunity cost of these expenditures when assessing the costs of drug development. In perhaps the most comprehensive analysis to date, DiMasi et al. estimated that the capitalized out of pocket costs at the point of market approval averaged $231 million (1987 pre-tax dollars).[3] This figure includes the cost of projects abandoned along the way. Thus, each individual marketed drug represents a substantial investment of resources for the firm. These investments are made in the anticipation of obtaining future profits on the manufacture and sale of the drug. Others have examined the profitability of these investments and have found that only the top 20 percent of the drugs had large enough returns to cover the average cost of R&D.

13.5   COMPETITION IN PHARMACEUTICAL MARKETS _____

The market for pharmaceutical products can be divided into three separate markets based on the purchasers of the product. The first market, which has traditionally been the largest, is through the retail drug store market. In this market, physicians prescribe a pharmaceutical product and consumers or insurers pay for the drug. Because the actions are separate, the payers have little influence over what the physician prescribes and as a result, this market is not very price sensitive. The second market, which has been growing in importance, is the managed care and hospital market. In this market, the drug is purchased directly by the managed care group or hospital, and a physician's choice of which drug to use is limited by a restricted formulary. Because the managed care group or hospital has the ability to shift a large number of patients from one product to another, it has some market power. Exercising this market power enables the hospital or managed care group to purchase from the manufacturer at a discount. The third market is the government market. The state and federal government are one of the largest purchasers of pharmaceutical products. The state and federal government jointly finance Medicaid purchases, and the federal government finances the Veterans Affairs, CHAMPUS, and military purchases.

The competition for consumers differs significantly across these markets. In the traditional market, where consumers are price insensitive, competition takes place between products on the basis of product quality and detailing. Detailing is a form of marketing that is unique to the pharmaceutical industry. A salesperson, or detailer, will provide a physician "detailed" information on the approved product indications. Detailers are prohibited from discussing "off-label" uses of the product.[4] Studies have consistently shown that detailers greatly influence a physicians choice of drugs. Moreover, once a physician becomes familiar with a particular product, its method of action and the potential side effects, they become reluctant to try a new product unless it offers a substantial advantage either in efficacy or side effects—price tends not to be an important criteria for this market. Thus, competition in this market tends to be on product quality, effectiveness, and detailing, and generics have not been able to make significant inroads into this market.

The managed care and hospital market is almost exactly the opposite. Since the HMO or hospital is directly paying for the drug, and restricting physicians prescribing patterns through a formulary, they appear to be primarily interested in the price of the product—or more recently, its cost-effectiveness. That is, unless a product can demonstrate that it is clearly superior, they will tend to opt for the cheaper product. Since most clinical trials are designed to compare the drug to placebo, most of the traditional research conducted by pharmaceutical companies is not suitable for establishing these superiority claims. A new field is emerging in the 1990s called **pharmacoeconomics.** This field is aligned with developing methodologies for evaluating the cost-effectiveness of individual products and establishing data necessary to support these claims with the managed care and hospital markets. Currently, managed care companies claim to represent nearly 25 percent of the U.S. population, and projections call for this to double by the year 2000. Thus, this is a large and rapidly growing segment of the market, and an increasingly important segment of a pharmaceutical companies business. Most of the large pharmaceutical companies have developed sales, marketing, and research groups specifically aimed at addressing the concerns of this market. In addition, pharmaceutical companies are beginning to explore new contractual relationships as a way of increasing sales and locking in specific customers. In addition, this is the segment of the market where generic products have had the most impact, since the generic is supposedly chemically identical to the original product and often sold at a much lower price (up to 60 percent less).

To date, government purchasers have chosen not to exercise fully their monopsony market power on a drug-by-drug basis, but instead have adopted a standardized discount policy that pharmaceutical firms can either accept or reject. Under this policy, the government is rebated an amount equal to 15.2 percent of the average wholesale price for Medicaid purchases, or equal to the "best deal" given by that company on that product. There are similar provisions set up for other government contracts. In exchange for agreeing to these discounts, Medicaid agreed not to establish restrictive formularies. Thus, although pharmaceutical firms must "cut" their prices to sell to this market, they are essentially free to detail the physicians on their products and do not face stiff competition from generic products.

13.6 CURRENT TRENDS _____

There are several important emerging trends in the way pharmaceutical products are developed, manufactured, and sold in the United States. These trends are a direct response to changes elsewhere in the health care industry, namely, the rapid growth of managed care and the increased use of restrictive formularies.

Restrictive formularies enable managed care to switch large numbers of patients from one drug to another in response to small changes in relative prices—that is, they increase the elasticity of demand. Pharmaceutical firms can choose from several immediate responses to this shift in market power.

The first is price reductions. Pharmaceutical firms can compete with each other through successive reductions in the prices of their competing products. Since much of the costs of drug development and manufacturing are sunk, short-term competition can significantly reduce prices. During the past few years one can point to specific instances where there has been increased price competition, particularly in areas where there are several branded products, such as antihypertensives and cholesterol reducers.

The end result of price reductions, of course, would be decreased profitability, increased consolidation of the pharmaceutical industry, and capital flight. As expected, there have been several significant mergers in the industry in recent years. From a societal perspective there could also be a huge cost to this short-term gain—namely, reduced prices decrease the incentives for future R&D and drugs that otherwise would have been developed are delayed or may never be discovered. Currently one observes a trend towards less R&D in the industry as a whole, and R&D activity that is more carefully scrutinized, focused in specific areas, and focused on being the first to introduce a new line of products, rather than developing a "me-too".

A second response to the increased elasticity of demand is the development of new ways to establish product differentiation. Outcomes research, pharmacoeconomics, and disease management are just some of the several ways the pharmaceutical firms are trying to differentiate their products from each other and develop "value" messages about their individual products. Fundamentally, these are attempts by the industry to not only demonstrate the safety and efficacy of their product, but also to translate the efficacy of treatment into measures that consumers value. For example, rather than simply showing that a cholesterol drug can reduce LDL by x percent, firms in the industry have undertaken studies to show what that percent reduction means in terms of reduced coronary events (heart attacks, strokes etc.) and to show that reducing these events saves future health care expenditures and improves the quality of patients' lives. New metrics, such as cost per life year saved and cost per QALY (Quality Adjusted Life Year) saved have been developed to provide more descriptive information for physician's consumers to assist in decision making (see Chapter 2). Nearly every major pharmaceutical firm has begun to develop expertise in this area and several new journals have developed to publish the results of these kinds of studies.

A third response involves developing contractual relationships between pharmaceutical firms and managed care companies. Possible arrangements include:

1. Basing discounts for specific drugs on specific performance measures (such as market share)
2. Establishing cost-sharing arrangements or warranties on specific products
3. Developing capitated contracts, whereby a pharmaceutical company agrees to provide all of the drugs needed for a fixed (per member per month) charge for a managed care population (e.g., specific drugs, drug classes, or even large bundles of drugs)

4. Developing complete disease management programs, whereby the pharmaceutical firm may assume some of the financial risk for the total costs of treatment, not just the pharmaceutical costs

A number of pharmaceutical firms have begun to explore these alternative contractual arrangements in attempts to "lock-in" customers to their products and services; and some firms have vertically integrated by purchasing or merging with PBMs.

In addition to these market changes, important trends exist in research and development. These trends include a broad shift from chemistry-based medicines to biology-based medicines. Again, changes in legal structures have played a role in this, as the courts have ruled that new organisms created in the laboratory may be patented. Much of the early development of these new "products" takes place in small start-up companies—so-called biotech firms. As these products move out of the laboratory and into clinical testing, the biotech firms often either take on partners from the traditional pharmaceutical industry; are bought out by established firms; or develop licensing agreements. Thus, much of the most basic research has shifted from the large firms in the industry to smaller, high-risk ventures. As health care in America continues to evolve, the pharmaceutical industry has begun to evolve in response to these changes. These responses have taken several directions, including shifts in the focus of R&D activities, consolidation of the industry, new measures of product value, and new contractual relationships between the industry and managed care providers.

SUGGESTIONS FOR FURTHER READING ____

Abbott, T. A. "Regulating Pharmaceutical Prices," In *Health Care Policy and Regulation*, Boston, Mass.: Kluwer Academic Press, 1995, p. 105–34.

DiMasi, J. A., R. W. Hansen, H. G. Grabowski and L. Lasagna. "Cost of Innovation in the Pharmaceutical Industry," *Journal of Health Economics*, 10(1991):107–42.

Frank, R. G., and D. S. Salkever. "Pricing, Patent Loss and the Market for Pharmaceuticals," *Southern Economic Journal*, October 1992, pp. 165–79.

Peltzman, S. "An Evaluation of Consumer Protection Legislation: The 1962 Drug Amendments," *Journal of Policitical Economy*, September 1973, pp. 1049–91.

Temin, P. *Taking Your Medicine: Drug Regulation in the United States*, Cambridge, Mass.: Harvard University Press, 1980.

U.S. Senate, Special Committee on Aging, *Earning A Failing Grade: A Report Card on 1992 Drug Manufacturer Price Inflation*, Serial No. 103-B. Washington, D.C.: U.S. Government Printing Office, February 1993.

SUMMARY _____

1. The pharmaceutical industry has undergone dramatic changes during the last fifty years as a result of **scientific discovery, regulatory pressures**, and, more recently, **market pressures**. It arose from makers of "potions and elixirs" to a scientifically based industry with research and development at its core. Along

the way, the requirements placed on the industry have also changed, from simply making patients feel better, to scientifically proving the safety and efficacy of their products, and now to providing value and comparative information for their products. These requirements were initially imposed by governmental regulations, but have increasingly been replaced by market pressures.

2. **Research and development** of new products is **a risky, lengthy, and costly process**. Only one in a thousand compounds initially studied eventually makes it to the market. On average, the time from discovery to successful market introduction is more than ten years, at a total cost of more than $231 million. **The most costly part of the process are the clinical trials** needed to establish safety and efficacy claims, which can take up to five years and involve thousands of patients. It is the hope of large profits made from discovering the next "blockbuster" product that keeps firms investing in R&D and fuels progress in the pharmaceutical industry.

3. Although pharmaceuticals represent only **8 percent of total health care expenditures** in the United States, they are almost 30 percent of out-of-pocket expenditures, and an even higher fraction for elderly Americans. Thus, there is a great deal of attention focused on the prices (and price increases) of pharmaceutical products, and several bills have been introduced to regulate these prices.

4. The pharmaceutical market can be divided into three major market segments: fee-for-service, managed care and hospitals, and government. The **fee-for-service market is very price insensitive because of moral hazard** (physicians prescribe—patients or insurance pays). **The managed care and hospital segment is very price sensitive** and has developed **restrictive formularies** to consolidate market power and extract significant price discounts from manufacturers. To date, the government sector has only exercised market power in the Medicaid program through the institution of mandatory rebates on single-source products.

5. **Generic** manufactures have increased in importance since the legal changes in 1984 enabled easier approval for generic versions of established products. Generic firms have been most successful in penetrating the managed care and hospital markets, which are most price sensitive, although they are making inroads in the fee-for-service market as well.

6. Pharmaceutical manufacturers have begun to respond to changes in their markets brought about by managed care and generic competition. These changes include the use of **discounts**, development of **pharmacoeconomics** and **disease management**, and the development of various forms of **risk-sharing contracts**.

PROBLEMS _____

1. {*flow of funds*} What fraction of the total cost of pharmaceuticals is paid for directly by patients? Does this mean that price is more or less important than for other types of medical care?

2. {*research, incidence*} How is most pharmaceutical research paid for? What is the most costly aspect of pharmaceutical research?

3. {*market segmentation*} How many distinct market segments exist in the pharmaceutical industry? How do these segments differ from each other?

4. {*competition*} On what basis do pharmaceutical firms compete in each market segment? Is price a more important factor for the choice of what doctor to see, or for what drug is prescribed?

5. {*insurance coverage*} The major form of health insurance coverage for the elderly is Medicare, and the elderly are much heavier users of pharmaceuticals than other groups. It would seem reasonable to expect that Medicare is the largest source of payment for drugs. Is it?

6. {*marginal costs, revenues*} Do hospitals have more of an incentive to control the costs of surgical implants, anesthesiologists' fees, or pharmaceuticals? In which case do they bear the highest fraction of marginal cost? In which case do they receive the highest fraction of marginal revenue?

7. {*patents*} How would a change in the length of the patent period affect the structure of the pharmaceutical industry?

8. {*competition*} Marketing accounts for a much larger portion of the cost of pharmaceuticals than of other forms of health care. Why? To whom are most pharmaceutical marketing efforts targeted?

9. {*capital investment*} If $50 million is invested in a drug that subsequently fails to gain approval from the FDA, what is the rate of return on this investment? Are pharmaceutical firms more or less capital intensive than hospitals? Than doctor's office practices?

10. {*anti-trust*} Since the FDA regulations limit the entry of new drugs into the market, do they constitute an "unfair restraint of trade" that reduces competition and raises prices to consumers?

11. {*price elasticity*} When a brand name drug loses patent protection after seventeen years and competing generic products enter the market, will the price of the brand name drug increase or decrease (hint: what changes occur in the brand-name drug's demand curve).

12. {*risk*} Which form of investment is more risky, developing a new drug or building a new nursing home? Which type of publicly traded for-profit firm would you expect to show greater variability in earnings, pharmaceutical firms or nursing home chains?

ENDNOTES _____

1. Peltzman, "An Evaluation of Consumer Protection Legislation: The 1962 Drug Amendments," *Journal of Political Economy*, September 1973, p. 1050–51.
2. Despite the relatively large sample sizes, many important adverse reactions can be missed during the phase III studies because they have a low probability of occurring. For example, a 1:10,000 adverse reaction causing death could easily go unnoticed in a phase III trial on several thousand patients, even though it could cause 30,000 deaths if the drug were released to all 300 million citizens. As a result, when a new drug is re-

leased, the FDA requires the pharmaceutical firm to conduct extensive post-marketing surveillance for any adverse reactions and to immediately report all deaths of people taking the drug, regardless of whether there appears to be a direct link between the death and the drug usage.

3. J. A. DiMasi, R. W. Hansen, H. G. Grabowski and L. Lasagna, "Cost of Innovation in the Pharmaceutical Industry," *Journal of Health Economics* 10:107–42, 1991.

4. As discussed earlier, although a product is approved by the Food and Drug Administration for a specific use or indication and some drugs may have multiple indications, physicians are permitted to prescribe the product as they see fit. At the same time, physicians and drug companies are always exploring potentially new (or related) uses for the drug. The results of these studies are often published in the literature long before a new indication is obtained from the FDA. As a result of these publications, many drugs are prescribed for conditions outside of their indications. This practice is called off-label prescribing.

CHAPTER 14

Introduction to the Macroeconomics of Health

QUESTIONS

1. *Why abstract from reality if one wants to study trading in the real world?*
2. *What is the "fallacy of composition?"*
3. *How should the wealth of a community be measured?*
4. *What determines how many people in a society are rich? How rich the richest 1% are? How poor the poorest 20% are?*
5. *Why does size make a difference? Is the behavior of a system different from the behavior of the individuals who make up the system?*
6. *Are "prices" the essence of trade, or just one aspect?*
7. *Does cheating hurt the individual, or the system?*
8. *Who makes the rules that govern the economy? Who challenges them?*
9. *Is community health the same as individual health?*
10. *Are some questions better answered using time series analysis rather than cross-sectional analysis, or vice-versa?*

14.1 WHAT IS MACRO HEALTH ECONOMICS?

Macro means large. Macroeconomics deals with large-scale properties and institutions that characterize the system as a whole. Individuals only become an economic system when they start to trade with each other, and in doing so they create a whole that is larger than the sum of the parts; develop a *government* to set the rules under which trade will occur; and create a special medium, *money,* for carrying out trade.[1] Macroeconomics evaluates Gross Domestic Product (GDP) as a measure of national economic activity, whether it is *growing* (expansion) or falling (recession), and the *dynamics* of the process by which change occurs (investment, trade, unemployment, bankruptcy). Rather than the income of any particular individual or firm, it is the *growth* and *distribution* of income that is investigated in macroeconomics. It asks how many are rich, how many are poor, whether they are always the same groups over time, and whether the gap is widening or being reduced toward more equality.

Macroeconomic (system) Properties:

- Growth
- Dynamics
- Distribution

Macro (system) Institutions:

- Government
- Money

The macroeconomics of health is concerned with a parallel set of large-scale system issues concerning (a) spending, employment, and other aspects of health as a part of the economy, and (b) the biological health status of the population as a whole and its relation to economic changes. Thus, it must address how GDP growth affects the number and income of physicians, as well as how GDP growth affects the health (longevity, morbidity) of the population, and in return, how an increase in longevity affects both spending on medical care and growth in overall GDP.

Health System Properties:

	Economic	*Biologic*
	Spending	Longevity
	Employment	Fertility
	Prices	Productivity

Health (system) Institutions:

- Medical professions
- Hospitals and caring organizations
- Financing (insurance and reimbursement) structure

14.2 PROPERTIES OF THE INDIVIDUAL VERSUS PROPERTIES OF THE SYSTEM_____

*Micro*economics is about how individuals choose, how they minimize costs or maximize profits (or wealth or utility) within a given trading system, subject to a set of rules and prices. Microeconomists examine how individual choices are altered when prices change, or when the rules change. *Macro*economics, on the other hand, is about the properties of the system as a whole (growth, unemployment, inflation), and how the system changes over time as people modify the rules to better satisfy their needs. One could say that microeconomics is about how the game is played, and macroeconomics is about how the rules of the game are changed to make it better, more fair, or to favor one group over another, as well as the keeping of statistics on league standings.

Systems may behave quite differently than individuals, even when exposed to the same forces. For example, if the government makes a mistake and sends me a $100,000 tax refund, then I am much richer, and can buy a fancy new car. What would happen if the government sent everyone a check for $100,000? There is no extra production, so as a society, we would not be any richer. What would happen is a burst of inflation that would disrupt prices and everyone's savings plans so that we would all be made worse off by this massive mistake. This difference between individual and system results is known as **the fallacy of composition**. Other examples are: If I push my way to the front of the line at a dentists office, then I get served quicker. If everyone pushes, then it will take longer for all of us to get served. If I cheat on my health insurance, then I am better off. If everyone cheats, then premiums, waste and administrative overhead will rise, making us all worse off. In part, the Great Depression was a painfully clear example of how the fallacy of composition can work in economics. One person can consume more in the future by saving now and spending less of their current paycheck, but when everyone got scared and stopped spending, it contributed to an already falling aggregate demand, so much that one-fourth of all workers were unemployed and everyone's potential future consumption fell as the economy spiraled downward.

There is an old anecdote among business journalists—"If my neighbor is unemployed, then we are in a recession. If I become unemployed, then we are in a depression." An individual is either working or not, but the rate of unemployment is a characteristic of the system as a whole. The rate affects what the individual does (if many people are unemployed, I will always be polite to my boss, not grumble about overtime, and think about joining the army when I graduate), but rates are system-wide properties, and have to be measured at the level of the system as a whole. Similarly, a particular individual might be saving to buy a car, or borrowing to make the purchase, but it is the aggregate actions of all individuals that determine the interest rate. Inflation is perhaps the best example of a system property. Every individual consumer or firm reacts to and sets prices, but it is the flow of money into the system, and the degree of public confidence in the value of that money, that determines how fast the average price will rise.[2] With regard to health, an individual is either dead or alive. Yet for the system as a whole, averages (mortality rates, longevity) become useful measures of system performance.

In moving toward a larger perspective, it is important to remember that all macro phenomena arise from individual maximizing behavior. The system exists to serve the people, not the other way around. Government, credit cards, and bankruptcy laws may become personally inconvenient to me, but they make the economy as a whole function much better. Similarly, all of the special features of medical care such as insurance, licensure, and so on are ultimately justifiable on a micro level as being part of a choice that people have made to make themselves better off. Adam Smith's 1776 book *The Wealth of Nations* expressed a fundamental insight into system behavior and individual motivation that has come to be known as the "invisible hand" of the market—that people make others better off not so much because they want to, or out of altruism, but because going to work, obeying the law, and discovering a cure for arthritis is profitable.[3] The primary way to make oneself better off in a society is to do something for someone else. However, those who have the power to write the rules often bend them in their own favor, and such individual maximization can lead to adverse social consequences. Inflation, unemployment, and war all occur because somebody benefits.

14.3 DYNAMICS: CHANGE OVER TIME _____

It takes much less time to make a deal than to change the way that deals are made. Some of the confusion between individual and systematic responses arises because it takes longer for the system to respond. If we all get checks in the mail, it will take a while for prices to rise and eliminate this apparent windfall gain. Similarly, if a gay person with AIDS charges a lot of fancy gifts before dying to repay the friends who took care of him, he may seem to be making his community better off, but behavior such as this will, if it becomes prevalent in the long run, mean that no one with AIDS can get credit. Standard supply and demand analysis uses "comparative statics" studying the change between one set of equilibrium conditions and another, asking only what the result was, not how the system got there, or how long it took. A question regarding the effects of a change (e.g., will expansion of the hospital cause nurses' wages to rise?) is microeconomic in scope. A macro perspective must also address the **dynamics** or process of change, why and how growth occurred, how long it took, and what things had to happen (bankruptcy, unemployment, war) before a new equilibrium was reached. A recession does not occur because GDP is $500 trillion, or $5 billion, or $990 quadrillion, but because GDP is falling, or less than expected.

Microeconomists can make comparisons between different individuals at one point in time and test their theories using **cross-sectional analysis**. Macroeconomists usually cannot. They must look at the economy as a whole and see how it has changed from one year to the next as the money supply rose, or the population got older. Even if they were not interested in dynamics, they would be forced to use longitudinal **time series** methods to test their theories observing the same groups or individuals at different points in time. When economists make comparisons between the economies of different nations, there are often so few observations and so many differences in government and culture that any conclusions regarding the effects of money supply, age, education and other variables must be very tentative.

The fallacy of composition operates over time as well. Perfect efficiency right now implies that all current waste be eliminated. All the excess staff sitting at their desks wondering what to do, indulgently impractical research schemes, half-baked management reorganization projects, and so on, must be cut away to minimize costs. Yet it is precisely from such wasteful slack and indulgent impracticalities that the creative energy for new technology and new managerial structures arise. In order to change and grow over time, every organization in the economy must "waste" some resources trying out new ideas that don't work, or don't work very well (yet). Dynamic efficiency, optimizing economic output over time, requires that there be some activities that look wasteful from a static perspective, which considers only current costs and benefits.

14.4 ABSTRACTIONS AND COMPLICATIONS _____

While the terms *micro* and *macro* can be applied to purely individual and purely systematic effects respectively, most of reality occurs between these polar extremes. The following diagram may be helpful in providing a conceptual map to the different levels at which an economic question can be addressed.

The simplest form of trade is that which occurs on a spot market. A one-dimensional good is traded, at a single point in time, for a specified amount of money (the "price"). A transaction, whether going to the supermarket for groceries or being admitted to the hospital for gall-bladder surgery, is an event that may bundle up a number of goods and take some time. Exchange is a broader concept that brings in the notion of reciprocity and balance, that each party be satisfied with what they got from trading. Thus, an exchange may include a third party (patients pay insurance companies who pay doctors) and involve relationships of long duration (the company owes me something for my years of loyal service). Exchange takes place within a trading system or "economy" that specifies ownership and the rules for exchange. There is an understanding on everyone's part about what you can and cannot do, what you should expect, and how a "fair" price is determined—even for something as nebulous and unexpected as a facial scar that results from a mistake made by a surgeon. In the current U.S. economic system, the patient would take the doctor to court and sue for malpractice. In another economy, it might be that the doctor who blundered would not get paid, or would get beaten up. Finally, the economy exists within a social structure that expresses our collective sense of who we are and how we are to live together (Figure 14.1). Even before considering the terms of trade, it is first necessary to determine who gets to have what, and how much they can trade away. Are you supposed to beg or pay for something you need? Who gets to order whom about, and how much do they have to pay? Is cheating allowed, and, if not, how much will it cost me if I get caught? Whose desires count the most, and are we to treat outsiders as customers or enemies to be looted? Creating the best set of institutions (government, laws, markets, nonprofit organizations) for satisfying people's wants is what politics and philosophy and economics is all about. More realistically, we try to make some small improvements in the system that we have without destroying all the benefits of the traditions that have developed over time.

FIGURE 14.1   The Context of Trade

Social Structure

Economic System

Exchange Relationships

Transactions

Prices

In order to simplify economics and make it amenable to abstract mathematical formulation, a neoclassical approach makes a sharp distinction between properties of the system (macroeconomics) and of individual trades and traders (microeconomics). Then, the complex set of relations involved in trade are collapsed down to one bare essential, price. Governments, laws, institutions, reputations, and other complex structures that arise in the attempt to organize trade in the face of uncertainty and costly information are all assumed away so that the workings of supply and demand can be more clearly revealed. In terms of the preceding diagram, neoclassical economics ignores social structure and takes as the appropriate subject of macroeconomics only those elements of the economic system that are common to all economies. (More precisely, it takes as a given the social and cultural context for trade that prevails in global markets and in the Western democracies, so that this set of institutions forms a sort of unconscious assumption). These simplifications, that macroeconomics is divorced from social and cultural context, and that supply and demand are separate domains communicating solely through prices, are extremely powerful and useful—yet, like all intellectual tools, they have a cost as well as a benefit. This abstract representation is much closer to reality for some economic transactions (timber, steel, retail food) than for others (art, insurance, medicine). We might be lured into the error of the proverbial motorist who spent the night searching the street for his lost car keys. The police asked why he spent so much time looking in the street, when he had probably lost the keys while walking through the bushes. He replied, "Because it was dark, and the light was much better in the street." Just so, we may be tempted to look in the well-lit neoclassical street of clearly separated supply and demand divorced from social and systematic complications because the concepts are much clearer there than in the dimly lit reaches where each transaction depends on tradition and trust as well as price. Yet already, in previous chapters, we have been forced to talk about the rules of system and how these institutions (professional licensure, insurance, regulation) change to apply the concepts of supply and demand to medicine. Consider how quickly a simple question, "What is the price of an abortion?" shreds the neat divisions between firms and households and reaches up through the explicit rules of international trade into troublesome unresolved questions of social order and obligation. The complicated features of medical markets do not come from a desire to make this textbook longer, but because the trades organized by doctors and hospitals are not simple. These exchanges do not merely touch, but must often in practice define, difficult social issues, such as what it means to be alive, or to be human. The special institutions of medicine are there to make people better off; they come from the complex nature of the good to be traded (medical care), and the shaping of the rules by the groups that have the power to do so in their own interest, subject to the controls of economic and political competition.

14.5   THE ROLE OF GOVERNMENT (OVERVIEW OF CHAPTERS 15–20) _____

Governments attempt to develop rules so that the incentives for individuals are in line with the good of society as a whole. Thus, we have laws against stealing, a social consensus to prevent people from standing in their seats at a ball game, the National Institutes of Health to carry out medical research, and a central bank to offset fluctuations in aggregate demand. One of the most difficult tasks of a government is to determine which activities are best left to people to work out for themselves (what to eat, whom to marry, what to wear, where to worship) and what activities require government control (what you own, when to fight, whom to protect). Health touches some very controversial areas where agreement over what is a public responsibility and what is private is hard to reach (what drugs you can take, how and with whom to have sex, whether you can take your own life).

The next set of chapters will examine the role of government in health from a macro perspective. Chapter 15 begins with a broad historical review of the relationship between economic growth and health status. The tools of demography will be used to attempt to determine how much of the great increase in life expectancy is attributable to public health activities, to private medical care, or to improvements in the prevailing standards of housing, education, nutrition and other aspects of general economic well being.

Chapter 16 presents a schematic outline for analysis of market failure and the role of governments in health. Regulation is seen to arise from dependency and difficulties in defining and transacting property rights. However, the incentives of regulatory bodies are not always in line with the interests of the public, and many medical institutions are neither purely market driven nor governmental, but rather "voluntary" private nonprofit organizations.

Chapter 17 examines "public goods," those things that can only be provided efficiently on a collective basis (national defense, air traffic control, securities regulation, control of infectious disease epidemics). It is seen that in order to carry out public health action, it is necessary to achieve a political consensus, and to find a method for making choices when government action supersedes market evaluation of costs and benefits.

Consideration of how the government responds to disruptions of the marketplace raises the traditional macroeconomic subjects of business cycles, unemployment, and inflation in Chapter 18. Analysis of how public and private health care spending reacts to changes in prices and GDP leads to a discussion of adjustment dynamics, and of regulation as a form of health care cost control.

That sets the stage for Chapter 19, an international comparison of health care systems in different countries. A final chapter briefly presents some projections for the future, identifying some economic issues likely to be contentious as the health care system for the next century takes shape. In that review, it is recognized that while the abstractions of price theory can explain much of the mechanics of the market system, there is no way to avoid the value judgments that lie at the foundation of the system—and that such values are ultimately responsible for the health of the nation.

SUGGESTIONS FOR FURTHER READING _____

James S. Coleman, *Foundations of Social Theory*, Cambridge, Mass.: Harvard University Press, 1990.

Mervyn Susser, "Ecological Analysis in Public Health," *American Journal of Public Health*, 1994.

Oliver E. Williamson, *The Economic Institutions of Capitalism: Firms, Markets, Relations*, New York: Free Press, 1985.

PROBLEMS _____

1. {*aggregation*} Since macroeconomics is just the large-scale aggregate effects of many micro decisions by individuals, is it possible to simply add up the behavior of all the different individuals, or to multiply the behavior of the average individual by the total number of persons, in order to determine system behavior?

2. {*fallacy of composition*} Give two examples of the fallacy of composition that are sufficiently plausible to fool some newspaper readers. Give one that illustrates the fallacy of projecting micro behavior on the basis of macro changes, and another that shows the fallacy of projecting macro behavior on the basis of individual decisions.

3. {*competition, welfare maximization*} Does the "invisible hand" work in health care markets? Give an example that clearly illustrates the welfare-maximizing effects of self-interested competition, and another that calls it into question. Is health care more or less nonprofit than other types of human productivity and exchange?

4. {*dynamics*} Explain the difference between the "comparative statics" and "dynamics" of a market such as physician services or long-term care.

5. {*transactions costs*} Do all economic exchanges have a monetary price? How would a politician pay the price of changing insurance legislation to cover

hospital-sponsored HMOs? To whom would the price be paid? Do laws regulating exchange make trade more or less expensive?

ENDNOTES _____

1. This chapter borrows selectively from a number of authors, including James S. Coleman, *Foundations of Social Theory*, Cambridge, Mass.: Harvard University Press, 1990; Douglass North, *Structure and Change in Economic History* (New York: W. W. Norton, 1981); and Oliver Williamson, *Markets and Hierarchies*, New York: The Free Press, 1975,
2. Mervyn Susser, "Ecological Analysis in Public Health," *American Journal of Public Health,* 1994.
3. Adam Smith, *An Inquiry Into the Nature and Causes of the Wealth of Nations,"* 1776, reprinted by Random House: New York, 1985.

CHAPTER 15

Economic History, Population Growth, and Medical Care

QUESTIONS

1. *Does economic growth cause population growth?*
2. *Is medical care the most important cause of increasing life expectancy?*
3. *Must a society be wealthy to invest in medical care?*
4. *Do economic failures cause plagues and other mortality?*
5. *Was Malthus right? Will populations continue to expand until food supplies are exhausted?*
6. *Why do families have fewer children today?*
7. *Does medical technology cause growth, or does economic growth create new medical technology?*

15.1   ECONOMIC GROWTH HAS DETERMINED THE SHAPE OF HEALTH CARE _____

In order for a modern health care system to develop and be economically supported, four preconditions must exist. There must be:

1. Effective medical technology
2. A sufficiently low risk of death such that improving health is worthwhile
3. Ample wealth to pay for advanced medical treatment
4. Financial organization/insurance to pool funds from many people

While medical care has been provided for as long as human society has existed, these four conditions have been met only within the last hundred years, and even then only for the more developed countries. Most of Africa and parts of Asia and Latin America are still characterized by high mortality, subsistence farming, and a lack of broad-based social and financial organizations so that the risks of dying are high and are heavily influenced by the amount of income available.[1] It is economic development that creates the foundation for modern medicine, the factor upon which all the others depend. As large numbers of people live longer and have more wealth, they become more willing to pay for medical care. They pool funds to finance care through insurance (chapters 3 and 4) and also to support medical research, so that collectively they can obtain the technological wonders that none of them could afford individually (see chapters 16 and 17).

To grasp the complex process by which economic development, population growth, and medical technology are linked, it is useful to consider a very simplified schema dividing the growth of humanity into four periods; the Stone Age, the Agricultural Age, the Industrial Age, and a post-industrial "Information Age." From the dawn of civilization until quite recently, the primary limitation on the number of people and their health has been the ability for them to get enough to eat. Thus, we are led to consider the growth in productivity over that time, with particular attention to the leaps brought about by the Agricultural Revolution (10,000 B.C.–5000 B.C.; development of farming), the Industrial Revolution (1750–1830 A.D.; development of power machinery), and the Information Revolution (1960–present; development of computers). A major theme of this chapter is that optimizing the use of technology through changes in economic organization, from simple tribes to complex multinational corporations and global markets, has been more important for increasing human health and welfare than the technological discoveries themselves.[2]

Initially, the focus is on those few facts that can be quantified all the way back to the beginning of history: total population and life expectancy. Demography, the study of population, is briefly introduced by providing a few formulas that are helpful in dealing with data spanning thousands of years. Then, each of the four ages is discussed in terms of population, technology and knowledge transmission, economic and political organization, and income distribution. The income uncertainty due to illness and medical expenses leads to a discussion of the value of risk reduction and social insurance. Finally, some aspects of the history of medicine discussed in previous chapters are reviewed to bring out the structural connection between economic growth and the development of medical care.

15.2 BIRTH RATES, DEATH RATES AND POPULATION GROWTH

Population growth is determined by the number of births minus the number of deaths (ignoring immigration, which just transfers people between different parts of the world). Stated in percentage terms:

Natural Rate of Population Increase = Birth Rate − Death Rate

If the birth rate is 4.2 percent and the death rate is 3.9 percent, then the rate of increase is 4.2 percent − 3.9 percent = 0.3 percent per year. As a first order of approximation, the death rate ≈ 1/(life expectancy), thus a life expectancy of 25 years implies that 1/25, or 4 percent, of the population will die each year.* Throughout most of history until the Industrial Age, birth and death rates fluctuated wildly, but were forced quite close to each other on average by the uneasy equilibrium between population and food supply. If births were high for a while, there would be too many mouths to feed in the winter, and starvation became more likely. If food was scarce for many years, people delayed marriage and so reduced the birth rate. On the other hand, years of bumper crops meant people were more likely to survive, and to have babies.

It is important to recognize the numerical effects of **compounding**, how small differences in rates turn into large differences in size over time. If births and deaths are both 4 percent per year, the population is stable, neither growing nor shrinking. If there is a slight increase in births, to 4.1 percent a year, the natural rate of increase becomes 0.1 percent and population will double in seven-hundred years, as it did through much of the Agricultural Age. If births rise further to 4.2 percent (i.e, 0.2 % net increase), the population will be four times as large after seven-hundred years. A growth rate of 1.0 percent a year means doubling every seventy years, a total population growth of 106,000 percent in that same seven-hundred-year span.**

15.3 THE STONE AGE

Time span:	5 million–10,000 B.C.	**Economy:**	subsistence hunter/gatherer
Total population:	beginning apx. 4 million	**Distribution:**	roughly equal
Growth rate (doubles):	*.0007% (100,000 years)*	**Medical care:**	shaman/witch doctor
Life expectancy:	20 years	**Medical $:**	*na*

* Note that this relationship death rate = 1/(life expectancy) is a stock:flow equation that is analogous to the relationship between interest rates and the value of an annuity; i = (coupon)/(total cost of bond) presented in finance texts.

** A rule of thumb for compounding is known as the "rule of 70." If you divide 70 by the interest rate, it gives the approximate length of time required to double. Thus 70 ÷ 4 = 17.5 years to double at 4% per year. 70 ÷ .35 = 200 years to double at 0.35%. 70 ÷ 0.1 = 700 years to double at 0.1%. This rule is quite accurate for rates of less than 5%, and can be done on your calculator until you can take the time to check the result with a spreadsheet.

The **Stone Age** began with the emergence of the first hominids in Africa about 5 million years ago. People lived in small bands as hunter-gatherers, with a simple family/tribal social structure and little physical or intellectual capital to improve productivity. Population was limited by the amount of food in the immediate foraging area. Life expectancy was only about twenty years, and more than half of all the children born did not live long enough to start a family, although some elders might live on into their forties.[3] For millennia upon millennia, the rate of growth was so slow as to be almost unnoticeable. It took about 100,000 years for global population to double, an annual growth rate of 0.0007 percent. At the end of the prehistoric Stone Age around 10,000 B.C. there were about 4 million people in the world, mostly in Asia, Africa, and the Near East, with only a few in the Americas. For stone age hunter/gatherers, everyone lived pretty much equally at a subsistence level. Violent death and starvation in the winter were constant threats, but during the good times, life was relatively easy. Studies of remaining hunter/gatherer tribes that rely on Stone Age technology in the Amazon, Philippine jungles, and Africa indicate that only two to four hours per day is required to obtain food and repair simple shelters and tools, with much of the rest of the time being taken up by socializing, singing, art, and other pursuits. Exchange between groups was rare, so there were no organized trading systems.

Population growth during the Stone Age occurred primarily by expansion into new territory. As a tribe got "too large" for the local area, some family groups split off and occupied new land. Evolution and new technology (i.e., bows and arrows, flint knives) meant better exploitation of the existing food supply, not increased productivity. *Homo sapiens* displaced *homo erectus* because they were more efficient at hunting and killing, gathering and storing food, and building shelter. That increased efficiency did not increase the productivity of the land, and in some cases even reduced it as large game species (mammoths, sloths) were exterminated. In this prehistoric world of hunter/gatherers, each additional person required more land, and the ultimate size of the population was limited by the area under settlement. By the end of the Stone Age those limits had already been reached in some fully populated areas. Indeed, the population pressure in long-settled lands that were overfilled with people may have contributed to the development of animal husbandry and plant cultivation to feed the excess population, initiating the Agricultural Age.

15.4   THE AGRICULTURAL AGE _____

Time span:	10,000 B.C. to 1800 A.D.	**Economy:**	farming and harvesting
Total population:	4 million to 400 million	**Distribution:**	top-heavy, unequal
Growth rate (doubles):	*.046% (1,500 years)*	**Medical care:**	empirical
Life expectancy:	24 years	**Medical $:**	maybe 1%

Population growth accelerated with the development of agriculture, but only slowly at first. Agriculture appears to have originated around 10,000 B.C.–7,000 B.C.

in the river valleys of the Tigris, the Euphrates, and the Nile, and subsequently developed independently in China and the Peruvian highlands. People began to settle permanently in one place. Irrigation canals were dug and roads were built. The same acreage could support a much larger number of permanent farmers than of roaming hunter/gatherers. The productivity increases that made agriculture a stable way of life depended on many separate and often incremental innovations occurring at different times and places. Furthermore, the geographic diffusion of ideas was slow, only about one kilometer a year. As late as 4000 B.C., global population was still growing at a rate of only about 0.01 percent a year (doubling in 7,000 years).

Investment and Trade

Farming takes investment. Seed must be saved, fields must be plowed, and animal pens erected. A hunter might have worked at making a sharper spear or better root gatherer, but the increase in output was small compared to the gains obtained from farm improvements (building an irrigation ditch, selection of superior seed, invention of the harrow or plows). In the **Agricultural Age**, many farm investments, such as building a road or a large corral, were collective, and benefited the whole town. The returns to investment became larger the more people involved. There is a synergy in bringing people together. While each one might know something about farming, a hundred would compare experiences and draw on the best ideas. Each one could make tools, but with a hundred together, the few who were best at it would spend more time making tools for others, and get food in return. Specialization, trade, and division of labor arose. Towns and cities were built. Trade between regions became a regular part of economic activity.

For trade and investment to occur, societies must develop property rights. In order to have farms, people had to be able to stay on "their" land and improve it from year to year. They had to "own" a portion of the extra grain that was stored for times of famine, or traded for tools, salt and other necessary items. The stored grain had to be defended against the marauding bandits who showed up at harvest time. Once an agricultural society formed an army, it quickly discovered that force was useful for things other than defense. Neighboring tribes were displaced from their more productive lands, or conquered and made into slaves. The leaders who successfully rallied the troops in battle gained power, and through a hierarchy of princes and priests effectively controlled most of the wealth of society. Yet the development of governance was more than a military necessity. In order to grow, agricultural societies had to have rulers who could accumulate and manage the excess output necessary for collective investments in irrigation, laws, and warmaking.

Civilization, War and Government

With the advent of the first great civilization—the Sumerians—population began to increase much more rapidly. Growth rates increased to .07 percent per year (doubling in 1,000 years), about a hundred times the hunter/gatherer growth rate.

Although the Sumerian empire soon fell, the Pharoic Theocracy established along the banks of the Nile in Egypt endured for centuries. Between 1,000 B.C. and 1 A.D. many other large and vigorous civilizations developed. The classical Greeks rose to unprecedented heights, and Alexander conquered the "world" before being displaced by the Romans. In China the Han dynasty unified 50 million people, and in the Americas the great Inca and Olmec/Maya/Aztec civilizations began. By 1 A.D. empires spanned continents and trade routes stretched for thousands of miles. World population exceeded 200 million and was growing about 0.12 percent per year (doubling every 600 years).

As cities grew, the population split into two classes: peasants who worked the land and stayed at subsistence level, and rulers who controlled all the wealth. While hunter/gatherers were all at the same level, working two to four hours a day to obtain subsistence plus a little extra, farmers had to work much harder, eight to twelve hours a day, to obtain the same amount of food. Why, then, did anyone become a farmer? This probably occurred out of necessity rather than choice. When a climatic change caused a succession of bad years, or a stronger band of tribes pushed people out of favored territory, they were forced to try to get more out of what was at hand: husbanding animals rather than just hunting them, planting roots and grain rather than just picking them wild, and so on. Many peasants were "recruited" as they were captured and placed under the domination of a warlord. Once the shift from hunting to farming had occurred, it acquired a momentum of its own and became irreversible. There were too many people in the valley to go back to the old ways and the kings did not want to give up the wealth that they obtained by ruling others. Even if doubling the size of the city did not make the average person better off, it made the king and the court twice as well off.

Prosperity depended on the willingness of the people to support (or at least tacitly cooperate with) the existing system, and even to work toward improving it. While the king might coerce peasants into paying taxes, he had to deliver order and a rising standard of living in return, or face rebellion. The taxes collected had to be directed toward appropriate public works and services to maintain progress. The rapid growth of population could only be sustained by new forms of social organization, by creating the cultural, political, and economic institutions that make up civilization. Having enough wealth left over to indulge idle priests and philosophers as they researched mathematics, astronomy, chemistry, physics and medicine also fostered the conditions for continuous technological advance. This process of economic development was mutually reinforcing, as growth requires more government and investment, and also makes it possible to free up the resources that can support them.

The Decline of Civilizations Leads to Population Declines

The amazing growth of classical civilizations was followed by almost equally sensational declines when social order decayed. There were more people in ancient Greece at its apex in 440 B.C. than at any time over the next 2,000 years, and it was not until 1850 A.D. that the population again exceeded 3 million. As the Roman empire shrank, the total population of Europe fell from 44 million in 200 A.D. to 22 million in 600 A.D. By 1000 A.D., European population had only partly recovered, to 30 million. Similar, though less severe, declines occurred in China and Africa. A recent example is found in the traumatic transition of the Soviet Union as communism disintegrated in 1990. The sharp drop in economic output, widespread moral and social disorder, and precipitous decline in life expectancy has been dubbed *Katastroika* (catastrophic construction) by some commentators.

The Plague

As European populations began to robustly recover toward the end of the Middle Ages (500–1500 A.D.), they were hit by a new and rampantly destructive force, the plague. Bubonic plague, or "Black Death," swept through Europe in 1347–1352 and repeatedly thereafter, wiping out a quarter of the population.[6] Half the citizens of Genoa and Naples died in the plague of 1656.[7] Although bouts of plague continued to appear until 1700, changes in immunity, social structure, the plague bacillus itself, or some combination of the above, reduced the impact over time, and population growth resumed after 1500 A.D. The peoples of the new world were not as fortunate. After contact with the Spanish Conquistadors, plagues of measles and smallpox spread rapidly, with devastating effects. The native population of Aztecs dropped from 17 million in 1532 to 2 million in 1580, and fell to just 1 million by 1608. It was not just disease, but the collapse of social order that caused the permanent decline in numbers. The repopulation of the Americas after 1600 came largely from the growth of immigrant populations from Europe and Africa.

Food Supply Determines Population

From 1500–1750 the European and World populations grew at an average annual rate of 0.25 percent (doubling in 300 years). Food supply was the fundamental constraint on growth, since the great majority of people lived at a subsistence

---

IMPLOSION OF THE SOVIET ECONOMY CAUSES A DRAMATIC INCREASE IN DEATH RATES, DECLINING LIFE EXPECTANCY.

Life expectancy in Russia in 1990 was 63.8 years for males and 74.3 years for females, slightly higher than it had been 30 years previously.[4] The reconstruction *(perestroika)* of the USSR under Mikhail Gorbachev brought hope, and then disaster. The Soviet economy crumbled, the USSR fragmented, and quality of life declined. For some people on fixed incomes, hyperinflation took food prices beyond their reach, causing malnutrition. More importantly, the loss of jobs, and hope, meant despair. In such a grim situation, deaths from alcohol poisoning and accidents soared. By 1993, life expectancy had fallen four years for males (to 59 years) and three years for females (to 71.5 years), a decline that is virtually unprecedented in modern industrial countries. Fertility dropped below replacement level and total population declined. In 1992, births exceeded deaths by 184,000. By 1993, there were 800,000 more deaths than births.[5] For every live birth, there were 2.2 abortions. Only now are the true dimensions of this contemporary social and demographic catastrophe being measured.

level. One aspect of the relationship between food supply and population is illustrated in Figure 15.1. Increases in the prices of grain in the Italian district of Siena during the years 1550–1715 were associated with malnutrition and death.[8] Each time grain prices rose, the meager salaries of the residents were stretched thinner, and mortality climbed. The cycle is self-correcting and self-reinforcing. As people die, there are fewer mouths to feed, demand falls, and so prices fall. When food is abundant and prices are low, peasants are more able to marry and have children, the number of mouths to feed rises, demand increases, prices jump, and the cycle starts over again.

As the Agricultural Age drew to a close and the transition to an urbanized industrial society began, scarcity of food continued to be a major issue. A salaried worker was little better off than a peasant, since it took 80 percent of that salary to get enough to eat. For example, France in 1790 was a highly developed country,

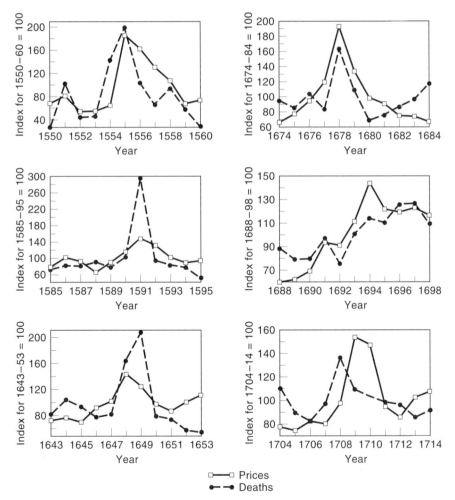

FIGURE 15.1   Sienese Grain Prices and Death Indices. Sources: Massimo Livi-Bacci, *A Concise History of World Population* Cambridge, Mass.: Blackwell, 1992, p. 80, G. Parenti, *Prezzi e mercato a Siena, 1546-1765*, Florence: 1942, pp. 27–28.

with perhaps the greatest cultural and political influence in the Western world, yet most of its citizens were still impoverished and undernourished. The average thirty-year-old Frenchman of 1790 had to live on 2,250 calories per day, stood just 5'3" tall, and weighed only 110 pounds.[9] The bottom 10 percent of society had so little food they were usually ill, and most people below the twentieth percentile did not get enough to eat to meet the caloric energy demands of regular work. Even relatively well-off people at the eightieth percentile were sufficiently stunted and wasted (height and weight below current U.S. standards) that they were at substantially higher risk of incurring chronic health conditions and premature mortality.

The Rise of Economics

The intellectual ferment of the Renaissance (1350–1650 A.D.) and Enlightenment (1650–1800 A.D.) brought advances in government, science, and commerce (although medicine was to wait until 1900 for major changes to occur). In 1662, John Graunt published his *Natural and Political Observations on the Bills of Mortality* in London, a work now recognized as beginning the science of epidemiology. In 1671, Sir William Petty made the first estimate of national wealth (GDP) in his essay *Political Arithmetik* (what we would today call "economic statistics"). As people moved from the rural estates, where they had been cared for (and/or owned) by the feudal lord, into cities where they worked at jobs for wages, the economic organization of society evolved from one based on tradition to one based on money. Only after exchange became standardized through the use of money could regularities be observed and statistical analysis (such as that of grain prices presented in Figure 15.1) be performed.

The development of accounting and statistics marked the emergence of a new "information technology" that revolutionized trade. Financial markets in London and other cities traded government bonds and shares in joint stock companies, shifting tons of gold with the stroke of a pen. Factories were built and thousands of people changed occupations and even changed nationalities to better their standard of living. Capital investment and labor mobility of this magnitude had been impossible during the Middle Ages because the necessary economic structure was not yet available, or still too rudimentary. Corporations, rental contracts, taxes, ownership and other property rights had to be refined before trade between individuals, firms, and governments could be carried out on a large scale. *The Wealth of Nations*, Adam Smith's insightful analysis published in 1776, is now recognized as the start of modern economics.[10] Yet Thomas Malthus's *Essay on the Principle of Population* (1798) has often been more influential. It more clearly presents the consensus opinion of thinkers at the end of the Agricultural Era, and was responsible for labeling economics "the dismal science."

The Malthusian Hypothesis

Malthus's hypothesis was that any increase in productivity could provide only a temporary boost to the standard of living.[11] Over time, increases in the number of people to be fed would use up all of the increase, so that on average people would be no better off than before—still living at a subsistence level. The **Malthusian hypothesis** is based on two key assumptions: (1) that *food supply* is a primary constraint on population growth, and (2) that any increase in the number of people would inevitably lead to more crowding, or to farming of less desirable land, so that the *declining marginal productivity* of labor (and hence, wages) would bring down the standard of living. Ireland became a natural experiment for testing the Malthusian hypothesis. The importation of a new crop, potatoes, lead to a tremendous increase in yields per acre. Using the new crop, the acreage that could support only one family in 1700 could be split up and support three families by 1800. Potato farming was so much more efficient than other types of agriculture that the peasants ate little else, consuming up to ten pounds per day. The population of this small and already fully settled island grew 50 percent in the half-century before Malthus wrote, and by another 50 percent over the next thirty years. Farms were chopped into smaller and smaller parcels, and the Irish people, with a diet now consisting almost entirely of potatoes, lived no better than before—there were just more of them. Then came the fungus blight that badly damaged the potato harvest of 1845, and destroyed the crop of 1846 entirely: 1.5 million people died, and another 1.5 million people emigrated, mostly to America. Those who were left tightened their belts and stopped having children (the women born before the blight who remained in Ireland were four times as likely to remain unmarried as those who emigrated to America).[12] Out of a population of 8 million in 1840, there were only 4.5 million left by 1900, and by 1950, only 2.8 million.

The assumptions built into the Malthusian hypothesis had been valid throughout the thousands of years spanned by the Agricultural Age, and continued to apply in countries that remained essentially rural, such as Ireland. The law of diminishing returns, as elaborated by Malthus, was a major intellectual contribution to economics. However, it applies only if the technology of production stays essentially the same. In England, Germany, France, and the United States, the same intellectual revolution that stirred Malthus to write his treatise led others to create a technological and commercial revolution so profound that productivity increases were continuous, and output grew much more rapidly than any natural increase in the number of people. A continuous excess of food and other goods became available for all to enjoy.

15.5   THE INDUSTRIAL AGE_____

Time span:	1800 to 1950 A.D.	**Economy:**	manufacturing
Total population:	0.4 billion to 1.6 billion	**Distribution:**	mixed
Growth rate (doubles):	*.65% (108 years)*	**Medical care:**	empirical
Life expectancy:	35 years	**Medical $:**	2% - 4%

Life was difficult at the start of the Industrial Revolution, and often got worse for those who moved into cities to work in factories. Crowded slums and harsh working conditions caused disease. Whereas diets on a farm could be supplemented by gardens and occasional hunting, in the cities food was monotonous and lacking in vitamins. As the countryside was enclosed (put under ownership of the lord rather than held in common) and people moved into cities, illness increased. Life expectancy in England, about 38 years in 1600 A.D., declined throughout the next hundred years, and did not regain earlier levels until about 1850.[13] Yet as the Industrial Revolution took hold, productivity increases caused the average person's standard of living to improve. There was a sharp rise in the rate of population growth to 0.43 percent from 1750–1800, almost twice the rate of the prior three centuries, rising to 0.53 percent per year for 1800–1900, 0.88 percent for 1900–1950, and surging upward to 1.8 percent a year since 1950. World population quadrupled from about 750 million to 2.5 billion. Overall life expectancy rose in those two hundred years by more than it had in the previous two thousand, going from 27 to 35 years. The rise is even more remarkable in the most developed countries, such as Sweden, where life expectancy rose from 37 years in 1750 to 71.3 years in 1950.

Why Malthus Was Wrong

There are two reasons Malthus' gloomy predictions were wrong. First, technological advance, rather than being a one-shot improvement, became a continuous process. Output expanded at an exponential rate as one invention led to another. In the Agricultural Age, the primary productive inputs were land and labor. The total supply of land is fixed, and any increase in the supply of labor meant more mouths to feed. In the **Industrial Age**, capital equipment, skilled labor, and knowledge became more important than land and unskilled agricultural labor. By 1950, a single farmer, sitting in an air-conditioned cab operating a combine, harvesting genetically engineered wheat, could feed more people per 100 acres than a dozen farmers in 1750. Although the rate of productivity increase during the Agricultural Era averaged about 1 percent a year, in the Industrial Era it rapidly tripled, and sometimes exceeded 5 percent a year. A second reason that Malthus's immiserating population growth failed to occur was that as death rates declined, birth rates also declined. With fewer children dying, parents chose to have fewer babies, and invested more in the education, medical care, and nutrition of each one. Parents acted in what they saw as the best interest of their own family as they made decisions regarding how many children to have and how to care for them. Cumulatively, these individual decisions brought about a social revolution. It also changed the character of labor and accelerated technological advance, leading to higher wages and a rising standard of living.

Why did Ireland suffer a Malthusian catastrophe and lose two-thirds of its population while most other European nations experienced surging growth during the Industrial Revolution? Ireland was not a self-governing nation, but a colony exploited by absentee landlords from England. Profits from Irish estates were not invested in Ireland, but used to build factories in England or sent overseas through joint stock companies. Irish farmers did not own their land, but were tenants working the fields for the benefit of the landlord. As crop yields went up, rents were raised, keeping workers in subsistence conditions typical of the Agricultural Era. With no claim on the profits, the tenant farmer has no incentive to innovate in order to raise crop yields, and little ability to save and improve the lot of the family in the next generation. The only way for the Irish farmers to capture any of the economic surplus created by increased agricultural productivity was to have more children, and so they did. An Irishman wishing to leave the farm and build a better life in the city had to leave his country and go to New York. The lack of property rights for citizens and restrictive colonial economic organization were largely responsible for keeping Ireland from joining the ranks of industrialized countries in the Nineteenth century.

Malthus's predictions were never quite so dismal or so wrong as his critics claimed. He hoped that by clearly laying out the logical conclusions of agricultural demographics, he could encourage people to delay marriage and have fewer children. Birthrates did, in fact, decline, but for other reasons. Women gained more opportunities, and spent less time on child-rearing. More children survived, so fewer births were needed to make sure that one or two lived to maturity. Dependence upon children in old age was replaced by reliance on savings. Perhaps most importantly, children went from being a form of supplemental income (as productive family farmworkers) to a form of consumption (bringing joy but costing money). All of these changes either raised the price or reduced the demand for children. Average total fertility per mature female in England fell from 5.3 births in 1750, to 4.6 in 1850, and 1.96 in 1900 (below the replacement rate of 2.0, so national population would actually have decreased over time without foreign immigration).

Demographic Transition

The process of economic development is linked to a dramatic change in national population known as the "demographic transition." In the agricultural stage many children die before reaching adulthood. High rates of mortality (4–5%) are matched by high rates of fertility (also 4–5%), so the total number of people is stable or just slowly increasing. This equilibrium between births and deaths is radically changed during the process of economic development. With greater material well-being, death mortality rates decline toward 1 to 2 percent. Since birth rates are still high, the rate of population growth (births−deaths) is very rapid, 2 to 4 percent a year, enough to double population in each generation (every 15 to 40 years). Such explosive growth does not continue indefinitely. Although with constantly increasing economic output there is no necessary reason that birth rates should have to fall, it is observed that in fact birth rates do fall in virtually every developed country. As children cease to be productive farm assets and become a costly form of family consumption, families decide to concentrate more care and investment on fewer children.[14] This decline in fertility does not require the use of modern birth control techniques. Delayed marriage, extended breast feeding, infanticide, and other methods have been used successfully to restrict population to desired levels in many countries without recourse to contraceptives. As economic development continues, low mortality (1–2%) is eventually matched by low fertility (1–2%) so that the total population is again stable or slowly growing, and the process of demographic transition is complete (see Figure 15.2).

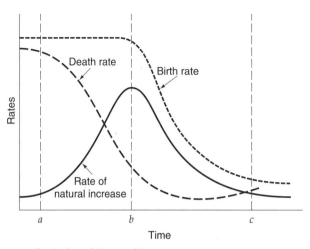

a = Beginning of the transition
b = Greatest difference between birth and death rates
c = End of the transition

FIGURE 15.2 *Demographic Transition: The period of Rapid
Population Increase*

Whereas Agricultural Era population growth spurts occurring during the settlement of new territory are caused by an increase in births, population growth during demographic transition is caused by a decline in deaths. These two demographic patterns have very different long-run consequences on the average level of individual wealth. When new territories are settled, the pioneers have much more land per person than in the country they came from, and thus initially enjoy a much greater marginal productivity of labor, and greater wealth. This advantage is eroded over time as more and more people are born in the new territories. Eventually, the new territories are just as crowded as the old country, the marginal productivity of labor declines back to the subsistence level, and the total population, although larger, is not much better off. In contrast, the economic advances that mark demographic transition, rather than fading over time, are reinforced with each succeeding generation. Healthier adults can work longer and harder, and thus accumulate more surplus for investment, while a smaller number of children means that each one receives more in the way of education, nutrition, and inheritance. These gains lead to even lower mortality, and even fewer children, and so on. Each generation is not only better off, it concentrates that material advantage among an ever-smaller number of offspring until transition is complete. By then, the amount of family income required to buy food has fallen from 80 percent to 20 percent. Getting enough to eat is no longer a significant factor in demographic change or labor productivity.

Demographic Change, Income Distribution, and the Rise of the Middle Classes

In a hunter/gatherer society, there are no wealthy people. The tribe as a whole is living at the subsistence level with only a little accumulated wealth in the form of weapons or religious objects. One or two bad years spells disaster. An agricultural society, in contrast, is hierarchical, and often has quite a bit of wealth, almost all of it concentrated at the top. Most of the agricultural population consists of rural peasants. As agricultural civilizations develop over time there are an increasing number of traders, soldiers, craftsmen, merchants, and other members of the bourgeois who live as free "citizens" in (mostly small) cities, but they are always a minority. The king's authority is absolute, and almost all of the wealth stays under his control.

In order to industrialize, the bulk of the population has to move into cities. People who leave the land are no longer under the control of the lord, and they enter into wage labor contracts with factories. As businesses and bureaucracies replace the feudal manor as a means of organizing production, the fruits of economic development are spread much more widely. While at first the wages of industrial workers are near the subsistence level, real earnings rise rapidly, for two reasons. The decline in the number of births during demographic transition means fewer new workers entering the market, thus the supply of labor grows much less rapidly than demand, putting upward pressure on wages. Second, the labor market becomes specialized. Whereas initially the threat of starvation drove the unskilled worker off the farm to take a subsistence wage in the city, the later movement of skilled mechanics, clerks, and managers required premium wages to create positive attraction. These well-paid workers and shopkeepers could afford some luxuries. They could also save for retirement, and in so doing, contribute to the pool of capital funds for investment and entrepreneurial ventures.

Although the feudal blacksmith had pride in his art, most of the benefits went to the lord. The master mechanic of the Industrial Era had a much greater incentive to improve his skills, since he got paid more for the increases in quality and productivity. Furthermore, he was apt to take the risk of innovating and starting a new business, since he might become rich. Even if his venture failed, he would only lose some money, not his life. He could still get another job and keep his family from starving.* In the city–states and empires of the Agricultural Era, lords and kings exercised centralized bureaucratic power to raise taxes, build roads, and support armies. Building factories and inventing new technologies in the Industrial Era required decentralized entrepreneurs who acted as managers on their own behalf, rather than on behalf of the king. Working independently or in small groups, entrepreneurs convinced investors to put up capital and attracted skilled labor with high wages. By the end of the Industrial Era, even people of modest means could go to school, start a business, or save for retirement. A startling change in the distribution of income and wealth had occurred—the bulk of the money was held by the large and growing middle class of laborers, tradesmen, and small business owners. In 1750 the market for art, education, travel, housing, and almost everything except food was concentrated in the upper 2 percent of families who were truly wealthy. By 1950, the market for such goods in the United States, England, Germany, and other developed countries was dominated by the middle classes. The wealthy bought luxury in a few shops, while the millions shopped in department stores (see Figure 15.3).

The hierarchies that dominated the Agricultural Era were broken up by tremendous increases in economic mobility and a general improvement in wages. The

---

* A surprisingly large number of successful entrepreneurs and inventors go bankrupt several times before and after they strike it rich. Such risk-taking is not feasible if two bad years means starvation.

	Hunter-Gatherer	Agricultural	Industrial	Informational
upper classes		$$$$$	$$	$$$$$$$
middle class	$	$$	$$$$$$	$$$$$$$$$
lower classes	$$$$$	$	$$$	$$$$$$$

FIGURE 15.3 *Distribution of Income at Different Stages of Development*

crowd at the bottom was replaced by a bulging middle class of people who actively participated in a monetary economy. This shift in social and economic structure, rather than the discovery of new technology per se, was the driving force that powered the growth of the Industrial Revolution. Many countries today remain poor and rural, struggling to make the demographic and economic transition to development. It is not because they lack technology (which can be found in many textbooks, ordered from a catalog, or shared in commercial joint ventures), but because they lack the property rights, social order, and administrative structure to create a context in which technology can be productively applied.[15] The deficit that allows starvation to remain a threat to the health of people is not a shortage of knowledge, or machinery or even of money for investment, but of economic organization.

15.6 THE INFORMATION AGE_____

Time span:	1950 to future	**Economy:**	services
Total population:	1.6 billion to ? 20 billion	**Distribution:**	not yet clear
Growth rate (doubles):	1.88% (40 years) but slowing	**Medical care:**	scientific
Life expectancy:	up to 80 years	**Medical $:**	6%–15%

The advent of a post–industrial **Information Age** is marked by the ubiquitous appearance of the television and the computer. The labor force is concentrated in "services" rather than agriculture or manufacturing. Information specialists, the dominant workers, spend their entire childhood and many years of adulthood in school investing in the skills required for active participation in a global economy linked by communications networks where massive amounts of capital flow between countries with a few keystrokes. Such training can be prevalent only in a population with long life expectancy and relatively few children per family. In this era the great majority of people are healthy and wealthy enough that personal income affects longevity and fertility primarily through lifestyle choices, rather than any material lack of food calories or shelter. What was a great rarity throughout history, the ability to retire with independent means and sufficient fitness to travel the world after age 65, has become not just attainable, but an ordinary reality of most people in post–industrial economies.

U.S. life expectancy was about 35 years in 1750, 49 years in 1900, rose to 68 years by 1950, and was 76 years in 1990. Although people will continue to live longer, incremental years of life expectancy are added at a slower and slower rate as infectious diseases and childhood maladies are removed as major causes of death. More important from a demographic point of view is that almost all the gains in longevity after 1950 occurred for mature adults who have already completed their families. Each generation may live longer, but will not have more babies. Additional increases in life expectancy will not increase the number of children, and so will have no long-run effect on the total size of the population.

During the demographic transition of the Industrial Era, and its final phase, the 1950s "baby boom," rapid population increase created expansive economic growth as more houses, roads, and factories were built. However, the rapid expansion due to demographic transition is a one-time occurrence. After transition, population returns to a steady state of slow or zero growth, typically a small natural decrease offset by immigration of those from less-developed countries seeking higher wages. It is important to recognize that the "normal" conditions of industrializing countries from 1770 to 1970 were in fact abnormal periods of spectacular but transitory growth. In comparison, the recent era's 1 percent to 2 percent growth rates can seem inadequate, particularly since most of the added value comes in the less visible form of service improvement and information content, rather than in the number of countable "things" (cars, houses, tons of corn) that are more readily measured for the GDP accounts.

Much of the world is still undeveloped, caught somewhere between an agricultural society and the modern information era. A world map shaded to show which nations in the 1990s have economies still dominated by agriculture is almost identical to a world map shaded to show which countries have the most premature mortality under age 30.[16] Such nations have the potential for fantastic growth as they industrialize (e.g., Korea, Singapore, Indonesia), but also for tragic population explosions without economic advancement, leading to starvation and social ruin (e.g., Somalia, Rwanda). In a still-developing country, such as Mexico, the average age of the population is about 17, longevity is below 70 years, many of the people still work on farms, and a sizable fraction still live at the subsistence level. Such countries have a tremendous "population momentum." Even if every family immediately limited fertility to the replacement level of 2.2 births, the total population would still double in size because so many young women have already been born. In the United States, as in most developed countries, the natural population growth is already zero to negative, so that the increase in national population is due to immigration from less developed countries. If current trends continue, almost every country in the world will be developed within a hundred years (by 2100 A.D.) and have steady or shrinking population.[17] Total world population will stabilize somewhere between 10 to 20 million, Mexico City will be many times larger than Los Angeles, and food supply will be a trivial health problem compared to pollution and congestion (see Figure 15.4).

15.7 REDUCING UNCERTAINTY: THE VALUE OF HEALTH AND ECONOMIC SECURITY _____

Economic development not only meant that most people had more, it also meant that the risks of losing it all were vastly reduced. For the first time, it was possible

	Stone Age	Agricultural Age			Industrial Age			Information Age		
	5 million - 10,000 BC	4000 BC	1 AD	1200 AD	1800 AD	1900	1950	1975	2000	????
World Population	beginnings to 4 million	8	250	400 million	950	1.6 billion	2.5 billion	4 billion	6 billion	stops @ 20 billion
rate of growth	.0007%	.01%	.09%	.04%	.14%	.52%	.88%	1.88%		
(time to double)	(100,000)	(7,000)	(800)	*varies*	(500)	(130)	(80)	(40)		
Life Expectancy	20 years		24 years			35 years			80 years	
Organization	family / tribe	fief - city - empire			national states			global village?		
Information	oral	written			statistics			electronic		
Economy	hunter-gatherer	farming & harvesting			manufacturing			services		
Incomes	subsistence	rich rulers / subsistence serfs			wages			wages & entitlements		
Equivalent $ per cap	$200	$300			$300 rising to $5,000			$25,000 (developed countries)		
% spent on food	all	almost all — 90%			80% falling to 30%			12%		
Income Distribution	roughly equal	highly unequal			mixed			not yet clear		
Type of Medicine	witch doctor / shaman	healer priest			empiricist			scientifically trained physicians		
Medical Spending	- - -	? maybe 1%			2% rising to 4%			6%	10%	?

FIGURE 15.4 *Timeline: Economic History, Population Growth, and Medical Care*

and reasonable for ordinary people to plan for the future—to decide how many children to have, whether or not to go to school or start a business, and to save for retirement. The improvements in health and income brought about by economic development had a powerful and somewhat paradoxical effect: the more secure the future became, the more afraid workers were of losing that security.

The Value of Risk Reduction

Consider how the value of reducing the risk of dying within the next ten years by 1 percent changes as workers become more well off. If the average person has a 50–50 chance of dying, it will not be worth much to change that to 51–49. Yet if a healthy person has only a 1 percent chance of dying, eliminating that risk, or just cutting it in half, will be worth quite a lot.* The value of risk reduction also depends on the level of income. In a subsistence economy where workers get paid only enough to buy food and rudimentary housing, they cannot afford to give up much of what they earn to buy medical care, even if it would help to avoid future illness and death. On the other hand, a skilled industrial worker with a $40,000 income can afford to pay $300 a month for health insurance, and another $100 for vitamin supplements and health-club membership. A rock star or corporate CEO earning $5 million a year can afford to spend hundreds of thousands of dollars just to keep looking young.

Social Security and Health Insurance

Whereas the poor agricultural masses were happy to get some chance to stay alive and maybe get ahead, the industrial middle-class expected progress. If their lives did not constantly improve, or if something went wrong, they expected their employer or the government to do something to correct the problem. Originally, coal miners went underground to work in order to get higher wages. As they stayed, they began to demand safety, compensation for accidents, and retirement plans for the disabled. As early as 1700, a few English industrialists offered health insurance to their workers. Such "employee benefits" made the workers loyal to those firms, and willing to work harder. The risks of disability and sickness were no longer born by the workers individually, but by the firm. This sharing of risk reduced the uncertainty and variability of wages to workers (chapters 3 and 4).

Industrialization and the change to wage labor also shifted the distribution of political power. Workers' revolts spread across Europe during the nineteenth century, stretching from Paris in 1798 to Russia in 1917. Economic, legal, and health security were fundamental demands of what became known as "socialism." In 1883, to forestall further labor unrest, Chancellor Bismarck created the first national social security system in Germany, providing pensions to workers over age 65, sick leave, and health insurance for medical care.[18] In the United States, private insurance provided by employers became the dominant mode of health care

---

* The value of risk reduction is also high at the other extreme, where a person faces near certain death. If you knew that otherwise you would die, you might well be willing to give up half of your money for just a 1 percent chance of continuing to live.

financing in the 1950s. These plans have been supplemented by the government Medicaid programs for the poor and Medicare for the elderly, so that today 77 percent of all health care spending, and 95 percent of hospital costs, are paid for through third-party financing mechanisms. In 1850, medical care was still largely a personal transaction. Workers paid, or did not pay, for what they thought they could afford, rather like they would buy clothes, musical entertainment, or education. By 1960, the economic organization of medical care had changed to encompass large pooled financing through government and private insurers. Now the shape of the health care system is determined by negotiations over benefit packages and government appropriations, not consumers' personal purchasing decisions.

Preconditions for Changing Medical Organization

This chapter began with a list of four preconditions for the establishment of modern medical care: effective technology, sufficient wealth, low risk of death, and insurance financing. These factors are not independent of each other, but mutually reinforcing. Increasing wealth meant more food, which reduced the risk of dying. Increased longevity also meant greater productivity, and hence even more wealth. As trade developed, financial markets increased in complexity, and insurance contracts were needed so as to better manage capital. Broad participation in pooled financing could only occur once most workers were relatively healthy and well-off. The development of medical technology was also the result of an interactive process, requiring advances in biology, chemistry, physics, statistics, and information science. Gaining knowledge and reducing the uncertainty caused by illness took both science and economics, and by the year 2000, it is quite possible that the most commonly used medical instrument will be the computer.

15.8 THE RISE OF MEDICAL TECHNOLOGY _____

Medicine is as old as humankind. One of the earliest-known written documents, the "Code of Hammurabi," contains references to medical price controls and malpractice in the laws of this Assyrian kingdom circa 2200 B.C. The Hippocratic oath, written about 1 B.C. and still quoted in medical writings today, put forth the principle that physicians should "first, do no harm." Good advice, since for thousands of years there was little that physicians could actually do to cure illness or reduce the risk of death. Despite the vast amount written about medicine, and the great store of practical knowledge transmitted orally in many cultures, this knowledge was largely unsystematic and did not create therapies that had a significant impact on the health of most people.[19] Medical theory, such as it was, usually consisted of a strange mixture of mysticism; serious looks and kind words; some sound advice about eating, sleeping, and fresh air; and a few favorite remedies, some of which might sometimes be useful in some cases. Hospitals were places where sick or disabled people were housed, and little was expected in the way of treatment. Physicians were counselors who could make someone feel better and preside over the deaths they prognosticated, but could do little to change the course of illness. Many were also priests, and the distinction between morality and medicine was often unclear. Plagues were more likely to be blamed on infidelity or blasphemy than on unseen organisms in the blood.

The change from mysticism and fear to scientific investigation was the defining characteristic of the enlightenment. Some notable milestones include the demonstration of proteins in urine by Paracelsus in 1500, the discovery of the microscope and "little worms" (bacteria and protozoans) by Athanasius Kircher in 1569, William Harvey's discovery of the circulation of blood in 1619, and Anton von Leewenhoek's microscopic description of red blood cells in 1668. The growing accumulation of knowledge presaged a form of medical practice that would eventually be able to provide effective treatments against disease. The crucial link, however, was organizational rather than technical, more a matter of changing the way knowledge was collected, used, and transmitted than any particular scientific breakthrough or discovery. The formation of "clinics" in the great hospitals of Paris around 1750 is particularly noteworthy.[20] These clinics were organized by what would now be called specialties: one for the eye, one for the hand, one for mental illness, and so on. Instead of trying to create a wholistic theory that covered all aspects of health, the clinics broke medical problems down into component parts. A single doctor would then become an expert in disease of the hand, or the eye, and then train others. The clinic provided the working classes with access to the services of trained physicians whom they otherwise could not afford. The physician was provided with a large group of compliant patients all suffering similar illness so he could experiment with new therapies, teach students, and perfect his techniques. Practicing on the masses of poor workers allowed him to charge higher fees to wealthy patients, and to collect tuition from students eager to learn the latest advances. The creation of clinics was a success because they provided a social exchange mechanism that yielded gains to both parties.

Organizational innovation was complemented by an intellectual innovation, statistics. Clinic doctors began to count how many people were treated, and how many got well. Numerical comparisons of outcomes began to replace doctors' personal assessments. Determination of which treatment was best had previously depended mostly on the reputation and experience of the physicians who vouched for it, but now experiments and statistical observation were used. The impact of this new approach to medical science is well illustrated by Edward Jenner's discovery of vaccination for smallpox in 1798. The act of making a healthy person sick (inoculating them with cowpox) to prevent possible future illness is a form of therapy that can only be defended statistically. No single patient feels better or gets cured because of what the doctor does.

Scientific advances accumulated rapidly throughout the latter part of the nineteenth century; Pasteur, Semmelweiss, and Koch determined that bacteria cause anthrax, childbirth fever, tuberculosis, and other infectious diseases; Eijkman discovered vitamins; and Roentgen discovered X-rays. Whereas France was preeminent in the eighteenth century, Germany was arguably the world leader in medical technology by the end of the nineteenth century when Bismarck provided the landmark social insurance legislation. American physicians tried to improve the quality of practice in the United States with the Flexner Report of 1910, promoting the "Johns Hopkins model" (actually, the German model, but we needed a local champion to make it more acceptable). By the end of the 1930s, a license and modern scientific education were required to enter the practice of medicine, and most doctors sought to treat their difficult cases in the hospital using a range of technical devices and nursing support (chapter 6).

Information systems and access to capital gave hospitals economies of scale, and made them necessary adjuncts to medical practice. As modern surgical techniques using anesthesia and antiseptics turned what were formerly warehouses for the sick into technologically sophisticated treatment facilities, written medical records became the locus for storage and communication of test results, diagnostic information, and treatment documentation that linked all the trained medical practitioners together. Florence Nightingale, through her work in military hospitals during the Crimean War, and subsequent books, is the person most often credited with developing the hospital as an organization. Her patients may have seen nurses as "angels of mercy," but she saw them as soldiers gathering intelligence and carrying out orders as part of a grand campaign against disease. As technology became more advanced and specialized, it also cost more—too much for any individual physician to purchase on their own. In 1816, Laennec invented the stethoscope to investigate the body, and every doctor bought one. In 1885, Roentgen's X-ray machines peered inside the body, but the equipment was so large and so expensive that most doctors had to join the staff of a hospital to use one. The CAT scan (Computed Axial Tomography), developed in 1973, costs millions of dollars, depends on software that few radiologists understand, and can transmit images through the Internet to be digitally enhanced and read by a specialist thousands of miles away in another country.

A long, historical perspective shows that although medicine was actively practiced since ancient times, only fragmentary technological advances were made until the end of the Industrial Era. In the eighteenth and nineteenth centuries, scientific discoveries came more and more rapidly, yet there was still little improvement in treatment outcomes. Only after 1900 did effective medicine start to become available, fully 150 years after the productive expansion that marked the beginning of the Industrial Era. Between 1900 and 1950, a virtual revolution took place, and medicine became one of society's most valued occupations.

Medical progress was more a result of planned effort and massive public investment than serendipitous discovery or any pre-ordained march of ideas: Florence Nightingale's scientific hospital was supported by kings who wished to cut the cost of putting soldiers into battle; Pasteur's discovery of bacteria was made under contract to the French wine and beer industry; Walter Reed worked to conquer yellow fever so that construction of the Panama Canal could be completed in tropical jungles. Rising incomes, falling mortality, and commercial organization were more than just contributing factors, they were the central forces driving the demand that created medical technology.

Although all four preconditions for modern medicine (technology, wealth, low mortality, organized financing) operate concurrently and reinforce each other, it is clear that medical technology is more a result of the process than a cause. Society's accumulation of the necessary prerequisites for modern medicine began with the rise in wealth brought about by trade and technology, which quickly led to a decline in mortality, and subsequently to a decline in the birth rate. The application of science and industrial technology to medicine not only took time, it took money and an independent profession dedicated to continuous improvement. Both organized medicine, with its schools and professional associations, and organized financing, with insurance risk pooling and government funding, were necessary to carry out that research and pay for years of trial and error as treatments were perfected. The development of integrated health care systems and decentralized contracting through managed care will bring medicine to the final stages of the Industrial Revolution's productivity enhancements, and set to evolve in new directions so as to meet the challenges of the new era.

SUGGESTIONS FOR FURTHER READING _____

Fogel, Robert W. "Economic Growth, Population Theory and Physiology: The Bearing of Long-Term Processes on the Marking of Economic Policy." *American Economic Review* 84(3):369–395, 1994.

McKeown, Thomas. *The Modern Rise of Population*. London: Edward Arnold, 1976.

Livi-Bacci, Massimo. *A Concise History of World Population*. Cambridge MA: Blackwell, 1992.

McEvedy, Colin and Richard Jones. *Atlas of World Population History*. Middlesex: Penguin, 1978.

North, Douglass C. *Structure and Change in Economic History*. New York: Norton, 1981.

Robert G. Evans, Morris Barer, and Theodore Marmor, *Why Are Some People Healthy and Others Not? The Determinants of Health of Populations*, New York: Aldine De Gruyter, 1994.

Mancur Olson, Jr. "Big Bills Left on the Sidewalk: Why Some Nations are Rich, and Others Poor," *Journal of Economic Perspectives* 10(2):3–24, 1996.

SUMMARY _____

1. Four preconditions must be met for modern medicine to develop:
   a. The risk of dying must be low enough (i.e., **life expectancy** long enough) that spending money to improve health is worthwhile.
   b. People must have **sufficient income** to pay for sophisticated medical care.
   c. There must be a way to pool funds and **organize financing** for large numbers of people through insurance or government programs.
   d. **Medical technology** must be effective enough at improving health to be worth paying for.

2. **Life expectancy** averaged about 20 years from 10,000 B.C. to 1 A.D., and populations grew slowly, taking 100,000 years to double in size. From 1 A.D. to 1750, life expectancy averaged 22–28 years, and population doubled every 1,000 years. From 1750 to 1900, life expectancy averaged 30–45 years, and population doubled every 200 years. Today, life expectancy in the United States is above 70 years, and births almost exactly match deaths so that total population is stable. In less-developed countries, life expectancy is still less than 50 years, and population growth is still very rapid, doubling every 30 years.

3. **Demographic transition** involves the movement of the population into cities, a rise in output per capita, a decline in mortality rates, followed by a decline in birth rates, to the stable and well-off populations characteristic of a developed country.

4. **Growth in population and increase in life expectancy have been much more influenced by economic development than improvements in medical care.**

5. Development has always had some adverse effects (crowding, pollution) even though its total improvements in nutrition, security and technology have made the overall effect of economic development positive.

6. The dismal hypothesis of Thomas **Malthus** was that any increase in productivity would bring on an uncontrolled increase in population, eventually making people worse off as the number of mouths to feed expanded faster than the food supply. While Malthus's analysis provided insight into forces that had previously governed population growth, he did not foresee the rapid and continuous rise in productivity due to the Industrial Revolution, nor did he understand how the newly emerging middle-class families would choose to have fewer children so that they could invest more in their care and education.

7. In the hunter/gatherer economy of the pre-historic Stone Age, no one had much more than basic necessities. In the Agricultural age, most people lived at a subsistence level, but the rulers controlled vast wealth and made major investments. In the Industrial age, workers' wages rose rapidly above the subsistence level, economic organization became more complex, and most income was held by a large **middle class**.

8. A 1 percent reduction in mortality is worth more to people with a 70-year life expectancy than to people with a life expectancy of only 25 years. With good salaries and savings, people can afford to pay more to protect their health than could their grandparents who earned barely enough to eat.

9. The **reduction in uncertainty** brought about by lower mortality and better jobs made it possible for ordinary people to plan for the future. Having a taste of freedom from fear and loss, they wanted more. In time, the demand for insurance and social security became universal.

10. The development of **medical technology** came only after the Industrial Revolution was already well advanced. Improvements in the productivity of medicine (ability to actually heal and extend life expectancy) began about 150 years after technological change had begun to raise industrial productivity. While scientific advances are to some extent fortuitous accidents, **the rate of technological change in medicine is largely determined by the economic resources** devoted to making new discoveries and applying them in practice.

11. The **economic organization** of medical care is rapidly evolving. From prehistory until 1900, most care was given by doctors practicing alone as independent practitioners. By 1950, the hospital and an organized medical staff funded through third-party payment had become common. By the year 2010, the majority of care will probably be provided by integrated health care systems with thousands of employees. **The most important medical advances are being brought about by improvements in information technology**, not pills and scalpels.

PROBLEMS _____

1. {*life expectancy*} What is the current average life expectancy? What was life expectancy one hundred years ago? One thousand years ago? Ten thousand years ago? Is life expectancy likely to increase more or less rapidly during the next 100 years?

2. {*population growth*} How rapidly is population growing in the United States? Is it growing more or less rapidly elsewhere in the world? Was it growing more or less rapidly one hundred years ago? One thousand years ago?

3. {*population growth, dynamics*} What were the causes of the "baby boom?" How long did it last? How long will it affect the U.S. economy? Which part of the health care system was (is, will be) most affected?

4. {*population growth*} If the birth rate is 5 percent and the death rate is 3.5 percent, what is the rate of population increase? What life expectancy is consistent with that death rate? That death rate is consistent with a life expectancy of approximately how many years? That birth rate is consistent with approximately what family size? (*hint, family size = number of children per year times number of fertile female years*)

5. {*population growth*} If population is growing 1 percent a year, how long will it take it to double? If it is growing 0.1 percent a year?

6. {*distribution*} Is the distribution of income per capita more or less equal now than in the past? Is the distribution of life expectancy more or less equal now than in the past?

7. {(*life expectancy*} Which has been more influential in raising life expectancy, economic growth or the development of medical technology? What evidence would support your answer? What evidence would tend to contradict your answer? What evidence would support either answer?

8. {*population growth*} What is the Malthusian hypothesis? How did Malthus link population growth to declining marginal productivity?

9. {*population growth*} What are the most common reasons for population declines in the world today? (give examples)

10. {*family dynamics*} Will a family with higher income have more or less children? What other economic factors affect choice of family size?

11. {*demographic transition*} Why do birth rates fall during demographic transition? How can population growth be accelerating if birth rates are declining?

12. {*demographic transition*} Why might death rates rise at the end of demographic transition? Can you give an example of a country where death rates might be rising now for this reason? Would such a situation imply more or less growth in per capita income? Why?

13. {*flow of funds*} Why is the development of a middle class a precondition for the development of medical insurance? Why is insurance necessary for the development of a modern, high-technology medical care system?

14. {*risk*} Does an increase in uncertainty, especially life-threatening uncertainties such as famine and plague, make medical care more or less valuable?

15. {*dynamics*} Did the productivity of medical technology start to increase before or after improvements in the productivity of industrial technology? Why? What determines the rate of technological change in medicine?

16. {*productivity*} Assume that you are writing a science-fiction book that takes place in the year 2050. Which would be more devastating to the health of the world, loss of the drugs that cure AIDS, or loss of computers?

17. {*productivity*} Which has grown more rapidly, the productivity of farmers, or the productivity of doctors?

18. {*statistics, productivity*} The application of statistics was necessary to improve productivity in which field: industry, agriculture, or medical care?

19. {*health production*} If the cities were the growing centers of economic opportunity, why did many of the families that moved to the city during the Industrial Revolution experience shorter average life spans than those who remained in the country?

20. {*industrial organization, dynamics*} Was it economic organization, social organization, political organization, medical organization, or technology that lead to the creation of a national medical insurance plan in Germany in 1883?

21. {*distribution*} Does health insurance make income distribution more or less equal? Who is favored by such income redistribution? Would a national health plan such as that proposed by President Clinton in 1994 be more or less redistributive than the current mixed public/private health insurance system in the United States? Which groups were most likely to benefit? Which groups were most likely to lose?

22. {*distribution*} What is the difference between income and wealth? Which has grown more rapidly in the United States?

23. {*social insurance*} What is the difference between "social security" and "insurance?"

24. {*pricing, productivity, risk*} To whom will a drug that provides a 1 percent increase in ten-year survival be most valuable? Try to list factors that will raise, increase, or be ambiguous/mixed/dependent with regard to effect upon market valuation.

ENDNOTES

1. *Mortality* is the death rate, the number of deaths per 100 (or 1,000 or 100,000) persons alive at the beginning of the period. *Morbidity* is the incidence of illness or ill health, the number of cases per 100 (or 1,000 or 100,000) persons. While clearly related to mortality, morbidity should also be clearly distinguished from mortality rates. While it is possible to obtain mortality rates from a variety of sources throughout history and so to create a reliable record, morbidity rates are available only under special circumstances (i.e., epidemics, aboard ships or in school or prison populations) until the advent of routine health surveys in the twentieth century, and are still lacking in many low-income countries with less comprehensive government statistical capabilities.

2. Douglass C. North, *Structure and Change in Economic History*, New York: Norton, 1981.

3. The demographic data in this chapter is drawn largely from the books and articles by Fogel, Livi-Bacci, McEvedy & Jones, and McKeown listed among the *suggested readings*.

4. Theodore Tulchinsky and Elena Varavikova, "Addressing the Epidemiologic Transition in the Former Soviet Union," *American Journal of Public Health,* 86(3): 313–320, 1996.

5. Barrie Cassileth, Vasily Vlassov, and Christopher Chapman, "Health Care, Medical Practice, and Medical Ethics in Russia Today," *Journal of the American Medical Association,* 273(20):1569–1573, 1995.

6. Johannes Nohl, *The Black Death: A Chronical of the Plague, Compiled From Contemporary Sources,* London: Unwin Books, 1971; Philip Ziegler, *The Black Death,* New York: John Day Company, 1969.

7. Massimo Livi-Bacci, *A Concise History of World Population,* Cambridge Mass.: Blackwell, 1992, pp. 47,106; Colin McEvedy and Richard Jones, *Atlas of World Population History* (Middlesex: Penguin, 1978), p. 25

8. Massimo Livi-Bacci, *Population and Nutrition,* Cambridge: Cambridge University Press, 1991.

9. Robert Fogel, "Economic Growth, Population Theory and Physiology: The Bearing of Long-term Processes on the Marking of Economic Policy," *American Economic Review* 84(3):369–395, 1994, p. 374.

10. Maurice Brown, *Adam Smith's Economics: Its Place in the Development of Economic Thought,* London: Croon Helm, 1988; E. G. West, *Adam Smith and Modern Economics: From Market Behavior to Social Choice,* Aldershot, Hants, England: Edward Elgar Publishing, 1990.

11. Thomas Robert Malthus, *An Essay on the Principle of Population,* 1803, new edition by Patricia James for the Royal Economic Society, Cambridge: Cambridge University Press, 1992.

12. Livi-Bacci (1992), p. 65.

13. E. A. Wrigley and R. S. Schofield, *The Population History of England, 1541-1871: A Reconstruction,* Cambridge, Mass: Harvard University Press, 1981.

14. Gary Becker, *A Treatise on the Family,* Cambridge, Mass: Harvard University Press, 1981.

15. Mancur Olson, Jr. "Big Bills Left on the Sidewalk: Why Some Nations are Rich, and Others Poor," *Journal of Economic Perspectives* 10(2):3–24, 1996.

16. The World Bank, *World Development Report 1993: Investing in Health,* Oxford: Oxford University Press for the World Bank, 1993, page 237.

17. United Nations, *World Population Prospects,* New York, 1989; The World Bank, *World Development Report 1986,* Oxford University Press, 1986, Livi-Bacci pp: 199–208.

18. Isidore S. Falk, *Security Against Sickness,* New York: Doubleday, 1936; Jesse George Crownheart, *Sickness Insurance in Europe,* Madison, Wisc: Democrat Printing Company, 1938.

19. Thomas McKeown, *The Modern Rise of Population,* London: Edward Arnold, 1976.

20. Michel Foucault, *The Birth of the Clinic,* New York: Pantheon Books, 1973.

CHAPTER 16

The Role of Government

"To do for the people what needs to be done, but which they cannot, by individual effort, do at all, or do so well, for themselves." Abraham Lincoln

"In the evolution of economic enterprise, the things which could be produced and sold for a price were taken over by private producers. Those that were not, but which were in the end no less urgent for that reason, remained with the state." John Kenneth Galbraith

QUESTIONS

1. *Is competition better than regulation?*
2. *Which parts of the health care system are paid for, or controlled, by government? Why?*
3. *Why is Medicare so much more popular than Medicaid?*
4. *Does the Food and Drug Administration, or any other agency that regulates health, operate in the interest of the public, in the interests of the people who work there, or for the special-interest lobbies?*
5. *Is it because health is "priceless" that medical markets are so heavily regulated?*
6. *Do people vote for what is good for society, or what is good for themselves?*

16.1   THE FLOW OF GOVERNMENT HEALTH FUNDS _____

State, federal, and local government will account for almost half of all health spending (45%) in 1997.[1] However, most "government" health care is actually third-party insurance payment to the highly regulated private health care industry composed of independent physicians, hospitals, nursing homes, and so on. More than 90 percent goes to such personal health care services, and less than 10 percent to core government functions such as medical research laboratories, infectious disease control, national health statistics, or other public health. Government's share of the rapidly growing health care sector has tripled, from 14 percent in 1929 to 45 percent in 1997. In earlier years, state and local governments were larger sources of funding than the federal government. In 1965, the biggest single category of government spending was state/local hospitals, institutions providing care for both general medical conditions and chronic mental illness. Since then, Medicare and Medicaid have grown to be much larger, and these two programs now account for more than two-thirds of all government spending on health care.

The bulk of the $532,300,000,000 in 1997 government funds came from general tax revenues. Premiums paid by enrollees for supplemental Medicare insurance (set to pay a quarter of costs) brought in $16 billion, and the designated Medicare Hospital Insurance tax of 2.9 percent on the wages and self-employment income of all workers brought in another $100 billion. These funding schemes shift the incidence of the tax burden, but do not change the total amount. Ultimately, all government spending must come at the expense of private consumption and investment.

Although the U.S. government provides the largest flow of funds into health care services, it has remained relatively passive. Both Medicare and Medicaid are **entitlement programs**, open-ended commitments for government to pay the bills incurred by any patient who qualifies as eligible (i.e., over age 65 or indigent, respectively). Unlike budgeted programs, where a fixed dollar amount is appropriated each year, there is no limit to the amount that can be spent on Medicaid and Medicare. Explosive growth in expenditures has been a major cause of deficits in state and federal budgets, and has "crowded out" spending on vital public health activities. From 1965 to 1993, the share of health care dollars devoted to public health declined from 8 percent to 6 percent, and spending for medical research to discover new therapies and diagnostics fell from 12 percent to just 3 percent. The future health of the U.S. population is being compromised to pay for uncontrolled and excessive use of resources today (see Table 16.1 and Figure 16.1).

16.2   THE ROLES OF GOVERNMENT _____

Government is Necessary, Even for Private Exchange

As people go about their daily activities, trying to stay happy and healthy and save a few dollars, they are usually not aware of government intrusion. Suppose that you get a headache and go to the drugstore for some aspirin. You are making

TABLE 16.1   Distribution of Government Funds

	1997	1965
Total *(millions)*	$532,300	$10,799
Medicare	42%	—
Medicaid*	31%	20%
Veterans/DOD	6%	18%
Workers' compensation	5%	8%
Maternal/child health	1%	2%
State/local hospitals	3%	22%
Public health	6%	8%
Research	3%	12%
Construction	1%	7%
Other	2%	3%

Source: HCFA Office of the Actuary.

* Medicaid category includes general assistance (welfare) payments for
health care, and in 1965 is composed of a variety of medical care programs for the indigent, as Medicaid was not yet enacted.

that choice individually, as a private citizen, and buying from a private company.
Yet this simple transaction could not take place unless a government had already
done many things to prepare for the welfare of you and that company. To begin
with, government provides a medium of exchange (money) and maintains its
value. Without money you would have to engage in barter and search for someone who wanted you to cut their lawn, or care for their children, or whatever, in
exchange for the aspirin. Not only is the value of money determined by the government, so are the measurements of what you buy. You don't ask for "some" or
"a handful," but for 500-milligram capsules. Furthermore, without government
policing, you could not be sure that the white pills were made of aspirin instead
of sugar or flour, or some noxious chemical. In fact, you depend on your govern-

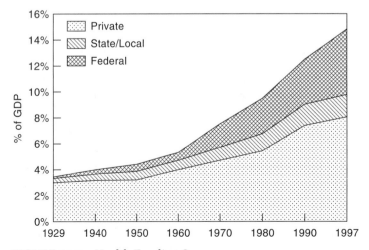

FIGURE 16.1   *Health Funding Sources*

ment to keep your local store from selling you anything that would kill you when ingested. Without this form of consumer protection you would have to spend a lot of time and money making sure that the drugs you bought were safe (just ask a few junkies). All of these government activities that make exchange easy and inexpensive are going on almost without notice.[2]

To make any transaction, you must be able to say, "I own this, and I will give it to you in exchange for that." The most fundamental function of government is to maintain law and order. Unless we can define and enforce rights, including property rights, there is no way for people to cooperate and move beyond the law of the jungle—each person for himself or herself alone. Being killed because somebody wants your house or your cow or your mate is the most basic of threats to your health, and it is in response to such threats that government arose. Families banded together into tribes to protect each other. To do so, they had to agree on how to work together—who would farm and who would fight, who would lead, and when it was O.K. to disagree with the leader. Douglass North, the 1993 Nobel Laureate in Economics, defines the state as "an organization with a comparative advantage in violence, extending over a geographic area whose boundaries are determined by its power to tax constituents."[3] The state monopoly on violence makes it less costly for citizens to defend themselves and their property. Government is there to produce those goods and services that it can provide more efficiently than the market. When we say *efficient* we do not mean that government has no waste, or makes no mistakes, only that it does the job on the whole better than private action—or competing governments.

The Efficiency of Markets Under Conditions of Perfect Competition

The best way to run the economy is usually to let people work, play, and consume what they want without restrictions. This interaction of supply and demand in the market leads to an equilibrium at the point where marginal benefits equal marginal costs. The prices that arise direct people to work at the jobs where their skills provide the most value to society, to find the most efficient means of production, to limit the consumption of goods that are most scarce, and to save and invest for the future. If there were no special problems or difficulties, the entire economy could be coordinated without any central control or directions from the government. The power of market prices to organize production and consumption in a way that maximizes welfare is expressed in the two fundamental theorems of welfare economics: that under "perfect" conditions, *(i)* competitive markets will always lead to an efficient allocation of resources for production and consumption, and *(ii)* that *any* efficient allocation can be obtained through a market system without any central government control by adjusting the initial distribution.[4] These theoretical results emerged during the early years of this century from a continuing debate among economists and politicians of all persuasions, from conservative to liberal to Marxist, during the early years of this century. They provide the prime intellectual underpinning for advocating the use of markets rather than government intervention to solve economic problems.

Economists' most frequent criticism of government intervention is that it distorts prices so that marginal costs and marginal benefits are no longer equated at the margin. In trying to make things better, government gives up some efficiency, and often makes things worse. Governments also inevitably tend to favor certain politically powerful interest groups (e.g., tobacco producers, the military–industrial complex, sons and daughters of senators), and by helping them, harm the rest of society and reduce the overall efficiency of the economy. Yet recognizing that government action is sometimes wrong or self-serving does not mean that it is not necessary. Conditions are not always "perfect," and there are things that only government can do. Examining carefully the conditions of theoretically perfect competition (i.e., many buyers and sellers, all fully informed, costless transactions, with free entry and exit into the market) provides some insight into the roles of government in the real world. **Market failures** necessitating corrective government intervention will arise if conditions are such that the market can have only one or a few buyers or sellers, if access to information is restricted or prohibitively costly to certain participants, if **transactions costs** are so high that many potentially beneficial agreements cannot be negotiated, or if the market is closed by constraints of technology, morality, or law. Sometimes the problems with competition are so extreme that they preclude a market from developing at all, so that government must step in to artificially create one. In the case of **public goods** (chapter 17), the technology is such that only the government can act as a buyer or seller. Finally, the second theorem of welfare economics states only that the desired outcome could in principle be achieved if income were initially distributed in a particular way—which it is not. Therefore, governments must act to bring about a desirable **redistribution** of income.

Government in a Mixed Economy

As just explained, government has four primary tasks in all economies.

1. Maintain law and order
2. Provide "public goods"
3. Deal with market failures
4. Redistribute income

In order to achieve these ends, a government may (a) *produce* the service, (b) *finance* services that are provided by private contractors, or (c) *regulate* the private market. In practice, programs usually serve several functions and use a combination of methods. The Medicare program, for example, deals with market failure due to adverse selection, and also redistributes income to the sick elderly. While mainly functioning as a financing mechanism, it also uses regulation to enforce compliance and participation. In the face of such complexity, a simplifying conceptual framework helps to organize the analysis and make the fundamental economic forces more evident.

16.3 LAW AND ORDER _____

National defense, and its complex domestic version—law and order—is the most fundamental task of governance. Without protection of life and property, society could not exist. A uniform interpretation of the law and a system of taxation must be enforced by the police and courts. If the law applies to some and not to others, people are split into two different societies, even if both are nominally within the same nation. Coercive powers of taxation and law enforcement are freely given to the state by the citizens—we agree to have the government take our money and punish us if we break the law because we are better off that way. For each of us to fight our own battles is more expensive than all of the taxes and parking fines and so on that we love to complain about. Government is expensive, but anarchy, while it doesn't cost anything, is ruinous.

Getting people to agree that there should be law and order is much easier than reaching agreement on exactly what those laws should be, who pays how much tax, and so on. The philosopher John Rawls, in his book *A Theory of Justice,* suggests a useful way of looking at the problem of reaching a social consensus.[5] Rawls argues that much of the conflict over what is right and wrong is due not to differences in beliefs, but differences in the positions that people are coming from. The old want governments to provide nursing home insurance, while young families think better schools are more important. The rich want taxes to be kept low, while the poor (who hope to benefit from redistribution and government aid) want taxes to be higher. People with AIDS favor a national health insurance system that insures everyone, while healthy workers tend to favor higher take-home pay and insurance premiums based on expected costs. In each of these cases, the supporters tend to be those who can expect to benefit, while the critics tend to be those who stand to lose (through higher taxation, less service, or loss of preference).

Consider the formation of policy with regard to disability. It is clearly expensive to provide home care, prostheses, therapy, and building modifications. Including disabled students in regular classrooms (mainstreaming) helps them to become integrated into society, but imposes costs on the other students in the diversion of teachers' attention, pacing of lectures, disruption, and so on. If everything that can possibly benefit the disabled is done, it will cost too much. Yet providing only those benefits that reduce costs (e.g., a prostheses to help someone return to work) is not enough. Whether someone focuses mostly on the costs or tends to emphasize the benefits depends mainly upon whether they are disabled or not (or do or do not care deeply about a child, parent, or friend who is). However, even people who are currently healthy also recognize that there is some chance that they might become disabled in the future (after an automobile accident, for example) and then switch preferences. Rawls defines justice as that set of policies people would vote for "behind the veil of ignorance." That is to say, what each person would consider an optimal balance of costs and benefits if they did not know if they were disabled or healthy, or gay or straight, or young or old. Formally, Rawls' notion is a lot like insurance, where people willingly contribute enough to cover their expected losses to a plan that will spread the risk. Most health care, disability, and pension financing systems in Europe and Asia are considered to be "social insurance" operating under principles of fairness and solidarity rather than the private actuarial principles (such as rating and payment according to risk category) used in commercial insurance.

Justice is more than an abstract notion; it is a practical necessity for the operation of society. Unless people believe that the system is fair and serves their needs, they will not trust the government, and it becomes prohibitively costly to force them to behave according to the rules. Pervasive cheating will cause the whole system to break down. If members of a group think that they are not being treated fairly, the group will lose respect for the law. At the extreme, they will revolt and perhaps set up a separate government that conforms more closely to their ideal of a fair system.

16.4 PUBLIC GOODS AND EXTERNALITIES _____

A public good is something that everyone consumes collectively. National defense is a public good. So is clean air, the discovery of penicillin, or publication of national health statistics. Pure public goods have two distinguishing properties. They are *inexhaustible*, so that once produced, there is no additional cost for having additional people use a public good (i.e., marginal cost of additional users is 0). Second, they are nonexclusive, so people cannot be stopped from using the public good once it is there. Private goods are "exhaustible" and get used up by consumption (a pill, an hour of a doctor's time), while inexhaustible public goods (the formula for the pill, the discovery that eating foods rich in vitamin C reduces certain diseases, clean air) are not. If one patient uses that doctor's time, then another patient cannot. Yet if one patient uses a formula, or clean air, or nutritional advice, that in no way reduces the amount available for someone else to use. Private goods are *exclusive*, so that if one person uses it, another person cannot. This makes it easy to charge for use, and so to pay the costs of production. Public goods, like clean air, tend to be nonexclusive and indivisible, so that if anyone gets the benefits, everyone does. Since no one can be prevented from using the public good, no one has any incentive to pay for it. Selfishly, it makes sense for me to wait for someone else to discover a cure for AIDS (or clean up the air, or build a highway), because whether I contribute or not will make little difference. This is known as the **free-rider** problem. If no one is charged for public goods and no one voluntarily contributes, then there is no way to carry out medical research, reduce pollution, or build highways. Therefore, governments are allowed to force everyone to "donate" taxes to pay for public goods.

Many goods are not purely private or purely public, but somewhere in between, and the extent of "publicness" may change with market conditions. For people in an isolated rural area, building and staffing a hospital is mostly a public good. Without the hospital, they have no medical care, but once it is built, as many people as want to can come and be patients without displacing or reducing anyone else's consumption because there is plenty of excess capacity (i.e, marginal cost of additional patients is near 0). However, if population increases and the hospital becomes full, then each additional patient is displacing someone else who might have received care, and care becomes more like a private good (marginal cost rises to approximately equal average cost per unit). Highways, parks, and movie theaters show similar congestion effects, being almost pure public goods when they are mostly empty, and more like private goods once they fill up.

Externalities

Often, the production or consumption of a "private" good may have social consequences because it affects other people. A firm that produces cars might not be paying for the smoke it emits into the air, an airport may not compensate neighboring houses for the disruption caused by jets taking off in the night, a person who cheats may not compensate classmates for the inconvenience caused by new rules about taking tests, and a person who comes to class with a cold in order to take an exam might fail to compensate classmates for exposing them to illness. Whenever a transaction has an effect on some other party that is not paid for, it is said that externalities exist. Goods that are only externalities with negligible private consumption are public goods. Although both terms refer to similar phenomena, they emphasize different perspectives. *Public good* draws attention to the collective concerns that face us all, a need for consensus, government control, and a universal tax system. *Externalities* focus attention on those cases where the costs and benefits of an action are born by different people, so that private and social costs diverge. Whether considering more purely public goods like national defense and scientific research, or action externalities like infection control and pollution, we end up with the same issue—how to design appropriate institutions and government rules to make individual incentives more in accord with social welfare.

There are positive as well as negative externalities. Governments subsidize schools and colleges because they think that young people will become better citizens (and able to pay more in taxes) if they are educated. A person who fixes up an old house increases the value of all the other houses in the neighborhood, a cook who washes his hands reduces the risk of infection, and a technological discovery that allows more efficient production by one firm creates external benefits for other firms that copy it. However, that same technology may create negative externalities for some corporations and people, because it puts an obsolete factory out of business, and those workers lose their jobs. In fact, whether an externality is "positive" or "negative" may depend solely on the perspective from which it is viewed. The cook may have thought that he was doing his patrons a favor by washing his hands. The patrons may well have felt that being clean is part of his job, and that not washing was an unwarranted burden to impose on them. This mirror-image aspect, that an action may be considered either a negative "cost" reduction or a positive "benefit" increase, depending on one's point of view, leads to an important insight.

The Coase Theorem: Transactions Costs and Property Rights

If transacting were indeed costless, as is assumed under perfect competition, then the factory would pay a fee for the smoke it emitted, the cook with dirty hands would have to pay a fee to the people who got food poisoning, and a student with the flu would not show up for an exam unless he or she were willing to pay each classmate $20 for exposing them to airborne viruses—all of the externalities would be internalized by market transactions. If one or two people are affected by an externality, individual transactions can be used to deal with the problem. A person who wishes to dump some dirt in a neighbor's yard, or who breaks their neighbor's window, or a doctor who negligently causes a leg to fracture, will pay for it. When many people are involved, the costs of arranging thousands of individually negotiated transactions becomes prohibitive, and **property rights** (who controls what, and who must pay whom to use it) become unclear. No market develops to handle the external effects at this scale. Therefore, government must step in to act collectively on behalf of many persons by creating rules and regulations. It is cheaper to deal with the problem once and for all, despite some inefficiencies, than to make thousands of individual transactions with everyone who might be affected by pollution, infection, or air traffic control.

Suppose that the socially optimal decision (where marginal cost just equaled marginal benefits) would be to have factories clean 80 percent of the pollution from their smokestacks. The **Coase Theorem** asserts that there is *no difference* in outcome whether the factory has a right to pollute, or the people have a right to clean air.[6] As long as all rights are well-defined and there are no transacting costs (a big if), and ignoring income distribution effects, then the same result will be arrived at through contracting, either way. If the factory has the right to pollute, then the neighbors will willingly pay the company a fee to install smokestack scrubbers until pollution has been reduced to 20 percent. If the neighbors have a right to clean air, the factory will pay each of the residents a fee to allow discharge of 20 percent of the smoke and will buy scrubbers to clean up the rest. Either way, the final result will be the same: air that is 80 percent clean. The ability to make mutually beneficial trades through the market guarantees that whoever values smoke more, whether positively or negatively, will buy it from the other party. Coase's Theorem is important, not because outcomes would be the same under some hypothetical perfect conditions, but because it shows how transactions costs and assignment of property rights affect distribution and efficiency in the real world, and how the distortions and difficulties increase to the extent that the characteristics of a good are more public than private.

Politicians: Entrepreneurs Who Try to Get Votes

Whereas markets operate through voluntary exchange, public goods can be provided only through political intervention. You cannot go to the store and buy more clean air, or better schools, or safer highways. We depend on politicians to act as entrepreneurs, to propose some plan of action that appeals to us so that we will put them in power. Like all entrepreneurs, politicians expect to be paid for their efforts, extracting rents in the form of influence, prestige, perquisites, and some salary. To an extent, the political arena can be seen as a market, with people "spending" votes or influence. However, the correspondence is very imperfect. People are not allowed to buy and sell votes, or borrow with interest, or set up joint-stock corporations. The property rights to votes are much less well-defined and enforceable, and thus the transactions costs are very high.

Since it is difficult to make a political bargain, a lot of the effort and money must be wasted. Millions are used to win support, or to try to keep some wavering supporter in line. Formally, economists talk about the problems of "rent capture." If an ordinary entrepreneur has a good idea, they can trade it to a firm for money. For example, an inventor, a biochemist, or a screenwriter avoids the hassles of marketing and production by licensing the rights to their ideas and obtaining royalty payments in return. These profits are called *rents*, because once the entrepreneur has the idea, no more work needs to be done to get the money. It is just like collecting rent on a piece of land. Also like land, the rent depends entirely on the demand for the idea. A good idea (Mickey Mouse, penicillin, mobile phones) is valuable the way land in downtown Tokyo is valuable; bad ideas are like acreage in the Gobi desert.

Rents and rent-seeking pose a major obstacle to providing an optimal level of investment in public health. Many of the good ideas (well child-care, counseling parents with a potential genetic defect, dietary change) offer no simple way for innovators to capture the benefits, and thus there is little incentive to produce. On the other hand, when large sums are made available so that all these good ideas can be put into practice, most of the money is not well spent. The new road ends up mostly benefiting Senator Northeast's brother-in-law's construction company, the new AIDS campaign is highly visible and impresses voters but doesn't affect sexual behavior, and the new "educational" drug program for teenagers is so dreary that they use it only to make jokes. Even if we knew exactly how much to spend on public goods, it is doubtful that the money could all be well spent. Since no single individual has much of an interest, those who are able to capture a piece of the action will distort the program to benefit themselves, and the objective of meeting the needs of the public will be compromised.

16.5 MARKET FAILURE

Monopoly

For public goods, the marginal cost of additional consumption is 0. The production of some private goods has such high fixed costs and low marginal costs that the average cost per unit continually falls as output increases. Such goods (telephone networks, power and water supply) are said to be **natural monopolies**. Declining average cost means that the biggest firm can underbid all of the others, and competition will lead to a single firm that dominates the whole market. However, in order to break even that firm must charge a price above marginal cost (the high fixed cost overhead means that average cost per unit is always above marginal cost). Since there is no competition, the monopoly firm may push prices up and up to extract extra profits from consumers, stopping only when the profits are so great that another firm is tempted to enter, even at an inefficiently small scale. In a rural area, ambulance transport, hospital services, even a doctor's office, may all be natural monopolies. In addition to the technologically induced natural monopoly, there are also monopolies created by political action. A Certificate-Of-Need law may give a hospital an effective monopoly in its local market by barring the construction of new competitors, licensure laws may give a profession monopoly control over supply, quality regulations may give a particular manufacturer monopoly control over a special medical device, and requirements to hold clinical trials demonstrating safety and efficacy can give a pharmaceutical firm monopoly control over a type of drug.

The desire to maximize profits and the lack of competition will lead a monopolist, unlike a firm under perfectly competitive conditions, to charge a price which is above average cost per unit, thus generating excess profits known as **monopoly rents**. Monopoly pricing causes the market to be inefficient. With prices above average cost, some consumers choose not to buy, even though the goods could have been produced and sold for an amount less than their willingness to pay. The amount of consumer welfare foregone is traditionally estimated by the "welfare triangle," which under appropriate conditions is approximately 1/2 the difference between the monopoly price and the average cost per unit ($P_{monopoly}$ − AC) multiplied by the number of units not purchased due to the excessive price ($Q_{optimum}$ − $Q_{monopoly}$). The magnitude of inefficiency due to monopoly pricing is shown by the shaded welfare triangle in Figure 16.2. Note that while the monopoly rents (shown as dots) due to high prices are a loss to the consumers, they are a gain to the seller, and are regarded by most economists as a pure transfer which does not in itself create any loss of market efficiency. However, consumers do tend to get upset about being charged extra just because this firm happens to have a monopoly. Also, there is likely to be some fighting between firms for the right to become the monopolist who takes home the rents, and this fighting *is* a waste of resources which generates inefficiency.

There are essentially four ways for government to deal with the problems created by a natural monopoly:

1. Take over the process and let government be the producer.
2. Subsidize the fixed cost overhead and set a government-controlled price equal to marginal cost per unit.
3. Set a government-controlled price equal to average cost, which causes some inefficiency but avoids having to use taxpayers' money to subsidize a monopoly firm.
4. Do nothing, and let the firm set a monopoly price.

Some economists claim that government production is so inefficient that the first option should always be avoided. Options 2 and 3 depend on government's ability to accurately estimate marginal and average cost, which is always difficult, and is inevitably made worse by firms' attempts to overstate costs and hide revenues

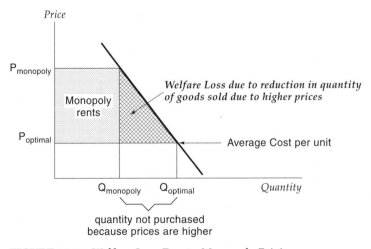

FIGURE 16.2   *Welfare Loss Due to Monopoly Pricing*

in order to make extra profits. However, allowing firms to become monopolies often costs much more than the traditional welfare triangle loss, since firms waste millions of dollars making donations to politicians, hiring lawyers, and otherwise competing for (and competing away) the potential monopoly rents. Natural monopoly is a cornerstone of applied welfare economics, but is relatively unimportant in health care. Most medical monopolies arise from government interventions (licensure, regulation, reimbursement rules) designed to ameliorate market failure caused by risk and information difficulties (discussed later), rather than technical market failures due to production conditions of declining average costs.

Paternalism

Market efficiency depends on consumers' ability to choose, to correctly balance their demands with prices and available income. Some types of consumers—notably children, the mentally ill, and addicts—are considered incapable of making reasonable choices. There is a biological necessity for parents to care for and make decisions on behalf of a child, forcing it to learn by doing many things it does not initially want to do (hence the term, *paternalism*). Market failure due to mental incapacity is dealt with by having a parent, legal guardian, social service agency, or government bureau make decisions on behalf of those individuals rather than allowing them to do so for themselves. Addicts are prohibited by law from buying drugs that they are clearly willing to pay for. To that extent, those people are wards of the state, and not fully participating citizens of the country.

Recently there has been a move to provide more freedoms and more rights to people who are mentally disabled. "Deinstitutionalization" emptied state mental hospitals as patients were released into the community. In principle, those inpatient hospital services were to have been replaced by community services, so that people who were previously in-patients could operate at a higher level of functioning and be integrated into the community. The rise of a new generation of homeless people on the streets is evidence that things have not worked out as planned. Economics, or rather, the *failure to consider* the economics of deinstitutionalization, was a contributing factor. The public was much more willing to recognize that people had rights, and vote for a change in the law that made it hard to keep people in mental hospitals, than to provide money for the community services that were to take care of those people. Once it cost something, voters approached the issue from a different perspective. Unlike a manager or a factory owner, voters are under no obligation to be consistent. Thus they could vote for principles on one day, and for their pocketbooks on another. Deinstitutionalization created a need for services, but not the taxes to pay for these services. Furthermore, the expected transfer of funding from hospitals to community programs did not occur. Employees at state mental hospitals fought to maintain their jobs and their budgets even though most of their patients were being discharged.

The initial proponents of deinstitutionalization were people who had worked with mental patients and were convinced that most of them could function better and enjoy more of life if they lived in the community. Like doctors, they were agents and even advocates for their clients. Yet they were not balancing the interests of *all* the parties involved. While living in the community might be beneficial to the mental patient, it might not be so beneficial to the community. Deinstitutionalization has had a large and unrecognized externality that we now call the "homelessness" problem.

16.6 INCOME REDISTRIBUTION AND CARE OF THE POOR _____

Every civilized society takes care of its poor. It is generally accepted that no one in the United States should die because he or she cannot afford a necessary operation, or medications to arrest a progressive disease. However, the poor cannot afford to buy insurance or medical care generally available to most members of society—not being able to buy is what being "poor" means. A country that provides health services as a public good just as it would provide water or mail delivery, as do Sweden and the United Kingdom, automatically provides medical care to the poor. In a pluralistic system where individual income affects access to the system, some more explicit mechanism to protect those least able to pay is required. In the United States, Medicaid is the most important of such programs to guarantee access to medical care by the poor. Originally directed toward impoverished families with dependent children, Medicaid has been broadened to include all classes of people who are medically indigent, and now pays for almost half of all nursing home care, even for the middle-class elderly (see chapter 12).

Medicaid and Medicare: Dependency or Rights?

Medicaid is fraught with ambiguity and compromise because of an unresolved conflict at its core: Is it charity or a form of social insurance? Is it a program for taking care of those who can't take care of themselves, and whose dependency, like that of the children, addicts, and mentally ill previously discussed, makes them inherently less qualified than other citizens to decide? Or is it the provision of a basic necessity of life, like safe water and national defense, that the indigent can claim as a right of citizenship, and therefore should not involve giving up any decision-making power?

Some people ("liberals") believe that most or all of the benefits of economic development should belong to society as a whole, and they favor very broad government activity to ensure a relatively equitable distribution of goods and services. In Sweden, for example, more than half of gross domestic product (GDP) moves through the government sector. Other people ("conservatives") believe that individual initiative and luck should determine who gets to consume what, and thus tend to want to limit the role of government to that of referee and provider of last resort. Medical care for the poor is caught between these opposing positions. Conservatives who believe in reducing taxes and the role of government as much as possible are willing to make an exception for medical care, but expect the indigent (like other dependent beneficiaries) to give up some autonomy and self-respect. Liberals want a more equitable distribution of all goods and services, but are willing to settle for a few (medical care, education) as better than none.

In general, rich people will rationally favor a conservative position since any redistributive government activity is likely to cost them more in taxes than they will receive in benefits. Conversely, the self-interest of poor people rationally favors a liberal position. The motivations behind these two positions are in conflict on several levels, and it is therefore almost impossible to design a practical program that satisfies both at the same time. This tension, and its policy implications, are well illustrated by comparing Medicare and Medicaid.

Medicare is a universal and popular program to pay on a national basis for the medical care of all elderly.[7] Medicaid is a much reviled and unpopular part-federal, part-state (local) program that requires each beneficiary to meet a means test, and covers a complicated patchwork of special programs. Even conservatives are not foolish enough to attack Medicare, and even liberals are not foolish enough to support an expansion of Medicaid. Why are these two programs perceived so differently? Medicare is constructed like a public good for all citizens, while Medicaid has the punitive elements of a qualified dependency assistance program. To qualify for Medicare, one need only be over 65, and it covers everyone, rich or poor, sick or healthy, black or white. Every voter expects to benefit from Medicare, and sees it as vital to their financial planning for old age. Medicaid is just the opposite. Applicants must submit to probing questions and must sometimes misrepresent their economic position to qualify for benefits. Most voters think that they personally will never benefit from Medicaid, and often feel shame when they help Grandma (and themselves) do so by transferring ownership of her car and her house in their name. Medicaid is not designed to provide satisfaction to its beneficiaries; it is constructed to force them to acknowledge dependence, and to serve as a necessary social backstop so that no one is deprived of minimal (but not comfortable) care.

The expansion of a Medicare-type program (universal access, no means testing, the same care for all) furthers liberal political goals by broadening participation in government activities seen to be helpful and of high quality. Replacement with a Medicaid-type program (means tested, differential standards of care by payment class) furthers a conservative political agenda by making government programs unpopular. Thus, the way in which a public health program is put together will affect not just the services different groups of people get, but also their future voting behavior and attitude toward government. Each political party fights to get programs that will make it easier for them to say, "I told you so," and favors the economic interests of its supporters as well. Attitudes toward public health activities and the design of programs thus depend on political ideology and self-interest as much as any objective evaluation of costs and benefits or morbidity and mortality.

16.7 HOW GOVERNMENT WORKS _____

Government influence on various parts of the economy ranges from watchful oversight to total control (Table 16.2). It is least intrusive when it confines its activities to creating a foundation of property rights and contract enforcement within which the market can operate freely, and is most controlling when it takes over production and replaces private ownership completely. Through regulation

TABLE 16.2   Varieties of Government Action

	Examples
Public Production	*Centers for Disease Control & Prevention* *Veterans Administration Hospitals*
Public financing	
• contract	*Neighborhood Health Center*
• producer subsidy	*Vaccine Liability Insurance*
• consumer subsidy	*Employee Health Benefits*
• entitlement	*Medicare*
Public regulation	
• for the market	*Financial Standards for Insurance Companies*
• superseding market	*Price Controls*
Private Production	*self-paid visit to therapist*

and third-party financing, the health care sector has a very high degree of government involvement. **Government production** is limited mostly to certain core public functions, such as setting and monitoring standards, infectious disease control, and medical research.[8] **Direct contracting** with production tailored to government specifications, such as occurs in military HMOs, Neighborhood Health Centers, immunization programs, and so on, offers extensive, yet not complete, public control, since the workers are employed by private firms. With **subsidies**, government can exert influence, but rarely control. For example, tax-exempt municipal bond financing can encourage construction of hospital facilities, but only rarely and indirectly affects the type of clinical services being offered. **Entitlement financing**, such as Medicare, may leave behavior essentially unconstrained since it is designed to be the equivalent of privately purchased insurance.

A large part of **health regulation** is intended *to make markets more efficient* by providing standard definitions, quality assurance, uniform insurance contracts, and other measures that reduce transactions costs. Other regulations attempt to change the shape of the market, *or to supersede the market entirely* and dictate prices and quantities. The regulatory apparatus can be tightened or loosened to allow government to exert more or less control, and can be made compelling without resort to legal action by combining regulation with financing. Medicare, initially a passive entitlement financing program that provided essentially private funding for purchase of physician services, now sets prices within a narrow range and may virtually prohibit the use of some medical technology by refusing to pay for it. Direct regulatory control is exercised by government only in a few areas where the threat to public safety is compelling: water and air quality, production and prescribing of pharmaceuticals, performance of surgery. For the most part, medical care is "regulated" through control over finances, rather than laws. Regulation is pervasive in health care markets, and specific examples have been examined at length in earlier chapters on physicians (licensure), hospitals and long-term care (CON). Federal price control regulations are reviewed in chapter 18.

The Voluntary Sector

The public good is sometimes best served neither by a government bureaucracy, nor by a private firm, but by an independent organization. Nonprofit status can free them from the dictates of profit maximization, and make it easier for such a "voluntary organization" (e.g., a hospital, a social service agency, a professional society) to pursue the goal of maximizing health. Independence from government often makes voluntary organizations more flexible and creative than the public sector in meeting social needs.[9]

Government as the Citizen's Agent

Government exists, to paraphrase the quote from Abraham Lincoln at the opening of this chapter, to do for the people those things that they cannot do for themselves. However, what guarantee is there that a government agency, once constituted, will act as the agency of the people, rather than of some special interest group, or of the bureaucrats themselves? When information problems cause market failure, and so preclude private action, governments will also have a difficult time collecting information, and voters will have a difficult time evaluating the performance of an agency to make sure that it is, in fact, operating in the public interest. Economists examine the performance of government agencies from four perspectives:

- Maximizing public welfare
- Capturing of regulators by profit-maximizing firms
- Maximizing bureaucratic objectives
- Balancing political interest groups

Public Welfare Maximization The starting point for the economic analysis of regulation is to assume that it does what it says it does—maximize public welfare. The British empire, the state of Pennsylvania, and other governments argue as much when they define themselves as a *commonwealth*. However, to define *public welfare* it is necessary to make assumptions about whose preferences are to count, and how much. Is everyone equal? Do people who act to harm themselves through drug use or lack of exercise deserve the same services as those who try hard to stay healthy? Do those born with a genetic defect that shortens their lifespan deserve more, or less, than others? Does a desire for life-saving heart surgery count as much as a desire for face-saving cosmetic surgery? Even if all of these issues are resolved, there may in fact be no way to reach a decision about which government policy is best, as demonstrated in the proof of the famous "Arrow impossibility theorem."[10] The theoretical problems of welfare maximization pale beside the practical problems of public incentives. Unlike a firm, which has an owner, there is no one who has an interest in working to maximize the benefits of government. Each person seeks to maximize his or her own welfare, and will usually act or vote to achieve that end, even when the benefits to that individual are far outweighed by the costs to other individuals. Many government programs are characterized by *concentrated benefits* and *diffuse costs*. For example, regulations that limit competition and raise the price of drugs a few cents per prescription could add millions of dollars to the profits of pharmaceutical firms, but be almost unnoticeable in the medical bills and insurance premiums of consumers.

Regulatory Capture   The concentrated interest of the firms most affected by regulations makes it worthwhile for them to lobby government and try to "capture" the regulatory agency. For example, a hearing on the safety of cardiac pacemakers is sure to be attended by lawyers for all of the device manufacturers, but very few patients will be willing to travel to Washington to testify, and they will not be paid $200 an hour for doing so. Political campaign contributions are an obvious means of attempting to exercise control, but usually are not the most effective. It is common for firms in regulated industries to appeal directly to bureaucrats, not with money or gifts (which are illegal), but by hiring the former regulators and holding informational seminars in Hawaii. It is natural for someone who has worked for years in regulating health to take a job with a company in the same field, but such a **revolving door** is held by most commentators to compromise regulatory objectivity. How can a junior analyst remain clear when asked to make a difficult judgment call if the person on the other side of the table is the well-respected former chairman of the agency? Even a bureaucrat who just wants to do a good job performing daily tasks can be influenced by the asymmetry between concentrated producer interests and diffuse consumer interests. Even though there are many more patients than producers, complaints to regulators, or complaints to politicians about regulatory decisions, are much more apt to come from producers because they stand to gain much more from any change in the rules.

Bureaucratic Objectives   Bureaucrats, just like consumers, profit-maximizing owners, union workers, and all other individuals in the economy, prefer not to be harassed. Most people get paid to do tasks that are occasionally unpleasant in order to maximize long-run gains (e.g., impose discipline on second-graders, redo a botched repair job for free, fire an incompetent employee, hold the HMO doctors within the budget). The difficulty of evaluating how well an agency is performing can reduce the competitive pressure to take on unpleasant tasks. This can lead to an organization that is bloated and excessively risk-averse. Unlike an owner, who can gain large profits from taking on a risk, a bureaucrat will continue to be compensated on a civil service pay scale. Any effort to make changes or take a chance could go wrong and cost them their job, so they tend to play it safe. An owner may eliminate an employee if that owner believes that the additional revenues gained are less than the additional cost in wages. A bureaucrat, on the other hand, has almost no incentive to reduce the number of workers. Instead, an increase in employment usually means a larger salary for the director (since they now run a bigger agency) and better working conditions (since the tasks are spread out among a larger number of employees so each one has more time to do the job). Unlike a profit-maximizing firm, there is no internal incentive to limit the size of a government agency, so control must be imposed from the outside. Unfortunately, outsiders are, by definition, less familiar with the tasks, workload, and performance of the agency than the inside employees and managers, or the industry experts who lobby them. This does not mean that most government agencies are too large, since the fear of "waste" may lead legislators to preemptively cut regulatory budgets. What it does mean is that the difficulty of evaluating performance, which is why those tasks were taken out of the market and given to government in the first place, also makes it much harder to tell if the agency is too big or too small, or to manage it so that use of employees and other resources is optimized.

Political Interest Group Balance   The actual behavior of agencies is not determined by the public interest, self-interests of the industry, or of the bureaucrats, but by some complex and shifting balance of all interest groups. Transactions costs shape politics just as they shape markets, and the costs of organizing are lower when interests are concentrated, or when they are quite uniform across a large class of people (e.g., all of the elderly may favor increased Medicare budgets). The outcomes are much less predictable, since political deals cannot be negotiated, specified, and enforced with the precision weighting of conflicting interests that dollar "votes" bring to the marketplace, and since politicians are rewarded for swaying emotions and mobilizing public opinion as often as they are rewarded for responding to the public interest. Economists and political scientists have devoted considerable attention to studying how the process of making decisions affects the decisions made. For example, a majority rule implies that 50–49 wins while 49–50 loses, and so provides politicians with a great incentive to seek the median (50th percentile) voter, rather than to maximize the average level of support. Other political structures favor different parts of the voting spectrum. In union representation, for example, seniority is important, so the desires of older workers for more health benefits and pensions tend to outweigh the desires of younger workers for fewer benefits and higher wages. Several recent critiques of the health care industry claim that it is dominated by an "iron triangle" of providers, insurance companies, and government agencies, all of whom benefit from higher health care spending rather than difficult, but potentially worthwhile, cost cutting.[11]

Winners and Losers

Although economists will try to evaluate how a regulation changes the overall efficiency of the system, most hospital administrators, physicians, and patients are far more concerned with how it affects them personally. Even if a change in Medicare reimbursement is good for the country, a medical equipment vendor will fight it with everything he owns if that regulation would force his business into bankruptcy. Changes in the regulatory structure often have more to do with finding paths that have less resistance, than the achievement of noble ends. Many issues have solutions that are nearly the same in terms of overall efficiency, but quite different in terms of who bears the costs or receives the benefits. For example, it may not make a great deal of difference in terms of economic efficiency whether an expanded Medicare drug benefit is paid for through increases in enrollee premiums or an income tax surcharge for the elderly, but the one will fall harder on the poor while the later falls mostly on the wealthy (who pay more taxes), with predictable consequences on the political support for these alternatives by different groups. Research suggests that when a necessary change in policy is seen as involving two mutually exclusive options, the wealthy, even if less numerous and initially less powerful than the poor, may be able to hold out longer and obtain a result more favorable to their interests.[12] A disproportionately large share of all benefits, from Medicare reimbursement to subsidized medical educations, goes to those in the highest income groups who have the power to make their demands on government effective. Yet, without government intervention, the poor would surely be much worse off.

16.8 EROSION OF THE
MEDICAL MARKETPLACE_____

The factors that make health care an interesting and challenging subject for economic investigation (uncertainty, information asymmetry, life-and-death choices) lead health care toward special institutions that supplement or supplant prices (insurance, licensure, nonprofit organizations), and erode the use of the marketplace to allocate resources.[13] Insurance severs the linkage between what the consumer pays and what the producer gets paid. In doing so, it distorts the market, and makes the "prices" charged by physicians, hospitals, and nursing homes almost meaningless as indicators of the value of services, or of the cost of resources used. Concern for unmeasurable quality differences leads to a reliance on voluntary organizations that lack the clear incentives of private ownership. Yet to say that insurance, licensure, and nonprofit status create problems does not imply that they do not improve public welfare. Indeed, the universality of medical institutions that modify or supplant the market across many groups in many countries, is compelling evidence that these are adaptations that increase welfare rather than reduce it. An inability to rely on markets does mean that some other mechanism must be found or created to carry out the economic functions that prices usually serve.

One creative attempt to reintroduce market forces into health care is an MSA, or **"medical savings account,"** an idea that has been championed by health economist Mark Pauly.[14] An MSA is a sort of combination of an IRA and health insurance. Each year, people could put savings into the MSA that accumulate and collect interest tax-free, in addition to purchasing a catastrophic insurance policy that pays only for bills above a high threshold (e.g., $3,000). The MSA account could then be drawn on to pay for all the bills each year under $3,000, and eventually used for retirement or long-term care. In this way, the consumer would face the full marginal cost of all ordinary medical expenses, and so be motivated to shop for lower prices, make value judgments about how much higher quality physicians or hospitals were really worth, and avoid technology that is high in cost but low in benefit. Although appealing, the MSA plan suffers from several failings, as will any policy designed to deal with such a difficult problem. Although it would restore market forces to the bulk of consumers—the 85 percent of the population that spends less than $3,000 on medical care each year—it would do nothing to control costs among the remaining 15 percent who are seriously ill and account for 80 percent of all health expenditures. Debate will continue, and the easy answers will continue to elude us.[15]

16.9 PROS AND CONS OF REGULATION AND COMPETITION _____

Even when markets are suppressed, there is always competition. Physicians try to attract patients with their reputation for quality and with evening office hours; hospitals try to attract physicians with subsidized office rentals, access to new equipment, and helpful staff; HMOs try to attract enrollees with special benefits, picnics, or free radios. Conversely, even the most open market in health care is highly regulated, with oversight over safety, professional qualifications, and long term side-effects, even when prices are freely set. The issue is not "regulation" or "competition," but what combination and compromises to make (Table 16.3).[16]

There are a number of problems created by reliance upon government intervention. First of all, regulation itself costs money: agencies must be staffed,

TABLE 16.3 Pros and Cons of Regulation and Competition

Limitations of Regulation
- Regulatory agencies are costly to operate.
- Government is sometimes an inefficient producer with inadequate customer service.
- Rationing must still take place, and without prices, deadweight welfare losses are larger.
- Suppression of prices distorts markets in inputs and substitute goods as well.
- Government responds to narrowly focused interest groups, not broad consumer interests.
- Regulators must "do no harm" and avoid losses (except the hidden kind).
- Bureaucracies rigidly impose uniformity, treating everyone according to the same standard.
- All regulation is based on the past as a precedent, not directed toward the future.
- No automatic adjustment is made to changes in supply or demand.
- There are no incentives to be an entrepreneur developing new technologies that anticipates demand.

Limitations of Markets
- Markets are costly to operate and must be policed.
- Entrepreneurs maximize profit, not health or social welfare (which are not paid for).
- Under competition, prices pay for services valued by individuals, not public goods (education, research).
- Health care is not very price sensitive, so it is difficult to control behavior through prices.
- Consumers are willing to pay to avoid using prices to make health care decisions.
- Somebody must still take care of the poor, the chronically ill, and the seriously injured.
- Adverse selection may cause private insurance markets to collapse unless government steps in.
- The ethics of competition do not blend well with the ethics of medicine as a *caring* profession.
- Licensure, insurance, and other erosions of the medical marketplace must do more good than harm or they would not be built into the health care system of every country.
- Even the U.S. government must be doing something right, since it has been given increased funding responsibility and control over the medical marketplace.

salaries paid, and information systems maintained. Many of these costs have to be paid for with taxes. Others, such as the compilation of mandated reports and time spent in preparing for regulatory inspections, are imposed on private firms, who then pass them on to the public in the form of higher prices. When government takes over production from private firms, it has sometimes proven to be inefficient and not adept at friendly customer service. Even if the market is superseded by direct government provision of services, some form of rationing must still take place. Since prices are not used to match demand and supply, the amount distributed will often be too large or too small, and the people served may not be the ones who value the services most highly. Both discrepancies cause deadweight losses of consumer welfare. Government suppression of the price mechanism prevents desirable trades from occurring, and will also distort related markets in inputs and substitute goods.

Government responds well, perhaps too well, to focused interest groups that are willing to lobby for their position in Washington. Markets are better able to respond to diverse and diffuse consumer groups, and prices are a superior mechanism for getting people to reveal publicly the true value of the services they use as they pay for them. Politicians are constrained by public scrutiny to "do no harm," and every dollar spent becomes a "federal case," so services that are valued by consumers and raise average health levels (e.g., mass immunizations, fluoridation, abortion) may not be available. Government is subject to so many attacks that agencies can become very risk averse. This exacerbates bureaucratic formalism. Of necessity, government programs designed to deal with the public impose universal standards, and are thus less able to respond to the variation in individual tastes, or to make individual exceptions. Legal constraints make bureaucracies rigid, and may stifle innovation. A central failing of regulation is its reliance on precedent for guidance. There is no flexible equilibration of supply and demand through prices to create automatic adjustments as conditions change, and little scope for entrepreneurs who are willing to make mistakes and go out on a limb to create the next generation of clot-dissolving drugs or continuous monitoring diagnostic technology based on cellular phone links.

Markets have their flaws as well. They, too, are costly to operate, requiring salespeople, billing systems, and policing mechanisms. Entrepreneurs are apt to push the newest and most expensive technology because it is the most profitable, rather than a more cost-effective substitute that would do more to improve health.[17] Markets reward those who provide what the individual consumer wants, not the providers of public goods such as medical research, infection control, and ethical standards of professional education. Furthermore, markets for health do not appear to be very price sensitive, perhaps due to information problems and the potential for death from even small errors, so reliance on prices to motivate behavior seems ill-placed. Even when people do get a chance to use prices and can afford to do so, they seem to want to avoid having prices influence their medical decision if they can, as with the 90 percent of the elderly who, though given extensive coverage through Medicare, obtain supplemental insurance that reduces the marginal price to zero.

Although advocates of competition emphasize the beneficial effect of creating incentives to win, what about the losers? Who will care for the mentally retarded, the alert but alone and alienated 92-year-old, the genetically defective, the truly unlucky accident victim? Although markets can enable socially beneficial risk pooling through insurance, adverse selection may be so severe that insurance is unstable or fails to cover many of those most in need of protection unless government intervenes. Medical *care* is so grounded in a concern for health of others that any competition sufficiently vicious to really cut costs and close all the unnecessary hospital beds may entail such a fundamental violation of human caring that it is socially unacceptable. One might well ask why, if the erosion of the marketplace due to licensure, insurance, and nonprofit organization is so terrible, that these anti-competitive features are an integral part of every health care system in the civilized world?

The United States pursues a path in health care that is among the most highly privatized and most responsive to individual rather than social concerns. Yet even in the United States, government is the largest funding source, paying 45 percent of the bills directly, subsidizing much of the remainder through tax relief, and regulating virtually every dollar that is spent. It is the mixture of competition and market forces, the matching of programs to needs, that must be evaluated, not the pros and cons of one or the other alone.

SUGGESTIONS FOR FURTHER READING _____

Ronald Coase, "The Problem of Social Cost," *Journal of Law & Economics* 3:1–44, 1960.

Paul Feldstein, *The Politics of Health Legislation: An Economic Perspective,* Ann Arbor, Mich.: Health Administration Press, 1988.

Douglass North, *Structure and Change in Economic History,* New York: W.W. Norton, 1981.

Joseph Stiglitz, *Economics of the Public Sector,* New York: W. W. Norton, 1986.

Burton Weisbrod, *The Non-Profit Economy,* Cambridge, Mass.: Harvard University Press, 1988.

Charles Wolfe, *Markets or Governments: Choosing Between Imperfect Alternatives,* Cambridge, Mass.: MIT Press, 1994.

SUMMARY _____

1. **Government accounts for 45% of health care spending**. The vast majority goes to pay for essentially private medical services of special populations (the aged, the indigent, veterans). **Only one-tenth goes for core public health** activities such as infectious disease control, research, and monitoring of drugs, food, air, and water.

2. Under certain conditions, it can be shown that a **purely competitive market allocation** of goods and services, where marginal benefits equals marginal cost, enforced by the price mechanism, is most efficient.

3. The conditions of perfect competition are rarely met in the real world. There are **market failures** due to uncertainty and information problems, transactions costs, **externalities**, and the existence of **public goods**. Government or some other **paternalistic** agency must step in when an individual is incapable

of making appropriate market choices due to immaturity, addiction, or severe mental limitations. Civilized societies also **redistribute income** to protect the poor and disabled.

4. Since most benefits of government are public goods available to all without restriction, many people would be **free-riders** who avoided paying unless forced to do so through **compulsory taxation**.

5. Government is formed to act as the agent of the citizens to **maximize public welfare**. However, the ability of special interests to exert undue influence may lead to **regulatory capture**, where government favors the industry rather than the public. Also, the employees of a government agency may pursue **bureaucratic self-interest**, avoiding risks and controversy, and increasing budgets to obtain higher salaries and easier workloads. The most realistic model of government action combines all three perspectives and a consideration of **transactions costs** in achieving political **interest group balance**.

6. Although people say that they want to do what is best for everyone, **in practice they tend to vote for what is good for themselves**. That is why some programs for which government is essential, like Medicaid financing care for the poor, are unpopular and only grudgingly supported, while the Medicare program, which could be privately funded but which most voters think will give them better benefits now or in the future, and incidentally helps to keep politically connected doctors and hospitals well-off, is very popular.

7. To some extent, **politics is a kind of market**, albeit a rather slow and imperfect one, with legislators trying to get elected by promising the best package of benefits and costs in return for votes. Special interest legislation benefiting a small group at the expense of the many is most apt to occur when large benefits are concentrated on that group, making it worthwhile for them to organize and lobby, but the costs are widely dispersed across all of society, and so get little attention from the millions of voters for whom that particular piece of legislation is just one of many minor concerns. **Prices change much faster than laws**. Public goods take longer to adjust because groups and individuals with many different interests must agree for any changes to occur.

8. The **voluntary sector**, composed of **non-profit organizations that are independent of government** whose objective is to foster the public good, dominates the ownership of hospitals in the U.S., and the important private disease control and medical research "firms."

9. Non-profit organization and the provision of universal public goods such as insurance and professional licensure tends to **diminish the importance of prices**, and to produce a gradual **erosion of medical markets**.

10. **For the most part, government works with the market**, regulating and financing private activities. Government supersedes the market when it tries to exert control over prices and quantities, or to prohibit certain kinds of trades. Direct government production is, however, always used for critical functions such as the maintenance of order (police and courts) and national defense (army). The important question is not whether government or markets are

"better," but how to **balance and blend regulation and competition** to best optimize social welfare and meet necessary constraints. To do so, it is necessary to have some consensus about what constitutes **a just society**.

PROBLEMS _____

1. {*flow of funds*} What fraction of total health expenditures in the United States are paid for by government? Which are the largest government programs? Were the same, or similar, programs at the top of the list for government funding in 1900?

2. {*market failure*} What aspects of the economic organization of U.S. medical care are due to market failure?

3. {*distribution*} In several marches on Washington, demonstrators have carried signs saying, "No Justice, No Peace." Explain what this slogan means, and how it relates to the level of funding for Medicaid.

4. {*incidence*} Why is so much more of dental care paid for privately while so much hospital care is paid for publicly?

5. {*welfare*} Which results in lower prices, competition or regulation?

6. {*incidence*} Why is Medicare so much more popular than Medicaid?

7. {*public goods*} Does the demand for public health increase or decrease as the size of city increases?

8. {*rents*} How are rents different from other input payments? Which of the following are rents:

    Royalties from a biotechnology patent

    Lease payments for use of laboratory

    Payments to subjects who are observed while sleeping

    Surgical fees

    A bonus paid to a research assistant who finishes an experiment ahead of schedule

    A bonus paid to a Nobel laureate for switching to another university

9. {*transactions costs*} What is the Coase Theorem? What does it imply about the extent of immunization among herds of cattle? What does it imply about the levels of immunization among classes of school children?

10. {*regulatory capture*} Explain how the FDA might be subject to regulatory capture. Who would favor, and who would be opposed, to regulations that limited regulatory capture?

11. {*regulatory capture*} Name several medical professional/trade organizations that have made large donations for political campaigns. Did they get their money's worth?

12. {*incidence*} Who benefits and who loses from "deinstitutionalization" of the mentally ill? What factors tended to thwart the original plans for transfer of funding to community treatment facilities?

13. {*flow of funds*} Which of the following are funded as entitlements?

    Medicare

    Medicaid

    Medical Research

    Public Health Statistics

14. {*voting*} Who counts for more in political calculus:

    the sick or the well?

    the old or the young?

    the rich or the poor?

15. {*incidence*} Medical Savings accounts will tend to favor which groups of people?

16. {*dynamics*} Why does it often take longer for a government program to change in response to shifts in external conditions than for a private company? Is this good or bad?

17. {*dynamics*} Which is harder to close, a public hospital or a private clinic? Why? Which is more likely to take advantage of information asymmetry to cheat patients?

ENDNOTES _____

1. National Health Accounts, Office of the Actuary, Health Care Financing Administration. See notes to Chapter 1.
2. Oliver Williamson, *Markets and Hierarchies,* New York: Free Press, 1975.
3. Douglass C. North, *Structure and Change in Economic History,* New York: Norton, 1981, p. 21.
4. Joseph E. Stiglitz, *Economics of the Public Sector,* W. W. Norton: New York, 1986, p. 77.
5. John Rawls, *A Theory of Justice,* Cambridge, Mass.: Harvard University Press, 1971.
6. Ronald H. Coase, "The Problem of Social Cost," *Journal of Law & Economics* 3:1–44, 1960.
7. Marilyn Moon, *Medicare Now and In the Future,* Washington, D.C.: The Urban Institute, 1993; Mark V. Pauly and William L. Kissick, editors, *Lessons from the First Twenty Years of Medicare: Research Implications for Public and Private Sector Policy,* Philadelphia: University of Pennsylvania Press, 1988.
8. A significant exception is the Department of Defense/Veterans Administration health care system. Although national defense is a pure public good, the fact that VA/DOD health is an adjunct to defense does not necessarily make it public, and indeed large parts of the VA/DOD health care are now being privatized through subcontracting.
9. Burton Weisbrod, *The Non-Profit Economy,* Cambridge, Mass.: Harvard University Press, 1988.
10. Peter J. Hammond, "Social Choice: The Science of the Impossible," pp: 116–134 in George R. Feiwel, *Arrow and the Foundations of the Theory of Economic Policy,* New York: New York University Press, 1987.
11. Lawrence R. Jacobs, "The Politics of America's Supply State: Health Reform and Technology" *Health Affairs* 14(2);143–57 (Summer 1995). See also Lawrence D. Brown, "Politics, Money and Health Care Reform," *Health Affairs* 13(2:II):175–84 (Spring 1994), and "Commissions, Clubs and Consensus: Reform in Florida, *Health Affairs,* 12(2):7–26 (Summer 1993).
12. Alberto Alesina and Allan Drazen, "Why are Stabilizations Delayed?" *American Economic Review* 81(5):1170–1188, 1991.

13. Kenneth J. Arrow, "Uncertainty and the Welfare Economics of Medical Care," *American Economic Review*, 53(3):941–73, 1963.

14. Mark V. Pauly, *An Analysis of Medical Savings Accounts: Do Two Wrongs Make a Right*, American Enterprise Institute: Washington, D.C. 1994; and M. V. Pauly and J. C. Goodman, "Tax Credits for Health Insurance and Medical Savings Accounts" *Health Affairs*, 14(1): 126–39, 1995.

15. See Deborah Chollet, "Why the Pauly/Goodman Proposal Won't Work," *Health Affairs* 14(2):273–74 (Summer 1995); and William Hsiao, "Medical Savings Accounts: Lessons from Singapore," *Health Affairs:* 14(2):260–66 (Summer 1995).

16. Charles Wolfe, Jr., *Markets or Governments: Choosing Between Imperfect Alternatives*, Cambridge, Mass.: MIT Press, 1994.

17. Eleena de Lisser, "Ready or Not, Firms Rush to Sell the Public on Laser Eye Surgery," *The Wall Street Journal* CCXVI(38):A1, A8, August 24, 1995.

CHAPTER **17**

Public Goods and Public Health

QUESTIONS

1. *Should treatment of syphilis be part of the public health system or private medical care? What about psoriasis? Psychosis? Scoliosis?*
2. *Why not charge people full price for vaccinations?*
3. *Why are new surgical techniques developed with public funds while pharmaceutical research and development is carried out privately by for-profit firms?*
4. *Who paid for Pasteur to discover bacteria?*
5. *Why pay for cost–benefit analysis to decide which public programs are worthwhile instead of using prices to let the market decide?*
6. *Do the preferences of smokers, mental patients, or unborn children count when assessing the efficiency of the public health system?*
7. *Is medical care for homeless and terminally ill AIDS patients a public good, or a waste of money?*

17.1 CHARACTERISTICS OF PUBLIC GOODS _____

It is not possible to charge for some goods because no one can be excluded from using them (e.g., clean air) and there are other goods no one wants to charge for because it does not cost anything to accommodate additional users (e.g., a news release reporting the discovery that eating oranges cures scurvy). How easy and how desirable it is to use market pricing to ration goods or to exclude people from using a service determines whether it is part of public health or private health care. The two dimensions of publicness i) ability to enforce exclusion with prices and ii) marginal cost of accommodating additional users are illustrated with examples in Figure 17.1. A knee brace is costly to produce, and it is easy to charge for use. Therefore it is a purely private good. Arthroscopic surgery for knees is somewhat intermediate. While the surgery itself has a relatively constant average cost per unit, the development of the techniques and the instruments is more like a public good. Once knowledge is obtained, it can be used over and over again. It is relatively easy to charge for the surgery, but a bit difficult to charge for the years of development work. Polio vaccine is more public. Once discovered, the cost of production, although constant, is so low per dose as to be almost negligible. Although it would be relatively easy to charge users for vaccination, it would not be economically desirable to do so, since the benefits of freeing the population of disease are externalities that benefit everyone, not just the user. The monitoring of infectious disease reports to look for epidemics by the U.S. Centers for Disease Control and Prevention (CDC) is a pure public good. If the agency is successful, there are fewer epidemics, and there is no way to charge individuals for having prevented some mass tragedy that does not happen. Also, once CDC's *Morbidity and Mortality Weekly Report* is printed, there is essentially no additional cost for having more physicians make use of that data to protect their patients. Publicness can vary with local conditions. A congested suburban hospital can readily charge for services, while a quiet rural hospital that sits three-quarters empty most of the time until there is a disaster cannot. Most of its benefits to the community come from being there in case of an emergency, "option demand," rather than from use of services. There are also goods that are publicly provided, even though some amount could be sold privately. Motor vehicle inspections are required and thus do not depend on the owners' willingness to pay because there is a compelling public interest in having a car's brakes and emission controls work properly to protect other people. A social calculation of costs and benefits must supersede market pricing.

Privatizing Public Goods

Prescription drugs are an interesting case of a public good being privatized. Once a discovery is made and validated through clinical trials, the actual costs of production are nearly zero. However, unlike vaccine, which benefits the public by inhibiting communicable disease, all of the benefits from a prescription drug accrue to the user. Patent law gives the firm a monopoly on the drug for seventeen years so it can charge users for all of the sunk costs of discovery and testing.[1] Geographic enclosure also privatizes public goods. Thus, residents of a resort

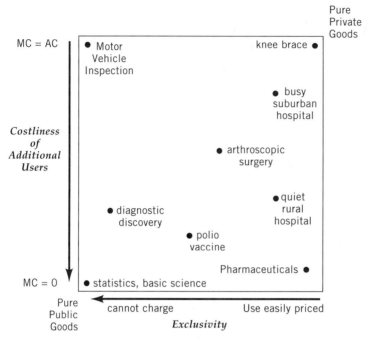

FIGURE 17.1 *Dimensions of publicness*

community will pay privately for maintaining the cleanliness of a lake, and have private agreements to limit noise and pollution. Externalities arise primarily because the costs and benefits are borne by different people, so that one or the other is external to the market transaction. Patent laws, enclosed communities, and membership clubs are all means of internalizing effects so that government intervention is less necessary.

Social Costs Depend on the Number of People

The extent of externalities depends on the magnitude of the costs and the number of people involved. For example, very strict sterilization procedures are followed for spacecraft because of the possibility that some extraterrestrial bacteria could threaten the health of the entire world. Airplane accidents are treated differently than automobile accidents, and nuclear power plant failures are even more closely scrutinized by government safety inspectors. The larger the number of people who could be hurt, the more thorough the investigation.

Garbage disposal provides a nice example of how the treatment of public goods changes with the number of people involved.[2] In prehistoric times people did whatever they pleased with their garbage and no one worried about a waste disposal system. The same is true today in isolated rural areas where people may toss the garbage out in the woods, or bury or burn it. Keeping one's own house tidy and the neighbors happy is sufficient incentive to maintain a social optimum, and no government rules are needed. However, as people move closer together, creating a town, the divergence between private and social costs widens. Dumping in fields, or in the yards of strangers (or people you do not like) rapidly creates a problem. Therefore rules are formulated designating when and where garbage can be dumped. As the town becomes larger, public spending is eventually required to handle all the garbage produced. Land is purchased and set aside to serve as a dump. As the town becomes a city, it is not enough just to have a dump; the city must actively collect all the trash and carry it to the dump. Taxes are imposed and trucks come around to collect garbage at people's houses. In this way the private costs of conforming with the social optimum are minimized. Garbage collection is a public activity that requires collective financing through taxes, but the actual work can be done by a private firm, and often is.

Insurance Makes Any Good More Public

Whenever a service is financed through third-party insurance rather than being paid for directly by individual purchasers, it makes that service more of a public good. When individuals purchase a good, one person may choose high quality, another low, one wants the color to be blue while the other wants it green, and so on. Within a risk-pooling group, they all become the same. Whether the person being treated is the head of marketing or the assistant janitor, the hospital gets paid the same amount. It is possible to have extensive coverage for plastic surgery and 200 days of mental health coverage, but everyone in the benefit plan must get it. The differentiation between individuals by payment is eliminated. The quality of services to be paid for by the insurance package is a public good. There is no benefit to the janitor of seeking out a cheap hospital, since even if the employer does obtain some savings, it won't make insurance any cheaper to the janitor personally. Thus, once medical care is financed on a group basis, any change in quality or standards of service affects everyone, and requires collective action.

17.2 INFORMATION _____

Research on new drugs, new surgical techniques, and new methods of diagnostic imaging is very popular and gets billions of dollars in public funding. However, it is the collection of statistics over many years and millions of patients that makes it possible to tell how medical discoveries actually work in practice. Statistics and scientific discoveries are both forms of information, and are almost pure public goods.[3] Once a set of statistics has been tabulated or a discovery has been made, there are no additional costs incurred as more and more people use it (zero cost); and once it is known, there is no way to stop anyone from using it, regardless of whether or not they have paid (zero charges). The discovery of bacteria by Louis Pasteur began a revolution in the treatment of disease. It also saved the wool industry from the plague of Anthrax, which had been decimating sheep (his original research project), the wine and beer industries that were having trouble with irregularities in fermentation, and the dairy industry, whose "unpasteurized" products caused diarrhea and many fatalities among infants.[4] Much of Pasteur's work was supported by a series of government grants, just as medical research is today. No single person or firm could obtain enough benefits to justify spending the money required to fund such a large research and development program. It was a collective enterprise. Note that there were still many free-riders. Although the costs were paid mostly by France, and to a lesser extent by some industrialists in Belgium and Germany, people in the United States, Africa, China, and the rest of the world all benefited. To the extent that those who benefit do not contribute, there will be under-investment in the development of knowledge.

Information is created not only through new discoveries, but through the compilation and organization of existing data as well. A landmark breakthrough in the history of medicine and public health was the printing of *Observations on the Bills of Mortality* by John Graunt in 1662.[5] Graunt went through the City of London death records and tabulated the number of persons dying each year, and the causes of death, thus creating the first modern work in the science of epidemiology. With the causes of death plainly laid out, the years of plague and the probable effects (or lack of effects) of government attempts to improve the health of citizens could be seen.

Measurement and statistics do not come into being just because it would be a good thing to have them; they must serve some economic purpose. The census that recorded Mary and Joseph at the birth of Jesus Christ was mandated to enable Caesar to collect taxes. Deaths have historically been recorded because they were necessary to establish inheritance, not to study the effects of medical treatment. It was the provision of universal public benefits, such as Social Security, that made it possible for the United States to easily enforce the requirement that all deaths be recorded. The fact that collecting information is costly explains why there are many more statistics on health care expenditures (which must be recorded on each transaction to pay employees, bill insurance companies, and so on) than on medical diagnosis or treatment effectiveness. The U.S. Health Care Financing Administration (which has power because it controls the funds) is setting standards for a "uniform bill" that will be submitted electronically by all hospitals and doctors, and thus provide an integrated database for comparing the costs and effects of all types of medical care. Potentially, this will not only reduce the administrative costs of running the system, it will also make it possible for researchers to tap into an on-line database with hundreds of millions of patient-years of experience, and therefore rapidly determine which treatments, types of hospitals, drugs, and so on, are most cost-effective for treatment.

The National Institutes of Health (NIH) has overall responsibility for medical research in the United States, and the National Center For Health Statistics (NCHS) is responsible for data collection and distribution. Its oldest and most important publication is its series of "vital statistics" on births and deaths. The NCHS also conducts surveys of the health and nutrition status of a sample of the U.S. population, insurance coverage, and the characteristics of patients treated in doctors offices, and collates statistics on patients discharged from hospitals using billing records. All of this information is made available in "public use data tapes" and in free publications (which you can order or get from the library for your term paper) because it is a public good produced with public money. Those running the agency want to maximize the value of this "free" good so that they can argue for more funding from Congress—and, not incidentally, benefit all of us.

Rational Consumer Ignorance

Why does the government have a better information base for making decisions than most citizens? Because it has paid for it. From the safety standards for seatbelts in trucks to the efficacy of vitamin supplements, millions of dollars have been spent to determine the best possible answers. For each consumer to try, individually, to collect such information would lead to massively wasteful duplication. If the consumers banded together to share the costs of gathering information, then that banding together would constitute a form of government. Consumers are rationally ignorant of many health and safety effects because it is more efficient to have the government do it, once, than for each of us to try to do it separately. Rational consumer ignorance is sensible free-riding. Even for a private good, such as a bottle of vitamins, it is cheaper to do quality control once in a government lab than to do it over and over again in each individual's home.

In many of the cases where it is argued that government should make the decisions because consumers are ignorant and are not qualified to determine what is best, consumers are remaining rationally ignorant by delegating their decision-making powers to government because it is more efficient to do so—they are being smart by staying stupid! Thus, we have the government getting the FDA to test the safety of food and drugs, the EPA to do studies on the effects of different levels of pollution, and the various transportation departments to monitor the safety characteristics of highways and vehicles.

Milk or Bread: Which is More Public?

Whether a particular set of health concerns should fall in the arena of public or private action depends on the characteristics of the good and the way it is produced and transacted. In general, if something is produced collectively, so that one person's consumption cannot easily be separated from that of another person, more governmental intervention is called for. If the relevant characteristics are readily observable by consumers at the time of purchase, then more reliance on private markets is appropriate. Consider two products that are consumed by almost everyone: milk and bread. Milk was subjected to government regulations over a hundred years ago, and public milk dispensing stations were set up in New York and other cities.[6] It is now illegal to buy milk that has not been inspected and processed according to government standards in most states. Bread, while under routine surveillance as a food, is largely unregulated. Why this difference in treatment?

Bread may be mixed in batches, but each loaf is baked separately, and the baking process kills most germs. When bread gets old after sitting on the shelf too long, it becomes stale and hard, and gets green and white furry spots growing on it. These signs of deterioration are readily visible to consumers. Milk from many dairies is mixed together when it is being processed for sale; thus, contamination at any one dairy potentially threatens thousands of consumers. Contamination is most likely to occur during the milking process, and can best be prevented by keeping the cows clean, the equipment sterilized, and all of the manure swept out of the barn. On-site inspection is the best way to cheaply enforce cleanliness, and can be performed at moderate cost by government agents, but it would be prohibitively costly for consumers to visit all the dairies their milk comes from each week and check the floors. Bacteria are killed during the processing of milk, but how is a consumer to know that the "pasteurized" label on the carton is to be believed? When the crucial quality control step can only be monitored efficiently during processing and is not easily discernable at point of sale, then government oversight and labeling are called for. Most of the dangerous bacteria that people can get from milk, particularly salmonella, do not make it curdle or smell bad, and are thus hard to detect. Milk is an ideal culture medium for many bacteria, so milk distribution is, in effect, a perfect way to spread diseases. Contamination from one farm cannot be determined later since milk from all the farms is mixed together. The bacteria will rapidly grow to infect all the milk and then are delivered invisibly, with much of the product going to the most vulnerable part of the population, children.

Many factors make milk more suitable for government regulation, but the crucial issue is what information consumers can easily obtain at the point of sale. Bad bread is visible to consumers, bad milk is not. The information necessary to protect the safety of the public is available at low cost if regulations are enforced *during production,* a process that would be prohibitively costly for consumers to carry out on their own. The asymmetry of information costs is what makes milk quality a public good, while the quality of bread is largely private.

Given the benefits of good information for both science and political management, it seems that there is often too little of it around. Problems frequently have to reach the crisis stage before the necessary information is collected, and decisions regarding thousands of lives or billions of dollars are made without adequate study. The difficulty lies in the conflict between individual and collective incentives. A lot of data may be quite useful in solving a public problem, but it is in the interest of no particular person to collect that data unless that person can benefit from it—and even if people can benefit, they will not be able to devote enough resources to the problem because their personal benefits are much less than the total benefits to society as a whole. To see more clearly why free-riding leads to persistent underproduction, it is necessary to consider the theory of pure public goods in more detail.[7]

17.3 THE THEORY OF PURE PUBLIC GOODS _____

Information is a public good, but it can be provided privately as well as publicly. For example, people may purchase cable TV by paying for each channel or show, or they may tap into a broadcast, which is a public good paid for through taxes, donations, advertising, or some other collective means. To more meaningfully address the question, "How much of a public good should society produce?" we will consider a simple society made up of three people: Ann, Bob and Carl, who can either purchase TV from the cable company at $5 per channel, or who can contribute through taxes to have the signal broadcast to everyone at a collective cost of $10 per channel. The private demand and supply for TV channels for Ann, Bob and Carl is shown in Figure 17.2a. The total private market demand for this three-person market is obtained by adding together horizontally the quantity demanded by each person at any given price, as shown in Figure 17.2b. For example, at a price of $10, Ann would purchase one channel, Bob would purchase three channels, and Carl would not purchase any channels, so total market demand at $10 would be 1 + 3 + 0 = 4. Similarly, at a price of $5 market demand would be 2 + 5 + 0 = 7, and at a price of $1 it would be about 3 + 7 + 4 = 14. The market

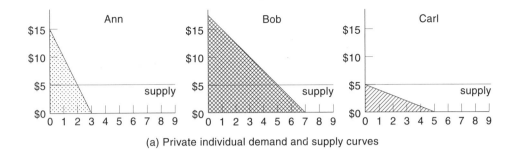

(a) Private individual demand and supply curves

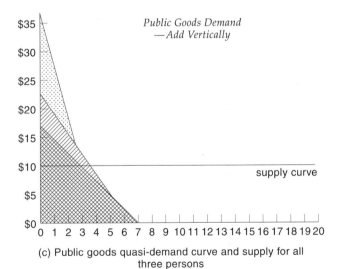

(b) Private market demand and supply for all three persons

(c) Public goods quasi-demand curve and supply for all three persons

FIGURE 17.2 *Public and private demand curves*

equilibrium with a perfectly elastic (flat horizontal line) supply curve at a price of $5 is for seven channels to be sold, two to Ann, five to Bob, and none for Carl.

The demand for a public good is quite different, since if the government provides one public channel, everyone gets to watch it. The value of that public good is the value of the service to each of the members of society all added together. In this example, the marginal value of the first channel is $10 to Ann, $15 to Bob, and

$4 to Carl, for a total social value of $29. Similarly, the second channel has a marginal value of $5 + $12.50 + $3 = $20.50, the third $0 + $10 + $2 = $12, and the sixth a marginal value of $0 + $2.50 + $0 = $2.50. Only Bob cares about having a sixth channel, and even he does not care very much. Whereas the quantities are added together horizontally in Figure 17.2b to find total market demand at a specified price for a private consumption market, the values are added together vertically at a specified quantity to find total social value for a public good as in Figure 17.2c.[8]

PUBLIC VERSUS PRIVATE DEMAND CURVES

Social Demand Curve for Public Goods: for each quantity Q,
$$\text{Value}_{\text{total}} = V_A + V_B + V_C$$

Market Demand Curve for Private Goods: for each price P,
$$\text{Quantity}_{\text{total}} = Q_A + Q_B + Q_C$$

The cost of broadcasting a channel to everyone is $10, twice as much as the price of providing it on cable to just one person. It is beneficial for society to produce more of the public good as long as the marginal cost is less than the additional value, so the social optimum is reached at the intersection of public good marginal cost "supply" curve and the public good quasi-demand curve. In this example, three channels would be supplied at a total cost of $30, since the marginal cost of a fourth channel ($10) exceeds the value to the members of society ($0 + $7.50 + 1 = $8.50).

Public Goods Make Most People Better Off, But Few Happy

In the private market, with channels selling for $5 each, Ann paid $10 for two and Bob paid $25 for five. Who will pay the $30 to broadcast three public channels? Suppose that a tax of $10 is collected from each person. Ann will be sort of indifferent to public versus private provision. Although giving up some flexibility, by participating in society she gets one additional channel for the same amount as she was previously paying. Carl is mad and wants to start a taxpayer's revolt. He paid nothing before and now must pay $10 for stations he barely wants. The consumer's surplus ($4 + $3 + $2 = $9) he obtains from getting three TV channels "for free" is worth less to him than the new TV taxes he has to pay. Carl has an incentive to understate his demand in order to get the government to provide less. He might say, "I hate the stuff, and as you can tell, don't watch it. If it has to be there, don't make me pay for it." If he could force the government to back down from the social optimum and provide just one channel, then he would be better off, although both Bob and Ann would then be worse off.

Bob loves TV and gets a large consumer's surplus. The value of three stations to him ($15 + $12.50 + $10 = $37.50) is far in excess of the new $10 TV tax. But he is not happy, either. He complains that he used to get five channels and now that the government has taken over, he only gets three! Bob wants to have five public stations. Although those two extra stations would cost $20, he would only get taxed to cover a third of the cost, or $6.67. To a certain extent, Bob would be a partial free-rider. He would push for even more TV channels than he would be willing to buy in a private market.

For public goods, cost–benefit analysis must replace market pricing as a mechanism for resource allocation and rationing. Voting and administrative procedures are used to make public decisions. In a private market, those people who value services more highly pay more to get them. Since a social optimum also depends on values, why doesn't government tax people more or less depending on how much they want the services? That not only seems unfair (imagine saying to a someone, "Since your accident forces you to stay immobile, we want to double your TV taxes"), it cannot readily be done because there is no way to tell how much someone values a public good. In a private market, the act of purchasing demonstrates a person's willingness to pay and reveals how much they value the good. With public goods, there is no purchase. In our example, both Bob and Carl watch all three public TV stations, but Bob values them much more. Suppose we sent out a questionnaire asking how much you like television in order to adjust each person's tax rates. Why should Bob be willing to reveal how much he likes TV and then pay more? His paying more will not increase the number of stations to watch. Conversely, Carl will say, "I don't care one bit, nothing, nada, zilch," since he would like to pay $0 and still be able to watch all three channels. That is why Figure 17.2c is only a *quasi* demand curve—it cannot show how people will behave, the choices they will actually make in a market, but only what we estimate they should do to optimize social value.

In order to get the government to provide more "free" services, Bob and people like him have an incentive to overstate their demand for TV if they do not have to pick up the extra tax personally, because most of the cost of expanding the broadcast will be born by the rest of the public. Since public goods are provided at no charge, there is no way to use market behavior to gauge demand. Everyone's self-interest would make them lie on a questionnaire in order to get more services. Conversely, when it comes time to pay, even Bob will claim that he doesn't like TV if checking off that box would lower his taxes—it will have no effect on the number of channels he gets to watch. Suppose that the number of channels broadcast is reduced if lots of people check "less" on their tax form. Won't Bob then have an incentive to reveal his true feelings and pay more? No. Whatever he does individually will have almost no effect on the outcome. If everyone else checks "less," the number of stations will be reduced anyway, so why should Bob sacrifice by paying more? The sensible thing for Bob (and every other interest group) to do is to act as a rational free-rider; always tell his congressperson that he wants more and his taxman that he wants less. There is no simple way to get everybody to agree on the social optimum once we consider not only the benefits, and who will get them, but also the costs, and who will pay them. The social value function is only a quasi-demand curve, because the voluntary actions of individuals will never allow society to reach the optimum, and lead only to name-calling, avoidance, and unstable coalitions (also known as "politics").

The provision of a public good poses two problems; how much of it to provide, and how to pay for it. Neither is solvable through individual action. For example, a swimming pool is a semi-public good after it is built; it does not cost very much to allow one more person in, yet people can be easily excluded. The pool could be paid for collectively through taxes, so that each person would pay the same, or would pay according to income. It is also possible to pay for the pool with user fees. This way the people who value swimming the most, and go often, will pay more. However, neither method will get us to the social optimum. If we depend totally on taxes, taxpayers will not be willing to build as many pools as the social demand curve would indicate. If user fees are imposed, then some swimmers (such as the poor ten-year-old who thinks she will be in the Olympics) will be denied entrance even though the marginal cost of using the pool is $0. The actual method chosen to fund a service depends on the transactions costs particular to that case. How purely public is the good? Can users be easily charged for use? (pools, yes; clean air, no; TV used to be no and is now yes, sort-of). Can we tell in advance what aggregate demand will be? Are people able and willing to acknowledge their demand up front and promise to pay or vote for the proposed program? (schools, maybe; venereal disease clinics, maybe not). Is a dedicated revenue source available? (like recurrent proposals to put a tax on hospital bills to fund indigent or preventive care, and the near-universality of room and airport taxes to extract money from tourists). Is anyone likely to sue?

Purchasing of public goods is problematic even if the money can be raised. Since no particular person has a comprehensive interest in making sure that all of the goods contracted for were delivered, or that the quality was adequate, a supplier may extract some of the social benefits by providing poor service or inferior goods. Even if we all want a good army, or hospital or national weather service, none of us individually is willing to spend our time making sure that those who are paid to provide those public goods are actually doing the job, and doing it efficiently. The free-rider problem goes beyond payment; it makes the enforcement of public contracts more difficult as well.

17.4 INFECTIOUS DISEASE EXTERNALITIES _____

One way of looking at the "publicness" of a good is to ask how much one person's action affects the welfare of other people. As discussed earlier, a mistake by the baker will have only a limited effect on consumers, while a failure in sanitary procedures at the dairy could cause illness or even death among thousands. Economists observe that milk shows more externalities than bread. There are more potentially harmful effects that are not part of the transaction. Infectious diseases are a classic example of externalities, and the basis for many public health laws as well. The author's first job was as a venereal disease (VD) investigator for the city of New York. Why were tax dollars used to pay civil servants to run around finding out who was infected, who they had sex with, and then to bring those people to the clinic for shots of penicillin? Didn't people who were infected already have sufficient incentive to come in for treatment? No. Infection creates externalities. The one who is infected bears the personal costs of disease and treatment, but does not bear the cost imposed on society of increasing everyone else's risk of infection. The divergence between private and social costs means that people are not sufficiently motivated to seek treatment. Consider what happens once you know that you are infected. Whether you get treated this week or next week may not make much difference to you, but may significantly affect the risk you impose on others.

Sexual transmission of diseases heightens the divergences between private and social costs of infection because social stigmatization makes information harder to come by. The desire for privacy increases transactions costs. With the flu, everyone knows when you are sick. With syphilis or gonorrhea, the symptoms are usually unobservable, even by your sexual partner. Whereas coughing is a costless signal of flu infection, you must be told that you have been exposed to VD. This is difficult for most people because it marks them as infected, and involves the admission that they have been having sexual relations with other people. While it is beneficial to society as a whole that all of your sexual partners be notified that you are infected, it is often quite costly to you personally—it may cost you some friends, a marriage, or a job. The U.S. Public Health Service (U.S.P.H.S.) developed a rule of anonymity to minimize the costs of acting in the interests of society. When sexual contacts are notified to come in for protective treatment, they are not told who has given their name. One client showed up with his wife and three girlfriends (yes, all at once, in the same room) and demanded to know who had been infected. While it may have been in his interest to know, violating confidentiality would have made it more difficult for the PHS to get people to cooperate by divulging sensitive information in the future. Part of the folklore of the Public Health Service is the story that Julius Rosenberg, who was charged and executed for treason for allegedly selling nuclear secrets to Russia, had reportedly been treated in one of the city VD clinics. When the FBI approached the PHS for his medical record, it was told that they were confidential and could not be used to try to find someone, even for criminal charges. Whether or not the story is strictly true, it served to build an ethos among investigators and a reputation for being uncompromisingly protective of patients' reputations that was very important to clients, and thus made private and social costs more closely aligned.

Day care centers provide a useful and familiar example of infection externalities. Parents with a child who is slightly sick, or might be coming down with a cold, face a difficult choice. If they stay home, they miss a day of work; if they send the child to day care, lots of other children may be exposed. The first cost is borne personally, but the costs of other children getting sick is a social cost borne by the other parents. Therefore, many busy parents faced with deadlines at work make a decision that is in their own best interest and drop the slightly sick child off at day care. Day care workers hate this and have developed a rule that if a child does get sick at school, the parents must come right away and take the child home or they will be fined and/or barred from the school. The school is deliberately trying to increase the costs of bringing in a sick child to force the parents to act in accord with the collective good, to take account of social costs.

Epidemics

Sudden upsurges in disease have had profound effects on the course of human civilization: the black death of the Middle Ages; the biblical plagues that afflicted the people of Egypt; tuberculosis, syphilis, a pandemic (worldwide epidemic) flu outbreak in 1918 that killed hundreds of thousands of young people; and most recently, AIDS.[9] The externality imposed by contagion was recognized long before germs were identified as a cause of disease. Quarantine was among the earliest forms of public health action. In primitive societies, those who were visibly ill were sometimes banished from the tribe. As early as 1400 A.D., ships from ports where plague had been reported were held out in the harbor for months to see if those on board started to die. Only after sufficient time had passed for the authorities to convince themselves that the ship was not carrying disease was it allowed to unload. Note how the public interest in disease reduction conflicted with the private interests of ship owners. Most of the costs of an epidemic (i.e., deaths) would fall on the population of the city, while the benefits of continuing to trade accrued to the merchants. The plot of the famous play "An Enemy of the People" by Henrik Ibsen centers on the disastrous consequences of ignoring the long-run risks of disease in order to pursue short-run profits.[10]

Leprosy may have been the first communicable disease to be brought under control by public health measures. Now known as Hansen's disease, after the scientist who discovered the causative agent, leprosy is a slow-growing virus that destroys the neural sheath and hence, sensation. The virus itself is often less damaging than the side-effects. Since a person with leprosy cannot feel pain in the affected area, they may scratch an itch until the flesh is gouged away, may get burned or be seriously infected without knowing it, and so on. The virus is hard to transmit from person to person, so that infection usually requires intimate contact over an extended period of time. People with leprosy were isolated from the rest of the population to halt the spread of the disease. Although the United States still had leper colonies until 1953, effective treatment with antibiotics has now removed the threat of contagion.

In the twelfth century, there were more than 200 hospitals for the confinement of lepers in France alone. Leprosy almost disappeared from medieval Europe as a health problem, and confinement or permanent quarantine in hospitals appears to have played a significant role in reducing the incidence of disease. But consider the cost. Leprosy is a progressive disease. Without treatment, the person sent to a hospital is being put away for life, without visitors. Indeed, the church would hold a funeral for the leper, the family would mourn, and all of the person's property would be passed on through inheritance just as if that person had died. Given that the signs and symptoms of leprosy (a scaly rash) are common to a variety of ordinary, non-serious disorders (psoriasis, scabies, skin allergy), making a diagnosis was difficult, and therefore many people without leprosy must also have been permanently confined in such hospitals (where presumably, they caught leprosy after a while, anyway). The uncertainty of diagnosis and the severe consequences probably made people very reluctant to visit the doctor or share information with neighbors. Claims of leprosy were more apt to be made against those who were not welcome within the society (gypsies, Jews), and a disgruntled family member or impatient heir might assert that the wealthy grandfather had leprosy purely out of self-interest. Permanent quarantine probably did help to protect the community, but at the cost of making the diseased individual a non-person. Only when explosive epidemics reached high rates of mortality did the interests of the community in disease prevention outweigh the interests of the individual in property and freedom to live.

AIDS

AIDS also provides illustrations of economic issues in disease control and public policy.[11] When first diagnosed, in the early 1980s, the costs of treatment were very high. The first official estimate, made in 1987, was $147,000 per case. Subsequent estimates became lower and lower over time. One reason for declining costs were economies of scale. As more cases were treated, unit costs went down. There was specialization of labor as dedicated AIDS units were set up, and movement down the learning curve as infectious disease specialists became better at managing the opportunistic illnesses that affect immuno-compromised persons. There was also a growing recognition that while medical care served an important humanitarian purpose, current treatment technology offered no effective cure and only a limited effect on length or quality of life. The marginal benefits of additional treatment were quite small.

AIDS also increased the insurance market failure, due to adverse selection. The association between frequency, type, and number of sexual partners and AIDS means that the individual may possess private information about risk not available to an insurance company. People who are HIV-positive know that they will need lots of medical care in the near future, so individual insurance policies covering AIDS offered in the open market would be swamped by buying from this 100 percent risk group. The inevitability of illness, given infection, makes it almost impossible for someone who is HIV-positive to change jobs and switch insurance plans if there is any exclusion of pre-existing conditions. The appearance of a fatal disease at an early age disrupts many kinds of economic relations. A bank might wonder why an 83-year-old man would borrow $250,000, and would be unwilling to lend without security since he no longer has a job, while a 33-year-old who is currently employed might want to borrow that much to buy a house and be readily approved. However, if this young man is HIV-positive, he might actually want the money to take care of his medical bills, and the living expenses of his partner, and figure that there is little that the bank will be able to do to collect on the debt once he has died. Therefore, the bank is inadvertently thrust into the role of supplying life insurance to people with high risks. (No life insurer is willingly going to write a policy for someone known to be HIV-positive). Developing the social mechanisms to deal with consequences of the AIDS epidemic for economic contracts will take a long while, and hopefully some cure will be available long before financial institutions have to make a full adjustment.

The Sanitary Revolution: A Moral Campaign for Public Health

The public health reforms that reduced the threat of cholera, diphtheria, typhoid, and other great epidemic plagues were part of the nineteenth century social revolution that imposed Victorian middle-class values on society as a whole.[12] The posters that attacked working conditions in the coal mines did not stress the fact that the workers had to eat stooped over while standing in pools of water that collected human sewage, but rather that women working underground were stripped to the waist because of the heat. Mandating that children under the age of twelve work no more than ten hours a day seemed an act of kindness, not an attempt to prevent premature disability. Above all else, Victorians hated dirt, and so the social reformers wanted cleanliness and light—which happened to be effective in reducing the spread of infectious diseases, although there was no way to know that given the science of the time. A belief in what was morally right, not scientific evidence, underlay the English sanitary revolution.

Not all of the attempts to remove dirt and immorality proved to be healthful. Sending women to maternity hospitals instead of having a midwife attend birth at home caused the spread of puerperal (childbirth) fever and a rapid increase in maternal mortality. The replacement of breast feeding with sterile bottles deprived middle-class infants of maternal immunities. Diseases of poverty, like pellagra, were so consistently blamed on lack of cleanliness and insects that the mounting evidence of dietary deficiency was ignored. The sanitary revolution did much to clean up the environmental mess created as industrial urbanization brought masses of people together in cities, but science was decidedly secondary to morality and ideology. The net result was beneficial overall, but quite unbalanced. These historical lessons are worth remembering as we attempt to evaluate the hazards of environmental carcinogens and other public health issues today.

Formation of the U.S. Public Health Service

The U.S. Public Health Service had it origins in the merchant seamen's hospital founded in 1798.[13] The rationale for government involvement was threefold. Seamen were engaged in international trade, and ships frequently carried diseases between countries, so the government had an interest in making sure that the seamen were willing to report any illnesses. Secondly, medical care was mostly provided at home by one's family, but sailors spent years abroad on ships and rarely had families to depend on. Ordinary laborers who were alone without kin and became sick or disabled were the responsibility of local communities, but sailors were travelers who might have been born in Boston or Chicago or Kankakee or anywhere, and thus could not rely on any town to support them in their time of need. Finally, international trade was vital to the economic growth of the nation. Unless the national government was willing to take care of those who became ill and disabled, few would have been willing to leave home and become sailors.

Public health activity was much more limited in the United States than England during the nineteenth century. American cities were not as old, or as crowded. There were fewer innovations in the United States, but the European social programs and sanitary reforms were quickly adopted. Massachusetts set up the first state board of health following the Shattuck report in 1850. By 1900, the New York City health department had become an active center with special supportive programs for immigrants, and free sterile milk distribution for young mothers and children. The Pure Food and Drug act was passed in 1906, and in 1920 the Shepard–Towner act provided the first national government-sponsored medical care for dependent mothers and children. Other milestones in U.S. public health history include the formation in 1952 of the National Institutes of Health, now by far the largest public health agency, to carry out medical research; the 1965 passage of amendments XVIII and XIX to the Social Security Act, which established Medicare and Medicaid; and the 1970 acts creating the Environmental Protection Agency (EPA) and the Occupational Safety and Health Agency (OSHA).

The establishment of Medicare for the elderly and Medicaid for the indigent are examples of government intervention to deal with market failure. The inability of the poor to buy necessary medical care is evident, and the public responsibility for doing so has already been discussed at length in the previous chapter, but why pay for the elderly? Medicare cannot be justified on the basis of poverty. Many young people are even more needy, and in fact, the wealthiest segment of the American population today are those aged 55–64. Universal public insurance for the elderly through Medicare was created to remove a major source of market failure—adverse selection (see chapter 4). For most people below the age of 65, health insurance risk pooling is based on employment, and there is little opportunity for people with above-average expectations of illness to select specific coverage—a worker just gets the health benefits that come with the job. Working people also have less reason to try and select special coverages since most of their illnesses are essentially random events. The situation is quite different for the elderly. They are not working, and do not naturally belong to a benefits group. Many of their illnesses are chronic. They may have a much better idea of their own expected expenses, relative to the average for all 70-year olds, than an insurance company can. Any attempt to offer coverage on an individual basis will lead to over-buying by those who know themselves to be sicker, and under-buying by those who know themselves to be healthier than average, that is, to adverse selection. With private information and no natural grouping, the basis for risk pooling breaks down. The market cannot provide insurance even though it would be beneficial. One way to eliminate the problem of adverse selection by the elderly is to insure everybody and pay for it through taxes. With Medicare, the risk pool is universal and no individual selection is possible.

17.5 SEX, DRUGS, AND WAR: PUBLIC HEALTH IN ACTION _____

Government uses police powers to enforce health and safety regulations. It acts as the agent of all citizens to carry out collectively beneficial activities more efficiently than any individual could on their own. Rules made by the people and for the people are not an intrusion on liberty, but a way of making the people more free by maintaining order. Government is not there to enforce public health standards because people are too ignorant to know what is in their own best interests. Instead, government exists so that citizens can remain rationally ignorant and devote their time to sports, making money, and art rather than checking the temperature at the pasteurization facility each hour. However, government does sometimes intercede directly against the will of the individual, overruling his or her own desires. Such paternalism is based not on ignorance, but on a determination that the individual is incompetent, and is thus reserved for certain classes who are assumed to be unable to make decisions on their own: children, addicts, the mentally ill and retarded.

Sexual behavior reveals some of the underlying value judgments that ultimately lie at the heart of any paternalistic decision to override individual decision-making authority. For centuries, children's sexual behavior fell under the control of parents because inheritance was a major form of economic exchange.

Thus, the rules regarding whom to have sex with for the aristocracy (who had inheritable land) were much different than for the peasantry, and aristocrats who were not allowed to have sex with the 17-year-old sons and daughters of neighboring lords could have sex with their serfs because any children born from such a union had no property rights.

Sexual preferences are quite value laden, with active debates over homosexual marriage, age of consent for sexual activity, and acceptability in the military or public office. Although difficult to imagine on a college campus with prominent gay organizations, the American Psychiatric Association until 1974 listed homosexuality as a disease, and young men and women were treated for having the illness of "abnormal" desires. The labeling of behavior as illness is not limited to homosexuality. Activities such as eating pork, piercing lips and noses, circumcision, lying down to sleep with the dead, taking hallucinogenic drugs, speaking in tongues, mortification of the flesh, and many other behaviors are seen as normal or exemplary in some cultures and as clear signs of illness in others. The line between use of power to "do something for your own good" and dictatorial thought control is not always easily drawn, and rarely more contentious than when it touches on the continuation of society through procreation. In one society, it may be routine for a young person to be taken to a prostitute or religious center for sexual initiation, while in another that would be seen as unbearably cruel.

Advocates for the mentally disabled are willing to push quite far for the fullest participation in "normal" activities, but are often placed in a quandary with regard to the desire of the mentally disabled to have children, especially when the disability is genetically related. Can that person understand the consequences? Is it fair to the unborn child? Even if the child has no genetic abnormalities, is it fair for them to be raised by parents whose capacity is severely constrained, or placed in a foster home? Externalities forcefully raise the question: Who counts, and do some count more than others?

Who Counts as a Citizen? Abortion and Other Dilemmas

Nowhere is the conflict over whose views are to count more apparent than in decisions regarding abortion. American society has been unable to achieve a clear resolution, and we shall not be attempting to do so here. What we can do is to see how abortion poses most critically a dilemma that affects many other problems in public health, and so use it to clarify the nature of a general issue: who is to be counted as a citizen, and do everyone's views count equally?

In the marketplace of third-century Rome, there was a law stating that no citizen could be sold a fish that was more than three days old (which, given the lack of refrigeration, seems plenty).[14] What happened to fish more than three days old? They were sold to noncitizens. Although this kind of blatantly discriminatory behavior seems inconceivable to us today, most countries, in fact, follow similar policies. Pharmaceuticals that are not approved for use in the United States are routinely sold overseas, and for years many of the drugs whose shelf life had been exceeded were disposed of profitably that way as well. The most forceful statement of who is not a citizen, and what the country is willing to do to protect and enrich those whom it does represent, is war.

Even more difficult questions are posed by pregnancy. The right of a mother to choose as the one most proximately involved seems reasonable, but it does notably elevate her rights over those of others. Could that position, if accepted logically, be used to claim that someone else was even more proximate (a grandparent for example, especially if the mother were incapacitated by addiction or illness)? It is also directly in conflict with the right to life of the unborn child—*if* such an entity can be said to be a citizen. In general, societies seem to accede that mothers have special rights over their infants, and this extends with even greater force to before their birth. Yet this interest is not absolute. Similarly, it is accepted that a fetus does not have the same standing as a child. Consider how differently a court would treat a pregnant woman who took heroin because she was anxious and upset from one who gave the drug to her baby to keep it quiet. There is no social resolution to these issues other than in crafting some new set of rules and in agreeing to live, however uneasily, within them. It is quite possible that for many years there may be two or more sets of rules in operation for different groups of people who can agree only not to talk about the issue, or to fight in the courts and the streets.

Ultimately the question of who counts as a citizen, and how much, is a moral one, but it is heavily conditioned by economic considerations, and transactions costs in particular. Experience has shown that it is virtually impossible to stop women who desperately want an abortion from having one. Making the practice illegal leads to many unsafe operations that cause infertility, disablement, and death. Furthermore, any woman who can afford an airplane ticket to a country where abortions are legal can do so; thus, the practical effect may just be to limit access for those who are young and poor and perhaps less able to care for a child. Indeed, the cost–benefit argument (that abortion is much cheaper than years of social services) may have sufficient appeal to some people so that their "moral" positions are influenced by it. How strongly we support another person's right to self determination depends in part on our own self-interest.

Addiction

Addiction, which is sometimes treated as a mental illness, also reveals the tensions surrounding overrule of the individual by the state. Economists do not really understand addiction, but then, neither do medical doctors. Many foods and substances are habit-forming, and many people have bad habits without engaging in self-destructive addictive behavior. Yet legally, a rather sharp distinction must be made between those substances that are legal (e.g., candy, coffee, cigarettes, alcohol) and those that are not (e.g., steroids, marijuana, cocaine, heroin). The distinction is sometimes as much social and historical as it is biological. Heavy alcohol use is probably more likely to impair judgment and lead to injury than marijuana, and heroin taken regularly over years has far fewer adverse physical effects than do cigarettes. Yet alcohol has been a part of human culture for thousands of years, and is thus not only well accepted, it is also subject to some social controls. Cigarettes are a relatively recent innovation. Only in the last fifty years have large numbers of people been able to afford to smoke many cigarettes daily. They are also a rather mild addiction and are cheaply available. Heroin, on the other hand, is such a powerful drug that some addicts will do almost anything to get it, and illegality raises the price so much that it becomes necessary to steal a lot each day to stay high. It is the externalities (stealing, dirty needles) rather than use that makes heroin so harmful to society. Cigarettes may be bad for your health, but they provide income to farmers, bring you all kinds of sporting events, elect senators and representatives, and contribute mightily to the profits of some large multinational firms. In trying to understand how morality is shaped by economics, it is useful to remember that the British Empire started a war with China to enforce their "right" to cross the border and sell opium to the Chinese workers, a practice that the Emperor wanted to prevent.

There is no way to fully separate the moral issues from the economic ones. Who is or is not a person, and how much their wishes are to be respected, is ultimately more than an economic decision, but is always conditioned by economic factors. Government usually acts as a collective agent to carry out the wishes of (most) people, not as an omniscient ruler dictating the standards of good behavior. Of necessity, borderline cases can never be solved to everyone's satisfaction, and there will always be conflict over the appropriate boundaries of action for criminal and social justice.

War and Public Health

A common wall poster during the 1960s read, "War is not healthy for children or other living things." Activity dedicated to killing seems obviously inimical to public health, and indeed, the American Public Health Association has passed several resolutions condemning war. Yet many advances in public health have been associated with war: Florence Nightingale's reform of field hospitals during the Crimean War led to modern nursing, malaria was eradicated during the Spanish–American War, and the campaign against venereal disease and development of rapid psychotherapy occurred during World Wars I and II. The number of times that medical breakthroughs occurred during or because of a war raises the question: How (un)healthy is war?

As economic historian Douglass North has pointed out, it is competition between states that forces them to meet the needs of the people.[15] A government with no rivals does not need to develop new technologies. When kings or countries are vying for people's loyalty, it is in their interest to build hospitals, clean up the water supply, and carry out all the other public health activities that are costly but also yield net benefits to society. North points out that we cannot understand the development of laws and political organization unless we recognize that rulers put their own interests first. War has a positive long-run effect on medical science because it heightens the interest of the rulers in the health of the population—sick civilians make lousy soldiers.

In every war throughout history, at least until the twentieth century, many more soldiers died from diseases than as a direct cause of wounds inflicted on the battlefield. Armies of 20,000 or more would gather and camp in an open fields with no toilets or running water. Contamination of food and drink were a more likely cause of death than enemy attack. Even in battle, it was often infection rather than bullets that killed, because lack of sanitation made minor wounds fatal. Conscripts were often drawn from isolated villages, and so had never been exposed to many common diseases. The result was uniformed disaster. Armies that spent any long period together were decimated by disease. Rulers' incentives for finding ways to keep large numbers of people living in close proximity without illness and epidemics were much greater than in peacetime.

When the United States entered World War I, the first thing it did was to call up an army of young, healthy men. To the chagrin of leaders at that time, one out of every four volunteers was found to be medically unfit for service. They had tuberculosis, or syphilis, or had vision so poor they could not shoot straight. Prior to this time, it had been assumed that Americans were much healthier than their European counterparts who lived in the old world under crowded conditions with less food. The 1917 mobilization was the first time that the nation had collected information on the health of its citizens on a large scale, and the results were appalling. After the war, campaigns for the control of diseases and malnutrition were promoted based on the data collected at induction centers.

The war also radically changed the practice of medicine. What had been a local trade practiced without a license was transformed in the army. Standards were set up to determine how diseases were to be treated, and which doctors should be in charge. Physicians who had never seen modern medicine were educated by three years of practice in an organized setting, with antiseptic surgery under anesthesia saving thousands of lives. New occupations were developed to assist the harried field surgeons, and the organization of medicine was decisively changed from solo individual practice to cooperative expertise centered in the hospital. Although most people had been quite skeptical of medical science at the turn of the century, the stories and living examples of what medicine could do were spread as the injured soldiers returned to homes throughout America.

War changes the calculus of individual costs and benefits. As the collective interest looms larger, massive investments in new knowledge and infrastructure are made. The attempt to place as many men as possible on the front lines leads to the rapid acquisition of knowledge on nutrition, surgery, psychology, and infectious disease. Without in any way ignoring the shameful horror of death and destruction that they impose on humankind, the fact that wars have been a powerful force in advancing public health must be recognized.

SUGGESTIONS FOR FURTHER READING_____

American Journal of Public Health and *Public Health Reports,* published monthly.

George Rosen, *A History of Public Health,* MD Publications: New York, 1958.

Paul Samuelson, "A Diagrammatic Exposition of a Theory of Public Expenditure," *Review of Economics and Statistics,* November 1955.

Institute of Medicine, *Public Health in Crisis,* Washington, D.C.: National Academy Press, 1990.

SUMMARY _____

1. A **pure public good** is something that is **consumed collectively** by all. It is indivisible so that **no one can be excluded** (0 charges), and one persons consumption has no effect on another's **(0 marginal costs)**. Examples are clean air, statistics, and the discovery of penicillin.

2. Many goods are mixed, both public and private. The degree of **"publicness"** of a good increases with **the number of people**, the use of **insurance**, and the **transactions, information, and measurement costs.**

3. Although decisions about private goods can be made through the market, the **indivisibility** of public goods **means that governments must make those decisions through voting,** political compromises, or cost–benefit analysis. Invariably, this means that there is a **moral or social justice** dimension, as well as an economic one.

4. **Externalities** are said to exist when the actions of one person affect another (e.g., smoking, disposing of garbage). Infectious disease externalities have shaped most of public health from the foundation of the U.S.P.H.S. as the homeless seaman's hospital to the pasteurization of milk. The increased risk of infecting others is a cost that the individual does not bear, and government intervention is required to achieve (or, get closer to) an optimum level of prevention.

5. In order to improve public health, it is necessary to determine exactly **who "the public" is**; whether some people or **some preferences count more than others.** Conflict over who is and is not worthwhile or able to decide lie at the heart of some of the most contentious public health issues: abortion, addiction, and care of the mentally disabled.

6. Peoples **attitudes toward a particular public good** are always affected by their **private interests**. Universal access to high-quality medical care health care and redistribution of income *may* be an important public good. Whether or not you think so depends a lot on whether you are poor or identify with those who are.

7. **Competition** between governments over the provision of public goods may be just as important as competition between people or firms in creating economic efficiency, and particularly in **forcing beneficial change over time.**

PROBLEMS _____

1. {*property rights, public goods*} Why is most drug research paid for by companies while most medical research is paid for by the government?

2. {*public goods*} Explain which item in the following pairs is more "public" and why:

   AIDS or lung cancer?

   Milk or bread?

   Saturday morning cartoons or Sunday night late show?

   Stroke or lung cancer?

3. {*externalities*} Why not charge people full price for vaccinations?

4. {*welfare*} Which type of good is apt to have a larger consumer's surplus, a public good or a private good? Why?

5. {*property rights, scale*} Why have wars often given rise to improvements in medical technology?

6. {*property rights*} Caring for the poor costs money, much more than they are able to pay directly or in taxes. Why would different government jurisdictions compete to provide medical care for the poor?

7. {*incidence, voting*} There are many goods that are desired by some people and not by others. Since diversity of tastes is universal, why does it create more problems for public goods than for private goods?

8. {*aggregation*} Draw the demand and supply curves for (a) a public good and (b) a private good for two people, Adam and Barbara, and also (c) the market demand for a two-person (Adam + Barbara) market.

9. {*exclusivity, marginal cost*} Some forms of health care are public because the marginal cost of serving additional persons is zero, while other types of health care are public even though marginal costs are positive, because it is impossible to exclude beneficiaries even if they don't pay, while some forms of care meet both criteria, zero marginal costs, and a lack of exclusivity. Give examples of all three categories (recognizing that no real goods or services are perfectly public or entirely in one category or another).

10. {*welfare*} Why pay economists to do a cost–benefit analysis if the market will show the value of some new medical technology to consumers?

11. {*public goods*} Which has more externalities, cigars or chewing tobacco? Guns or knives? Laptop computers or portable telephones?

12. {*externalities*} What are the externalities of heroin addiction?

ENDNOTES _____

1. After seventeen years, other firms can manufacture the drug in generic form if they meet certain standards and obtain approval from the FDA. See chapter 13 and also Sam Peltzman, *The Regulation of Pharmaceutical Innovation: the 1962 Amendments,* Washington, D.C.: American Enterprise Institute, 1974.

2. Elizabeth Fee and Steven Corey, *Garbage: The History and Politics of Trash in New York,* New York: New York Public Library, 1994.

3. Donald A. Dunn and Aristides C. Fronistas, "Economic Models of Information Services Markets," in Robert Goldberg and Harold Lorin, editors, *The Economics of Information Processes,* New York: Wiley, 1982, Vol. 1, pp:141–162; Michael R. Rubin, *Information Economics and Policy in the United States,* Littleton, Colo: Libraries Unlimited, 1983.

4. Bruno Latour, *The Pasteurization of France,* Cambridge, Mass: Harvard University Press, 1988.

5. John Graunt, *Natural and Political Observations on the Bills of Mortality,* London (1662), see Charles Creighton, *A History of Epidemics in Britain,* 2nd Ed., New York: Barnes & Noble, 1965, p.532.

6. George Rosen, *A History of Public Health,* New York: MD Publications, 1958, pp: 354–60.

7. The classic paper setting out these results is Paul A. Samuelson, "A Diagrammatic Exposition of a Theory of Public Expenditure," *Review of Economics and Statistics,* November 1955.

8. Note how difficult pricing is in the real world of broadcasting. The network stations are in effect "priced" by making the consumer watch advertisements, while the "PBS public broadcasting" uses a mixture of taxes and voluntary donations. Such pricing problems, and the blandness of much government programming, may also explain why cable and satellite TV are doing so well in newly developing countries.

9. David Rosner (ed.), *Hives of Sickness: Public Health and Epidemics in New York City,* New Brunswick, NJ: Rutgers University Press, 1995.

10. Henrik Ibsen, "An Enemy of the People" (1882) in *Henrik Ibsen, The Complete Major Prose Plays,* translated by Rolf Fjelde, New York: Farrar, Strauss, Giroux, 1978, pp: 277–388.

11. Paul Farnham, "The Economic Cost of HIV/AIDS," in J.M. Pogodzinski, ed., *Readings in Public Policy,* Cambridge, Mass.: Blackwell, 1995. Recently there have been a number of press reports that a new type of treatment using protease inhibitors may be effective against the HIV virus, but only under such strict treatment regimens and at such great cost that a new set of economic issues is raised.

12. George Rosen, *A History of Public Health,* New York: MD Publications, 1958.

13. Odin Anderson, *Health Services as a Growth Enterprise in the U.S. Since 1875,* Ann Arbor, Mich.: Health Administration Press, 1990.

14. George Rosen, *A History of Public Health,* New York: MD Publications, 1958.

15. Douglass North, *Structure and Change in Economic History*, New York: Norton, 1981.

CHAPTER **18**

Dynamics of National Health Spending

QUESTIONS

1. *How does a person decide the right amount to spend each year?*
2. *How does the nation decide the right amount to spend on health?*
3. *Why do general tax revenues pay for so much of personal health care? Who will pay when the Medicare trust fund runs out of money?*
4. *Which is more important as a determinant of health care spending, how sick people are or how much money is available to spend?*
5. *What determines the level of wages in the health care industry?*
6. *Is it easier to adjust to growth or to a recession?*
7. *Does professional licensure, third-party reimbursement, and nonprofit organization make it easier or harder to adjust to changes in prices? Would delays in adjustment cause any real problems?*
8. *Will inflation affect health care spending? Permanently or only temporarily?*
9. *Do price controls work? If not, why might people think that they do?*

18.1 THE CONSUMPTION FUNCTION _____

How much should we as a nation spend on health care? This is the central public policy issue of health economics. It cannot be determined once and for all, but must be decided over and over again each year as conditions and opportunities change. The amount that individuals spend varies, primarily because their health status changes. For the nation as a whole, individual changes in health status tend to average out; for every group of people getting sick, there are patients getting well; for every group of people dying, others are being born. Thus, at the aggregate (national) level, there is little change in the biological need for medical care. What does change is the condition of the economy, which affects the ability to pay for medical care, and the state of medical technology, which determines what we get for all of the billions of dollars spent.

The factors that affect how much one person spends, and the factors that affect how much the nation spends, are not necessarily the same. Thus, the answer to the question, "What determines how much will be spent?" depends on the framing of the question. This chapter uses a macro perspective, but will make connections with the individual perspective to point up both similarities and disparities between the micro and macro economics of health.

The determination of how much people spend is known as the *consumption function*. If we include all possible uses of income, including savings, then people must spend exactly as much as they earn. A 10 percent increase in income will be exactly matched by a 10 percent increase in spending. By construction, the budget-weighted average income elasticity for all goods is unity, 1.0. Economists are interested in why a particular component such as food, or entertainment, or medical care, increases more or less than proportionately as income increases. Although required as one of the categories to arithmetically close the unit elasticity equation, "saving" is quite different from all other consumption categories, profoundly affecting interest rates, growth, the price level, and many additional macroeconomic variables.

When the Great Depression struck in 1929, there did not initially seem to be any reason for it. The country had just had ten years of prosperity following the first World War, the stock market was booming, and money was everywhere—but people were not buying enough to keep things booming. As demand went down, firms began to cut back, people were thrown out of work and could not afford to buy, then firms cut back more, or went bankrupt. This downward spiral and its causes were the most immediate concern of economists in the 1930s. Prior to 1929, it had been speculated that recessions and depressions were caused by droughts, floods, plagues, and other disruptions of supply; this depression, however, seemed to spring from a deficit in demand. John Maynard Keynes, whom many credit as the greatest economist of the modern era, developed a plausible theory based on an analysis of the consumption function.[1] While Keynes's theory was ultimately shown to be incorrect, his work began a chain of analysis and debate that led to a useful theory of the consumption function that does largely explain how and why national health expenditures respond to macroeconomic changes.

Surveys of consumption carried out in many countries had consistently shown that people in the higher income categories saved a larger fraction of their incomes than those with less income. The empirical generalization that the percentage of income saved rises as income rises was first articulated by Ernst Engel in 1853, and became known as Engel's Law.[2] Although these consumption studies had all surveyed individual behavior, Keynes generalized to a macroeconomic context and asserted that national savings also followed Engel's law: the higher the income, the larger the proportion saved. He put this concept into mathematical terms as:

$$\text{Consumption} = \alpha + \beta Y \quad (\text{Keynes})$$

The cefficient, β, is the fraction of income (Y) spent on goods and services, which Keynes termed the *marginal propensity to consume*. The regression constant, α, is the amount that would be consumed even if income were zero. Looking at Figure 18.1, we can see immediately the implications of Keynes's formula. Even though the marginal propensity to consume is constant, the *average* propensity to consume falls as income rises. At low income levels, consumption is greater than income, whereas at higher income levels, savings accumulate. As income becomes higher and higher, saving grows even more rapidly because the fraction of total income is growing. Keynes thought that, under certain conditions, this growing pool of savings available for investment could lead to a collapse in demand and an increase in unemployment.

Unemployment, bank failures, and all of the other dislocations caused by the recurrent boom and bust business cycles made it imperative to develop measures of macroeconomic activity so that these new theories could be tested, and so that forecasts of the economy could be developed. A whole generation of economists devoted much of their professional effort to creating the measures of gross domestic product (GDP), money supply, inflation, and employment that we now take for granted. The phrase *gross domestic product* was first used in 1937 by Simon

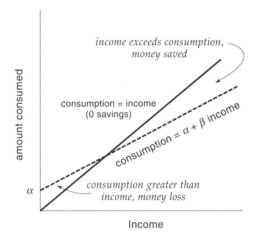

FIGURE 18.1 Keynesian Consumption Function. *People consume some constant amount α plus a percentage β of their total income. Therefore, people at low incomes consume more than they earn, and so have negative savings (loss), while high-income people consume less than they earn, and so accumulate savings.*

Kuznets, who played a leading role in developing not only the concepts, but also the data collection and statistical measures. Kuznets's studies of savings rates over the period 1869–1941 showed that while average per capita income for the nation as a whole had increased threefold over this timespan, the average fraction of income saved had remained constant.[3] These results regarding aggregate national consumption contradicted the results of studies on individuals and the Keynesian consumption hypothesis. Whereas analysis of consumption across individuals at a point in time (cross-sectional analysis) showed an income elasticity of less than 1.0, which is to say that individuals with higher incomes saved a *higher percentage* of their incomes, analysis of aggregate national data (macroeconomic time-series) gave the contrary result that income elasticity equaled 1.0 over a broad range. Thus, the nation's average propensity to consume and the fraction of income saved *did not change* as income rose. How could these disparate results be reconciled?

The answer came from the efforts of one of Kuznet's assistants, Milton Friedman. In the project of constructing a GDP accounting system during the 1930s, he had been given the task of measuring the income of doctors, lawyers, and engineers.[4] For most workers, if income data were missing, it could be replaced by an estimate using the amount spent on food and housing. Yet this group of self-employed people was causing great difficulty because their spending did not correspond to their income. What Friedman discovered was that professionals whose income varied greatly from year to year did not match spending and income in each year, but over the longer term. They tended to spend in accordance with what they *expected* to earn on average, which he termed their **permanent income**, rather than their actual income for any particular year. The apparent overspending of "low" income lawyers was actually a rational response of those lawyers continuing to spend at an average level even during a bad year, and the heavy savings of "high" income lawyers was the corresponding effort to put extra aside during a good year. Friedman generalized from the behavior of these self-employed professionals to explain why average consumption would appear to fall with income even when it really did not, using the graph shown below in Figure 18.2.

The low-current-income group earning $10,000 this year is made up of some people who are truly poor, but also some who are only temporarily poor—lawyers waiting for their big case to settle, for example. Thus, their true "permanent income" should be higher. On the contrary, the high-current-income group earning $90,000 this year contains some people who are usually average or even low income, but just happened to have one good year (e.g., got a big court settlement), thus their expected permanent average income is lower than their current income. Hence, measuring income by surveys imparts a systematic bias: "low"-income people will, in the long run, actually have a bit more than is measured, and "high"-income people a bit less. Therefore, what appears to be too much consumption by low income people is actually a result of misclassification based on survey responses. Similarly, the excess savings of apparently high income people is also a rational response to one lucky year. Once adjustment is made for the difference between people's actual long-run permanent income and the survey-measured-income at a point in time, analysis shows that *the average propensity to consume permanent income does not decline as income rises.* Thus, we arrive at Friedman's permanent-income (y^*) formula for consumption spending.[5]

What is actually happening in the **long run**   What *appears* to happen in the **short run**

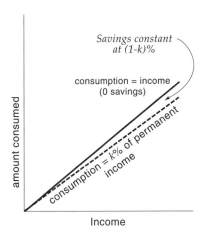
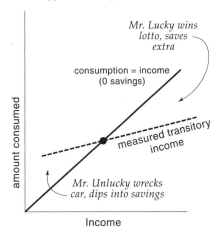

FIGURE 18.2   Friedman's Permanent Income Hypothesis. *People consume a constant fraction* k *of their permanent long-run income. Average income people who temporarily have high incomes (won lotto, just got a bonus, peak earnings before retirement) put aside excess savings for the bad years. Average-income people who temporarily have low incomes (lost lotto, made no sales this month, still in school or retired) use savings to maintain average*

$$C = k\mathbf{Y}^*   \text{[Friedman]}$$

The marginal propensity to consume (labeled β in Keynes' formula) is signified by "k" in Friedman's formula. Friedman asserts that there is no fixed consumption without income (i.e., that the constant α in Keynes' formula is equal to zero when permanent rather that temporary measures of income are used), and therefore the marginal propensity to consume is the same as the average propensity to consume at all income levels (Figure18.2, left panel).

Friedman's central point is that consumption is determined by what people expect to earn over the long run ($\mathbf{Y}^*$), not by current income. Franco Modigliani extended this insight when he observed that people's income varies predictably over the course of their lifetime; they earn little until age 25 or so, reach peak earning power at age 55, and then taper off until retirement.[6] Consumption is not matched in each period to earnings, but spread over the lifecycle. During peak years, people save extra so they will not starve during retirement. Similarly, young people are willing to go into debt, to travel, and to buy a house during their twenties, because they expect their earning power to increase over time. This "lifecycle" hypothesis yields the same empirical result as Friedman: people whose measured income at this point in time is low (retiree's, medical students) may actually have quite high expected long run income, and hence consume more than would seem to be justified by their current incomes. Conversely, some of those whose income is currently high at this point in time are actually at a temporary peak and trying desperately to pay off debts accumulated when they were young, while also attempting to save enough for retirement. The logic of the Friedman and Modigliani theories are parallel, since both are based upon the fluctuation of income over time. Hereafter, the term *permanent income* is used to refer jointly to both ideas. After five decades of research, the **permanent income hypothesis** has been repeatedly verified and is a cornerstone of modern macroeconomics.

18.2 SHARED INCOME _____

The divergence between individual and national income elasticities is much larger for health care than for most other types of consumption. Studies of individuals show that utilization of medical resources is only slightly related to income (elasticities of 0.0 to 0.4), but studies of nations always show that rich nations spend much more on health than poor nations (with income elasticities always greater than 1.0). The reason for the divergence is that an individual's ability to consume medical care is based not on his or her own personal income, but on the average income level of all the people in their community, in their insurance plan, and in the nation as a whole. Consider two people within an insurance plan that pays 95% of all hospital bills. Of course there is a tremendous variation in hospital use that depends upon whether or not a person is sick (health status), but we will assume that both members of this insurance plan, a file clerk and the chief financial officer, have the same illness. These two people will probably not live in the same type of house, drive the same type of car, or take the same vacations, but they will get pretty much the same hospital care. Even if the clerk is not making much money, most of the hospital bill is already taken care of. It would be foolish for him not to take advantage of his employee benefit package when he is sick just to save a few dollars. Now consider the head of finance. There is very little more medical care that he can buy, no matter how much he is willing to spend. If he wants to have the new gene therapy or positron scans he has read about, that decision is up to the medical staff, not him. Indeed, every effort is made to keep such medical decisions from being influenced by payment considerations. This is not to say that there are no differences in the treatment of the rich and the poor, but the differences are deliberately kept small by the professional ethics within the system. Government provision of care for the poor, and tax subsidies of health insurance, are a part of that system. Their consequences are not an accident, but is a reason that these policies receive wide public support. *Insurance converts personal medical care into a public good*, and as a society we have collectively decided that reasonable access to quality health care should be available to all citizens.

For public goods, like immunization or clean air, it is society's willingness to pay that determines how much is to be provided (see Figure 17.2). Since everyone is able to consume the same amount of a public good, individual income is irrelevant except insofar as it contributes to the total tax base. For a public good, or within a group insurance plan, the individual's income is not a binding budget constraint. It is possible to spend more curing one child than that child could earn in three lifetimes, and the spending to clean up the air in Los Angeles is hundreds of times greater than the money earned by any Hollywood star. It is the resources available to the group as a whole that determines the average level of spending.

The "shared-income hypothesis" implies that income will become more and more important as a determinant of spending as the unit of observation is increased to match the budgetary unit. For individuals, income is relatively unimportant, and income elasticities are near 0. For small areas, such as a census tract, average per capita incomes are somewhat more important, with income elasticities rising to perhaps 0.4. For counties or states, their budgets are a constraint, but it is still possible to obtain money from the federal government. Per capita income is significantly more important than health status, and elasticities are about 0.9. For the nation as a whole, the budget constraint is binding. No other country is going to reimburse our medical bills. Every dollar paid to doctors, nurses, or drug companies must be collected in taxes, insurance premiums, or direct fees. Income thus becomes the dominant determinant of spending at the national level, with elasticities greater than one, usually about 1.3 (see chapter 19, Figure 19.2).

18.3 DYNAMICS

If per capita income falls, then health care spending must also inevitably fall. However, it is impossible to make the adjustment all at once. Usually the country goes into debt during the transitional period. Even for an individual, adjustment to changes in income are not instantaneous. If you were to lose your job today, you would not immediately move into a smaller apartment, drive an older car, or wear less fashionable clothes. In fact, if you lose your job today you will probably go out and spend a little extra money to keep up your spirits. Next week you will cut back, but not too much, because you probably expect to find another job soon. If the recession drags on, and you are still out of work six months later, then you begin to find that your clothes and your house and your car start looking worse. Once you do get a job, it will take years to build your savings back up.

When college students graduate and begin to earn good wages, they find it easy to live and save part of their salary because their consumption lifestyles are still somewhat geared to being a student, and have not moved upward as quickly as their incomes. During this "I can't figure out how to spend it all" period, savings accumulate. Later on, with the fancy lifestyle appropriate to a young stockbroker or lawyer, it is hard to see how one could have lived on so little money as a student, or even on what one made three years ago. Consumption is geared to expected income, whether $5,000 or $50,000. The amount of income saved depends not so much on how high the income is, but on transitional (permanent income/lifecycle) factors, and to what extent a person desires to give up current pleasures for future consumption.[7] If a young lawyer who has just bought a new Mercedes loses his job, he will discover one of the underlying asymmetric truths of human behavior: it is a lot easier and more fun to adjust upward rather than downward.

The dynamics of adjustment for individuals (micro) and for nations (macro) are similar, except that it usually takes longer for macro adjustment, because the system itself must undergo structural change. We must convince people who have not lost their jobs that it is necessary to cut back, to reduce the provision of public goods, or to change the tax code. Achieving a consensus to alter organizations and revise institutional structures is very time-consuming. The health care system, being based on a shared public understanding of professional ethics and obligations, and heavily dependent on complex public and private financing mechanisms, is more difficult to change than other sectors of the economy. In the stock market, expectations of the future are traded every day, and prices change by the minute. Commodity sectors, such as farming and metals, are also forced to respond quickly due to market discipline. Although the housing stock cannot change rapidly, housing sales are very sensitive to macroeconomic conditions. The decision to buy is based on the individual's assessment of job prospects. The effective price of a house is the monthly mortgage payment, and that depends on interest rates, which are volatile and forward looking. For both of these reasons, housing tends to be one of the sectors that leads the economy into or out of a recession. Health care is slow to change, and lags behind other sectors in adjusting to macroeconomic conditions.

How long does it take for health care to adjust? From one to five years on average, but some parts take even longer. Even if everyone in Congress decided today that we need more or less health care, those decisions could not be carried out for months, and their full effects would take years to work their way through the system. A decision to expand the supply of doctors was made in the early 1960s. For a medical school to accept more students takes at least a year, and the building of new medical schools takes much longer. Once the students are there, it takes them four years to graduate and another three or four years to do a residency and enter practice. Thus, eight years after a decision to expand has been made, there are still no extra doctors in practice. Something could be done to slightly reduce the rate of retirement, but effectively the quantity of doctors in practice who graduated in year "19xx" is fixed once they leave school. It took twenty years for the impacts of the 1964 decision to expand physician supply to be felt in force—and by then Congress had changed its mind. It takes forty years, until all the graduating physicians have retired, before the full effects work through the system.

Not everything in health care takes as long to adjust as physician supply. Nurses are much more flexible because there are typically a large number who are licensed but temporarily not working, or only working part-time, and so any increase or decrease in demand is quickly translated into a change in the numbers employed. Clerical, maintenance, and other less-specialized labor adjusts even more smoothly and rapidly since people can move between health services and other sectors of the economy in response to changing conditions. Although we do not have data to look at each segment of the health care sector separately, the National Health Expenditure Accounts maintained by the U.S. Health Care Financing Administration to track aggregate health care spending (that is the analogue to the National Income and Product Accounts maintained by the Department of Commerce to track GDP and the economy as a whole), do categorize spending into hospital, physician, dental, nursing home, and so on, and enable us to examine the patterns of adjustment separately for each of these components.

Hospitals, the largest component of health care expenditure, are quite rigidly institutionalized and dependent upon public or third-party financing. As one would expect, they took a bit longer to adjust, 3.0 years, than the average for all medical spending, 2.7 years.[8] Physician services are somewhat more flexible and adjust a bit more quickly, with a lag of 2.5 years. Spending on drugs, much of which depends on direct consumer decisions and is paid for out-of-pocket with current income, takes only 1.3 years. Long-term care, which is a mixture of flexible personal spending and rather inflexible Medicaid spending, adjusts in 2.5 years on average. The component that takes the longest to adjust is construction, at 3.5 years. This makes sense, because capital must be accumulated in advance to fund new construction, and the decision to build depends on long-run future economic considerations, not just revenues and expenses today. The estimated average lag for adjustment of dental spending, 2.5 years, seems longer than one would expect since most dental bills are paid by individuals with limited third-party reimbursement, are a result of personal decisions, and occur in an office setting rather than within the large institutions. However, this estimate is the least reliable statistically, and may just reflect how hard it is to pinpoint the timing of adjustment in a complex area with many segments and sub-segments. Consider hospital expenditures again. Because of the way the NHE Accounts are kept, construction was listed as a separate component so we could see that it took longer to adjust than labor. If supplies had been listed separately, they would probably be seen to adjust even more quickly. The "average lag" is just that, an average. Some parts are moving faster, and some slower. It is also an average over time—in some periods the organization may respond more quickly than others. In particular, it appears that managers are quicker to step up purchasing when the economy expands than they are to cut back when the economy contracts. Everyone hopes that a slowdown is just temporary, and delays firing people or closing clinics. The time required to adjust also depends on the magnitude of the change. The statistical techniques used here can only pick up changes in the one-to-ten year range, but a truly massive revision of the system, such as occurred in 1965, may take several decades to complete. It can be argued that one reason health spending is so high in the United States is that we are still stuck with a health care system constructed on the lines of the Great Society envisioned during the 1960s, when economic growth was steady and strong. This system is not appropriate to the more constrained conditions prevailing in 1996.

Permanent Income and Adjustment of Health Spending to GDP

Adjustment is slow because the nation makes commitments that change the structure of the health care system, and affect spending for many years. Indeed, the reliability of government is based on a stable set of rules that are rigid, changing only slowly and with the consent of the citizenry. Once we have created a medical care financing system for the elderly through Medicare, it is a contract whose amendment must be worked out through the courts, the legislature, and public opinion. What are the dynamic consequences of slow and lagging adjustment? Most importantly, it buffers the economy. During a downturn, Medicare and Medicaid spending tend to continue so that workers are less likely to lose jobs in health care than in farming, housing, or financial services sectors. Conversely, any increase in employment during a recovery is also delayed. This has some adverse budgetary consequences. Since spending continues to rise in a recession even though government tax revenues are falling, a deficit builds up. In theory, such periods of excess spending average out over time with underspending during boom periods of rapid growth. The difficulty is that it is easier to gain agreement to pour money into the health sector and save jobs during a recession than it is to hold back and save money during good times. In a recession, everyone hopes that normal growth will soon return, and they will bend the spending rules to temporarily soften the impact of macroeconomic disorder. A boom feels so good that people do not want to remember that such high growth rates are abnormal, that another recession is bound to come eventually. It is more popular to claim that this time is different and we never need to go hungry again—and therefore, that we do not need to save up for bad times, or even give up much current consumption to pay off old debts.

Consideration of the costs and benefits to politicians makes this argument even more compelling. Politicians want to get elected. They need results that will affect the economy and the voters in the near term. Extra government spending during a recession meets those needs; extra savings when the economy starts to grow again do not. The benefits of a balanced budget—a reputation for prudence and a trust in the currency leading to price stability and steady or falling foreign exchange rates, stable conditions that allow business to invest long term in productivity improvement, and a modest but sustainable path of optimal growth—are long term. But none of these benefits can be realized quickly enough to help the politician worried today about the next election. In a pinch, a politician (or a professor) will sacrifice the long-run good that falls mostly to others in favor of the near-term benefits they can capture for themselves. It is hard to get politicians to behave in the long-term public interest, because it is hard to get voters to behave that way. One consequence of the asymmetry in political adjustment costs are well known to all economics students—a U.S. deficit of a trillion dollars. Eventually, just like the out-of-work lawyer running up his charge cards, we will have to bring spending back into line and balance the budget. But that is in the long term, and the elections keep coming up fast.

Adjustment to Inflation

Adjustment to inflation is an area that shows how micro and macro can differ. The slow adjustment of the health care sector to inflation means that during a period of rising prices, spending is less than expected rather than more.[9] To see why, trace carefully through the process of adjusting spending to changing price levels as illustrated in Table 18.1. Suppose that a hospital spent $100,000 in the year 2000, and wanted to spend the same amount in real terms (FTEs of manpower, gallons of fuel, square feet of office space, etc.) in each succeeding year. If the anticipated rate of inflation is 5 percent, then 105 percent of year 2000 spending will be budgeted for the year 2001; that is, $105,000. If actual inflation equals the expected 5 percent, then the same quantity of all inputs can be bought with the year 2001 budget. Inflation for the year 2002 is again expected to be 5 percent, so $110,250 is

TABLE 18.1 Adjustment to Inflation

	2000	2001	2002	2003
nominal spending	$100	$105	$110	$123
price index	100	105	117	123
real spending	$100	$100	$94	$100

Table 18.1: Hypothetical example of adjustment to inflation. The hospital tries to spend exactly the same amount ($100 in year 2000 dollars) in each year. In the first year, inflation is 5% and spending increases 5%, so there is no change in real deflated expenditures. In the second year, spending increases by 5% again, but inflation is 12%, so the real spending power declines. In the third year, inflation is 5%, and the hospital catches up by increasing spending 12% (7% to catch up and 5% for current inflation).

budgeted. However, actual inflation turns out to be 12 percent in that year. The budget does not buy $100,000 in constant inflation-adjusted dollars, but only $110,250 ÷ (105 + 12) = $94,000. With a 12 percent rise in prices, the budgeted 5 percent wage increase given to employees leaves them worse off, with less purchasing power. The budgeted 5 percent increase in the supply budget is not enough, and so some equipment purchases will have to be cut back. In the year 2003, inflation is expected to be 5 percent, and does actually turn out to be 5 percent. However, the hospital has to make up for the lost purchasing power due to underestimating inflation the previous year, so the budget for 2003 will be up 12 percent to $123,480. Having caught up, spending will once again be $100,000 in real (year 2000) terms (see last line of Table 18.1).

National health spending shows this type of lagging adjustment to unexpected changes in the price level for several reasons. First, the government and nonprofit organizations like hospitals usually set a budget at least a year in advance, which limits their flexibility. Second, most wage contracts run for at least one, and usually several years. A set of inflation adjustments is already built in to those raises, and any difference between what the negotiators expected to happen to prices and what actually happens falls on the workers. If inflation is less than expected, they are lucky and can buy more. If inflation is worse, then they have to tighten their belts. Estimates taken from the U.S. Bureau of Labor Statistics data on average wages for the health care sector indicate that for any 1 percent change in the rate of inflation, only about 0.5 percent shows up in the first year's wages, and another 0.3 percent in the following year. It takes three years for wages to fully adjust to a change in inflation. In the long run, all wages do adjust so that inflation is neutral—neither raising nor lowering real health care spending. The government can only temporarily trick workers and firms into accepting a dollar that is only worth $0.90. Any government that tries to "save" money by printing lots of currency ends up with chronic inflation like Brazil, or Russia after Gorbachev. Therefore, most governments aim for price stability and a sound currency. Yet the year-to-year fluctuations caused by temporary inflation adjustment problems may be larger than any real changes in health spending due to GDP growth or changes in health care policy.

The distorting effects of a surge in inflation are shown in Table 18.2, which traces prices and employment for Canada during the oil price shock of 1973. Inflation, which had previously been averaging 3 to 5 percent, suddenly leapt to 9

TABLE 18.2   How Inflation Distorts Reported Health Expenditures

CANADA	Inflation	Employment		Ratio	Health Share of GNP
		Nurses	Total		
1972	5.6%	152,005	8,447,000	.0180	7.3
1973	8.9%	159,274	8,860,000	.0180	7.0
1974	14.4%	168,530	9,220,000	.0183	6.9
1975	9.8%	177,182	9,364,000	.0189	7.4

Table 18.2: Inflation rates, nurses and total employment, and health spending as a share of GNP show how sudden price increases distort budgetary measurement of the relative size of the health sector. *Source:* OECD 1990.

percent in 1973, peaked at 14 percent in 1974, and remained high at 10 percent in 1975. However, by this time the health sector had begun to build in expectations of high inflation. It looks as if spending, measured by the fraction of GDP devoted to health care, fell during 1973 and 1974. However, real resources, as measured by the number of nurses working in the Canadian health system (there are unfortunately no comparable data on all health care employees) continued to rise throughout this period. Indeed, employment for nursing rose not only in absolute numbers, but as a fraction of total employment. In terms of real manpower, spending was rising. It only *appeared* to decline because the nurses were temporarily underpaid—getting raises smaller than the rate of inflation. Their wages had gone up somewhat during 1973 and 1974, but not as rapidly as the prices of the things they bought with those wages. Thus, the nurses' real purchasing power fell, and that is why the fraction of GDP spent on health declined. This "decline" was entirely transitory, because the nurses were not willing to make less than everyone else, and were able to get their wages revised upward to take account of the increase in inflation during the next set of contracts. Over the long run, whatever was taken away by a delay in adjustment had to be given back. When this was done, in 1975, there appeared to be a jump in the share of GDP spent on health. Actually this rapid rise is accounted for by the removal of the earlier distortion— eventually the health sector had to catch up with the rest of the economy.

Although expected inflation is built into contracts, any surge in the overall price level is not immediately matched by the health sector. To the extent that wages are slow to adjust, workers bear the burden by being made temporarily worse off. To the extent that budgets are slow to adjust, those organizations must make do with fewer supplies, drugs, buildings, and so forth, or temporarily go into debt. However, in the long run inflation has no effect on real health spending. After about three years health care wages and other contracts have fully taken account of earlier shifts.

A Dynamic Model of U.S. Health Expenditures

Using the permanent income hypothesis and the lagging inflation adjustment hypothesis allows us to create an econometric model of U.S. national health expenditures. Analysis of the correlation between actual spending and fluctuations in prices and per capita income indicates that health expenditures are a function of the average percentage rate of growth in real per capital GDP over the preceding five years (but not the current year), and lag by 60 percent of the change in inflation for this year compared to last, and 20 percent of the change in the previous year. This model can then be used to project future national health spending, and is shown in Figure 18.3.[10] The solid bars show the projected effects of previous GDP growth, which is always positive. The open bars show the effects of lagging adjustment to inflation, which is negative (dollars buy less than expected) when inflation is rising and positive when inflation is falling. This forecast, made at the end of December 1995, can use actual figures for GDP growth to make a forecast for 1996 spending (because only previous years 1990 to 1995 are required) but must make assumptions about the rate of inflation for 1996 based on the consensus opinions of economic forecasters. For years 1997 and beyond, more and more assumptions about macroeconomic trends are required,

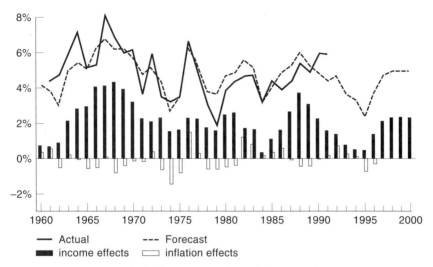

FIGURE 18.3 *Annual % Change in U.S. Health Expenditures Econometric Forecast: 1960–99*

and the forecast becomes increasingly less reliable the farther into the future projections must be made.

18.4 GOVERNMENT COST CONTROLS: SPENDING GAPS AND THE PUSH TO REGULATE _____

The lagging response of the health care sector to macroeconomic changes makes management easier in one respect—budget forecasts are usually very good, since the system is inertial and slow to change, and much of the movement over the next few years will reflect what has already occurred in the broader economic indicators such as the consumer price index (CPI) and GDP. However, this same inertia also makes it difficult to balance the budget. In a recession, expenditures will continue to climb even as revenues fall. The budgetary gaps created by delays in the adjustment of spending to changing macroeconomic conditions may force governments to put cost controls on health care. Almost every inflationary spike or sharp recession is followed by some new attempt at hospital rate regulation, rationing plan, price controls, revenue capping, or some other method to stem rising costs. For example, Figure 18.4. shows the progress of a recession in the state of Washington, and the legislative implementation of a hospital cost control commission. In 1965, Washington was a robustly growing state with above average per capita income (PCI), 108 percent of the U.S. average. Growth continued in 1966 and 1967 with PCI rising above 110 percent of the U.S. average, and state population growing 3 percent a year as people migrated in for good jobs, particularly in the aerospace industry. Growth slowed in 1968 and again in 1969, before the recession caused real per capita incomes to fall in 1970 and 1971. Boeing,

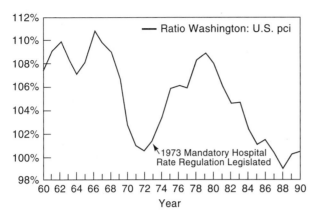

FIGURE 18.4 *Washington State per Capita Income Relative to U.S. per Capita Income*

which accounted for one in four jobs in metropolitan Seattle, eventually laid off half of its work force. Local businesses were devastated, and many retail stores closed. In 1972, state population declined, and per capita income had fallen to meet the U.S. average. The state suffered a fiscal crisis as tax revenues fell. In 1973, the legislature passed an act creating a mandatory Hospital Rate Review Commission that was among the toughest in the nation. In 1974, hospital expenditures per capita declined 2.8 percent in real inflation-adjusted terms.

Because of the recession, hospital expenditures would have declined anyway, even if the legislature had failed to pass any acts. Using a dynamic model that incorporates lagged income and inflation effects, it can be shown that the decline resulted from a delayed response to the severe state recession, not regulation. Eventually, the state legislature came to the same conclusion, and the hospital rate council was disbanded. Had the researchers responsible for the initial analysis of the program been able to wait ten years for more information, then they would have concluded that controls did not cut costs in Washington state, since the level of per capita hospital expenditures was essentially unchanged relative to projected levels or the U.S. average in 1990 compared to 1973.

The ineffectiveness of rate controls in Washington state does not mean that no state regulatory program can reduce costs. The Maryland cost-containment legislation, passed without the pressure of a severe fiscal crisis, did reduce costs.[11] Prior to implementation, Maryland costs were 111 percent of the U.S. average, and by 1990 they had fallen to just 95 percent of the U.S. average. Other state mandatory cost-control programs in New York, Massachusetts, and Connecticut may have had some impact, but the evidence is less clear.

Much of the ability to control costs is built into the existing government administrative mechanisms. Consider the state of California, which has never proposed or enacted hospital rate regulation. The combination of strict limits on taxation imposed by Proposition 13 and a massive recession caused what had once been among the most generous of health care systems to tighten down so much that by 1990, hospital expenditures per capita were 9 percent *below* the U.S. average.

Legislatures don't get together to pass cost-control measures for health care because the economy is going so well. Macroeconomic crises bring about a call for the legislature to "do something," but they also eventually push spending down, regardless of whether or not the legislature acts. Although the legislation has some incremental effect, the underlying macroeconomic trends largely control the path of health care spending. The ability of politicians to dictate spending independent of the rest of the economy is quite limited, particularly during the next one to four years, which are usually all that remain before the next election. The process is best conceptualized as shown in Figure 18.5. Incomplete adjustment to inflation and recession is apt to simultaneously exert pressure on legislatures to "do something" about excessive health care costs and force future spending downward, and thus will often create a spurious correlation between the enactment of regulation and the temporary moderation in costs.

Price Controls: The "ESP" Program

Economic growth slowed toward the end of the 1960s, and a recession occurred in 1970. Unlike previous recessions, there was no moderation in prices. This combination of slow or negative GDP growth with high inflation, called *stagflation,* rudely ended the dream of permanent stability and prosperity. The inflation of the 1950s and 1960s, low and relatively constant, had been perceived as a beneficial financial lubricant allowing for steadily increasing wages and a reduction in the burden of debt. This was different. "Cost-push" inflation threatened the whole economy with runaway wage and price increases that could destroy economic rationality. In response, President Nixon boldly stepped in to impose shock therapy in the form of wage and price controls with the "Economic Stabilization Program" (ESP) on August 15, 1971. All prices were frozen for ninety days in Stage I, with rules and procedures for Stages II, III, and IV to follow. In retrospect, U.S. experience from 1971 to 1975 served mostly to confirm the lessons learned from wage and price controls imposed by other governments around the world over the last twenty centuries. The underlying pressure created by excess monetary growth and the fiscal imprudence of waging a war without raising taxes could not be contained, controls were routinely evaded, and prices shot up as soon as controls ended in April 1974. Paul Ginsburg, an economist who worked with the Price Commission responsible for implementing the ESP, wrote an article that provided a detailed look at the practical difficulties of writing and enforcing regulations.[12] The problems of ambiguity in the definition of "price" (per item, per day, or per admission), crudeness in the construction of adjustment indexes, use of a "fudge factor" for technological change, arbitrariness in implementation, and the inability to provide a consistent and fair mechanism for determining exceptions, became cumulatively worse as time went on. Price control rules were frequently

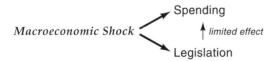

FIGURE 18.5 *Macroeconomic shock simultaneously causes spending reduction* <u>and</u> *passage of legislative cost controls. Any independent effect of legislation on spending is very limited.*

changed, became administratively complex, and lost credibility. Ginsburg also points out that cost-based reimbursement insulated many hospitals from the effects of controls over charges, and that hospital price inflation had already begun to decline even before controls were imposed.

Yet at the time, the public, government officials, and even many economists thought that price controls on health care had been successful. They thought so because there was a clear moderation during 1971 in both nominal and real health care costs from the 1966–70 trends (which fell from 11.1% to 9.3%, and from 6.1% to 3.5%, respectively). The dip was even more pronounced for the narrower measure, hospital costs, which grew 8.3 percent in 1970 but only 3.4 percent in 1971. A simple comparison of trends before and after ESP makes it appear that the controls were "effective" in reducing spending, yet most of the decline could have been predicted to occur anyway as a result of the slowdown in GDP growth and lagging adjustment to a rapid increase in inflation. To get a true picture of the incremental effect of ESP price controls, we need to compare the actual rate of increase in health care costs with the predicted value from the dynamic macroeconomic forecasting equation model above explained as shown in Figure 18.6. Spending was indeed 1.5 percent below expectations in 1971, and ESP could have been responsible for this decline, but ESP was in effect only for the last three months of the year. In 1972 spending was slightly above expected, 1973 below, and 1974 and 1975 slightly above again, but none of these differences are significantly different from the residual variation in the series. Econometric estimates of the "ESP effect" show that it may have reduced costs, but the evidence is inconclusive, and at most the reduction was perhaps 1 percent over the four years price controls were in effect—far less than the 10 percent and greater reductions that were claimed at the time.

The VE "Voluntary Effort"

After the expiration of ESP, health care costs were freed from external economy-wide controls, although they continued to be regulated by the rules of cost reimbursement (see chapters 3 and 4). Medicare, in particular, attempted to constrain costs, but without notable success. Then came a period of voluntary hospital reg-

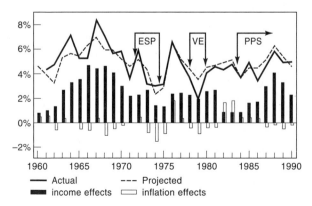

FIGURE 18.6   *Annual Change in Health Expenditures Actual v. Projected: 1960–90*

ulation known as the "Voluntary Effort," or VE. Its genesis lay in President Carter's April 1977 legislative proposal to regulate hospital revenues. The hospital industry was strongly opposed to the measure, and formed the VE coalition of providers and payers in December 1977. Flyers and buttons were printed to promote voluntary efforts to reduce the rate of cost increases. A national target, that cost increases be held to 2 percent less than the previous rate or 3 percent above the rate of inflation (the 1978 target was 13.6%), was promulgated. More buttons and flyers were printed as industry representatives lobbied Congress. After several modifications by the legislature, a new version of the Carter bill was voted on by the House in November 1979 and decisively defeated, removing the potential threat of federal regulations which had sustained the VE.

This tale of voluntary regulation would normally have been forgotten and relegated to footnotes, particularly since the effectiveness of even strongly supported legislation with comprehensive administrative regulations has been difficult to establish, yet the story lingers on because claims of its effectiveness were uncritically accepted. Three reasons for the persistence of the impression that VE "worked" are (1) that hospital price increases did moderate in 1978 and 1979, (2) that claims of VE's effectiveness were loudly voiced, and (3) that these claims were cited by Congress in the debate that led to defeat of Carter's legislation. It is difficult to understand how flyers and buttons could accomplish the force of law when government reimbursement rules could not, but the claims of effective voluntary regulation appear plausible until a closer examination of the data is made. Hospital costs had already begun falling in 1977 before VE. The rate of increase declined further in 1978 and was below the target (12.8% versus a target of 13.6%). Even believers at that time referred to the American Hospital Association's "luck," since the VE program, which was still mostly concepts and exhortations and did not convene a meeting until December 1977, could not have had time to directly affect hospital behavior. The financial reports upon which the 1978 national health expenditure figures were based came mostly from hospitals with July 1, 1977–June 30, 1978, fiscal years (FY), and for these hospitals, FY78 was already half over before the committee even met. For hospitals that operate on a calendar year, the FY78 budget would already have been up and printed by December. Once a budget is drawn up, allocations made, and labor hired, the ability of administrators to reduce expenses in the current year is very limited (chapter 9).

Luck, however, was but one factor in the fortuitous "success" of VE. The main reason that nominal expenses came in lower than expected was that hospital wages and supply prices, since they lag the CPI, had not yet caught up with the surge of inflation that had begun in 1977. There was no decline in hospitals' use of real inputs (labor FTEs, supply items), just a delay in price adjustment that made them temporarily cheap relative to the CPI (as in the Canadian example in Table 18.2). In 1979, however, there was a real decline. Nominal expenditures per capita rose by only 10.8 percent, 0.5 percent less than the year before. This drop placed spending almost 2 percent below the predicted value. Is this the real VE effect? Probably not. VE was a program to control *hospital* expenditures, and was promoted by the hospital industry. Therefore the effect of VE should have been greatest in the hospital sector, so hospitals would have had a lower rate of increase than the non-hospital spending, which was not under VE. In fact, the opposite was the case—non-hospital expenditures rose more slowly in 1979, less than half the rate of hospital expenditures.

PPS (Prospective Payment System) with DRGs

In October 1983, Medicare radically changed its method of paying hospitals from cost reimbursement to a new Prospective Payment System (PPS) based on the expected cost for each admission, categorized into diagnosis related groups (DRGs). This new cost control plan did work, sort of. There was a significant reduction in the rate of increase in Medicare part A (inpatient) expenses, and in hospital expenses generally. However, this was accomplished primarily by hospitals shifting services to outpatient and day surgery categories that were covered under part B of Medicare. Total health care expenditures per capita continued to rise at historically high rates (see Figure 18.6), and there appear to have been no net savings in federal health spending, despite the fact that deficit reduction was identified as a major reason for implementing PPS. In 1985, 16.9 percent of the $407.2 billion spent on health care was paid for by the federal government, and by 1990 the fraction had actually increased to 17.7 percent of the $643.4 billion spent in that year. PPS clearly had a large effect on the health care system. Administrators and doctors panicked, employment was (temporarily) held below trend, and the average length of stay (ALOS) for patients fell sharply. However, there were no long-run reductions in the total costs of health care.[13]

Why Do People Think Cost Controls Work?

The idea that ESP, VE, and PPS regulations were "effective" in reducing expenditures lingers on because a superficial before-and-after comparison in each case showed a decline in spending that the public and legislators could understand, and that was quickly reported in the newspapers. It is not so easily recognized that these declines were a delayed effect of the adverse macroeconomic conditions that had caused the regulations to be proposed in the first place. Also, the declines in spending in one reimbursement category (part A) due to regulations look like effective cost controls, until it is realized that those costs have just been shifted to another area (part B). A more human reason for the persistence of this belief is that many analysts and politicians worked thousands of hours to draft and implement these regulations, becoming so personally committed that it may have then been hard for them to accept that so much well-intentioned effort would have so little ultimate effect over the long run.[14] Only by examining the aggregate total of all spending with a dynamic model that shows how health care adjusts over time to macroeconomic changes is it possible to objectively assess the actual effects, or lack of effects, of regulation.

   Health care expenditures are never "too high" or "too low" in some timeless absolute sense; rather, they are out of line with the spending that can be afforded under current economic conditions. A theory of health care cost regulation must start with the realization that shared costs, and governmental expenditures in particular, are always regulated even when no external regulatory agency is in operation. Furthermore, costs can be ratcheted up or down within the existing framework by making administrative procedures tighter or looser, even if no legislation has been passed. Regulation is always an integral component of health care system management in a modern nation. It is part of the process, not an external shock. What an economist can evaluate is not regulated versus unregulated health care, but a change in the regulatory regime. To do so, one must first ask why the change took place, and why at this particular time.

What Will Happen to Spending in the Long Run?

The process of health expenditures increasing one and a half times as fast as GDP cannot go on forever. That would imply that eventually the entire national budget would be spent on health care. Not everyone can be a doctor or a nurse (or health economist), since somebody must work in the rest of the economy to pay for all this medical care. At some point, there must be a break in trend—a structural reform. That it will occur is virtually certain; when it will occur is totally unknown. For most of the last thirty years, economists and politicians have been giving their opinions that "health spending as a fraction of GDP could not go much higher without meeting significant public resistance." A few, frustrated by the failure of all these learned predictions to come true, have asked "why not?" at least for a while longer.

There is a tendency for analysts to study thoroughly only the most recent past as a guide to the future, since the data get less detailed and less reliable the farther back in time one goes. Yet the system may stay very constant for twenty, thirty, or forty years, and then suddenly undergo a marked change. Many of the structural problems in health care arose because policy makers assumed that the economic growth that had prevailed in twenty postwar years, 1949 to 1969, would continue for the next twenty years. Stability—and change—characterize the economy and its organizing institutions. Figure 18.7 presents a *very* long-run picture of health care spending (although some fairly obscure and shaky data must be used to do so)[15]—and the trends look very different from a perspective of two hundred years. Although the growth trend has been steeply rising since about 1950, health care spending appears to have been almost constant at 3 to 4 percent of GDP for 150

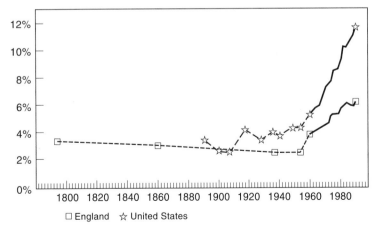

FIGURE 18.7 *Medical Care Share of National Income Historical Series 1795–1990*

years prior to that in England (even though per capita incomes were growing more than five-fold over this time), and to have been only gently rising, from about 3 percent to 4.5 percent, during the previous sixty years in the United States. There is clearly a significant change in the health sector of the economy after 1950. The trends are startlingly different, but we do not know the reason why. Technology? Tastes? AIDS? The cold war? There are more plausible explanations than data, and so we must be content to record that a structural shift did occur about forty years ago, and to predict that another one will come along sometime, perhaps within the next four years (there is too much inertia for it to happen much quicker than that), and probably within the next forty (before health care takes one out of every four dollars earned, 25% of GDP), and that this restructuring will reduce the rate of increase in health care expenditures, but will probably not bring about an absolute decline in amount spent.

18.5 "SPENDING" IS MOSTLY MANPOWER

What would it mean to control costs? Since health services are mostly labor, costs are primarily a function of the number of people employed in the health sector, and the wages (or professional incomes) that they are paid. Cost control must be manpower control. Yet it is a lot easier for a politician to say that they will control costs than to say that they will have people laid off or reduce wages, which is one reason that there is so much more rhetoric than action in health care cost control.

The most significant government interventions in the health care labor markets have been (1) cooperating with the medical profession in the formulation of effective licensure laws and making medical schools the restrictive gateway for entry into the profession during 1910–30; (2) extending of the medical licensure model to other health professions throughout the remainder of the twentieth century; and (3) enacting the Health Professions Education Act of 1963 to expand health manpower (see chapter 6).

Every occupation within the health services field has its supply and demand most strongly influenced by the particulars of licensure statutes and relations with the dominant medical profession. Yet what is true of each of the parts is not true of the whole. Most of the growth in health employment comes from the addition of new occupational categories rather than by expansion of numbers within an existing occupation. Therefore, to study how health manpower is related to the economy as a whole, it is necessary to look at aggregate employment in the health sector rather than any single occupational category.

Employment

There are two separate sources of data on U.S. health care employment. The decennial census began recording information on the occupation of respondents in 1850, and so can be used to create a long series of "health related occupations" with fifteen observations over the last 140 years, as presented in Table 18.3

and shown in Figure 18.8. The Bureau of Labor Statistics records employment within industries by Standard Industrial Classification (SIC) codes, and has identified health care (SIC 80) as a category since 1958, providing 33 annual (or 396 monthly) observations from 1958–90, presented in Table 18.4. The conceptual base of the two series is quite different. The census data is based on *occupation of the individual* so that a secretary, chemist, or accountant employed in a hospital would not be counted as being in a "health" category. The BLS data is based on the *SIC code of the employer,* and so a nurse, med tech or doctor employed in a manufacturing firm would not be counted as being a health care employee, but the hospital secretary would.

Employment in health has grown more than twice as rapidly as total U.S. employment over the last hundred years, 3.8 percent versus 1.6 percent for the period 1890–1990. Consequently, the share of total employment accounted for by health has increased from less than 1 percent at the turn of the century, to more than 7 percent (1 out of every 14 workers) now. Yet the percentage of total employment accounted for by physicians, 0.5 percent, has been essentially constant (see Table 18.3 and Figure 18.9). The health sector (SIC 80) has enjoyed positive employment growth every year for the past three decades. The average annual growth rate of this sector between 1958 and 1990 was 5.5 percent—more than double the annual average growth of total U.S. employment. During this period health sector employment never contracted (see Figure 18.10), in contrast to total employment, which experienced several minor and two major contractionary episodes. Total U.S. employment contracted in the early and late 1960s and especially following the oil price shocks of the middle and late 1970s. Although health sector employment grew more slowly during the mid-1970s and early 1980s, annualized year-on-year growth never fell below 2 percent. Health care employment shows less fluctuation because it adjusts more slowly and gradually to macroeconomic shocks. When total employment is shifted upward or downward 1 percent from trend, health care employment moves by only 0.2 percent after one year, 0.17 percent after two years, and so on (see Figure 18.11).[16] The cumulative rise or fall in health care is proportionately larger, about 1.2 percent for each 1 percent shift in total employment, but spread out over the entire decade that follows, so that on average shifts in health employment lag by 2.6 years.

The slow rate of adjustment to government intervention is shown in Figure 18.12, which presents the estimated impact on health employment due to the enactment of Medicare and Medicaid in 1965. Even though this legislation created a fundamental change in reimbursement and the flow of money into the system, and was ultimately responsible for a rise of more than 10 percent in the number of health care jobs, it had no visible effect on health employment during 1965 or 1966. Not until 1967 did employment begin to soar, leaping 3.7 percent above trend in that year, 2.4 percent in 1968, 1.2 percent in 1969, 0.6 percent in 1970, 0.4 percent in 1971, and so on (see Figure 18.12). The average lag between the enactment of Medicare and the creation of an additional job was 3.5 years.

Wages

Health care wage data for the United States are available from the BLS for hospitals from 1968 on, and for all health employment from 1972 on. There were rapid

TABLE 18.3 U.S. Health Sector Employment Statistics, 1850–1990 (thousands of persons)

Year	1850	1860	1870	1880	1890	1900	1910	1920	1930	1940	1950	1960	1970	1980	1990
Population	23,192	31,443	39,818	50,156	62,948	75,995	91,972	105,711	122,775	131,669	150,697	179,323	203,235	225,739	249,924
Employed Civilians	5,372		12,925	17,392	23,318	29,073	37,371	42,434	48,830	51,742	59,230	67,990	79,802	104,058	123,473
all Health Occup.	46	61	103	114	170	346	486	634	900	1,020	1,450	2,064	3,277	5,403	7,580
fraction	0.8%		0.8%	0.7%	0.7%	1.2%	1.3%	1.5%	1.8%	2.0%	2.4%	3.0%	4.1%	5.2%	6.1%
H/pop	1.97	1.93	2.58	2.26	2.70	4.55	5.29	6.00	7.33	7.75	9.62	11.51	16.12	23.94	30.33
MD/pop	1.76	1.75	1.62	1.71	1.66	1.73	1.66	1.43	1.33	1.33	1.31	1.30	1.46	1.92	2.35
aid/MD			0.2	0.2	0.5	1.0	1.4	2.1	3.2	3.7	5.1	6.7	8.7	10.1	10.6
Physicians	41	55	64	86	105	131	152	151	163	175	198	234	297	433	587
Dentists	3	6	8	12	17	30	40	56	71	71	76	83	95	125	156
Diagnostician, NEC							8	22	38	40	53	68	40	54	132
Pharmacists	2		18			46	54	64	84	83	89	93	116	146	182
nurse (practical)					47	120	166	212	236	200	224	276	267	435	429
RN-nurses			13	1	1	12	51	104	214	284	406	592	762	1,285	1,885
Att-Hosp/Nurse Aides, Orderlies									41	102	212	409	951	1,378	1,860
Att-Phy/Aides, Orderlies							4	7	14	35	42	73	134	292	249
Dent Asst							2	7	14				100	158	216
Dent Hygienist													17	46	72
Opticians, Lens Grinders						6	9	11	13	12	20	21	31	47	38
Therapists (licensed)									14	18	25	37	78	224	332
Psychologists											5	12	30	93	192
Dieticians											23	27	43	67	90
Med Tech											78	141	260	508	927
Managers, Medicine & Health													58	111	234

TABLE 18.3 U.S. Health Employment: Annual % Rates of Growth

Year	1850	1860	1870	1880	1890	1900	1910	1920	1930	1940	1950	1960	1970	1980	1990
population		3.1%	2.4%	2.3%	2.3%	1.9%	1.9%	1.4%	1.5%	0.7%	1.4%	1.8%	1.3%	1.1%	1.0%
Employed Civilians				3.0%	3.0%	2.2%	2.5%	1.3%	1.4%	0.6%	1.4%	1.4%	1.6%	2.7%	1.7%
all Health Occupations		2.9%	5.4%	1.0%	4.1%	7.4%	3.5%	2.7%	3.6%	1.3%	3.6%	3.6%	4.7%	5.1%	3.4%
Physicians		3.1%	1.6%	2.9%	2.0%	2.3%	1.5%	-0.1%	0.7%	0.7%	1.3%	1.7%	2.4%	3.8%	3.1%
Dentists		6.7%	3.6%	4.4%	3.6%	5.4%	3.0%	3.5%	2.4%	0.0%	0.6%	1.0%	1.4%	2.8%	2.2%
nurse (practical)				1.9%	11.9%	10.0%	3.3%	2.5%	1.1%	-1.6%	1.1%	2.1%	-0.3%	5.0%	-0.1%
RN-nurses					7.2%	28.0%	15.6%	7.5%	7.5%	2.9%	3.6%	3.9%	2.6%	5.4%	3.9%
Att-Hosp/Nurse Aides, Orderlies										9.6%	7.6%	6.8%	8.8%	3.8%	3.0%
Att-Phy/Health Aid								5.5%	7.1%	9.7%	1.7%	5.6%	6.3%	8.1%	-1.6%
Therapists (licensed)										2.5%	3.3%	4.0%	7.7%	11.2%	4.0%
Psychologists												9.4%	9.3%	12.1%	7.5%
Dieticians												1.5%	4.9%	4.5%	3.0%
Med Technicians												6.0%	6.3%	6.9%	6.2%
Managers, Medicine & Health															7.8%

Sources: Comparative Occupation Statistics for the United States, 1870 to 1940 (Edwards, 1943), U.S. Public Health Service (1969) and U.S. Bureau of the Census (1855, 1985, 1992).

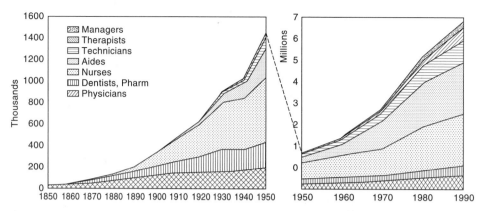

FIGURE 18.8   *Growth in U.S. Health Employment, 1850–1990*

TABLE 18.4   Trends in Total Employment and Health Sector Employment

	Total U.S. (1000s)	SIC 80 (1000s)	SIC 806 (1000s)	SIC 80 (% of total)	SIC 806 (% of total)	SIC 806 (% SIC 80)
1958	51,293	1,365	908	2.7%	1.8%	67%
1959	53,244	1,454	967	2.7%	1.8%	67%
1960	54,171	1,548	1,030	2.9%	1.9%	67%
1961	53,981	1,640	1,087	3.0%	2.0%	66%
1962	55,530	1,739	1,145	3.1%	2.1%	66%
1963	56,638	1,837	1,217	3.2%	2.1%	66%
1964	58,266	1,963	1,295	3.4%	2.2%	66%
1965	60,749	2,079	1,357	3.4%	2.2%	65%
1966	63,879	2,204	1,420	3.5%	2.2%	64%
1967	65,793	2,434	1,554	3.7%	2.4%	64%
1968	67,885	2,639	1,654	3.9%	2.4%	63%
1969	70,375	2,862	1,770	4.1%	2.5%	62%
1970	70,883	3,052	1,863	4.3%	2.6%	61%
1971	71,205	3,238	1,935	4.5%	2.7%	60%
1972	73,667	3,412	1,980	4.6%	2.7%	58%
1973	76,778	3,641	2,051	4.7%	2.7%	56%
1974	78,280	3,887	2,160	5.0%	2.8%	56%
1975	76,946	4,134	2,274	5.4%	3.0%	55%
1976	79,379	4,350	2,363	5.5%	3.0%	54%
1977	82,468	4,584	2,465	5.6%	3.0%	54%
1978	86,693	4,792	2,538	5.5%	2.9%	53%
1979	89,824	4,993	2,608	5.6%	2.9%	52%
1980	90,416	5,278	2,749	5.8%	3.0%	52%
1981	91,157	5,562	2,904	6.1%	3.2%	52%
1982	89,566	5,812	3,014	6.5%	3.4%	52%
1983	90,128	5,973	3,037	6.6%	3.4%	51%
1984	94,487	6,122	3,004	6.5%	3.2%	49%
1985	97,516	6,299	2,997	6.5%	3.1%	48%
1986	99,507	6,536	3,038	6.6%	3.1%	46%
1987	102,196	6,805	3,143	6.7%	3.1%	46%
1988	105,579	7,121	3,295	6.7%	3.1%	46%
1989	108,584	7,551	3,472	7.0%	3.2%	46%
1990	110,327	8,114	3,680	7.4%	3.3%	45%

Source: Bureau of Labor Statistics, *Employment and Earnings.*

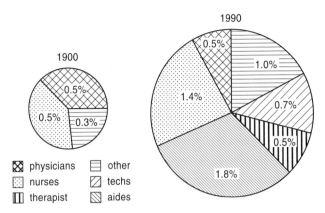

FIGURE 18.9 *Health Manpower as Percentage of Labor Force*

increases in real (deflated) wages of more than 5 percent per year in the late 1960s post-Medicare period. During the 1970s, health care wages were essentially flat, just keeping pace with wages in other industries and with inflation, and growing less than 0.5 percent per year. Since 1980, real average wages in the rest of the economy have actually fallen, and were 2 percent *lower* in 1990. Average health care wages rose by 19 percent over the decade, and the increases for hospital employees (27%) and self-employed physicians (33%) were even greater. There does not appear to be any correlation between economic growth (GDP) and health care wages, but the data cover only twenty years, and there is not enough to be certain of this. Other than the apparent surge due to Medicare (which occurred before health care wage data was collected) no government policy appears to have significantly affected the health care wage trend. The adjustment of health care wages to changes in the rate of inflation is slow. More than 60 percent of the rise (or fall) in inflation from one year to the next was not incorporated in health care wages until the following year, and 11 percent was still missing after two years, indicating substantial contractual rigidity in health care wages.

Real health expenditures per capita in the United States grew 5 percent a year from 1960 to 1990, outpacing the 2 percent rate of growth in per capita incomes

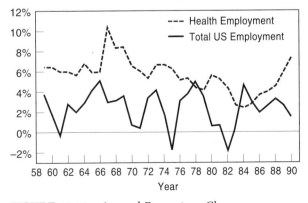

FIGURE 18.10 *Annual Percentage Change in Employment*

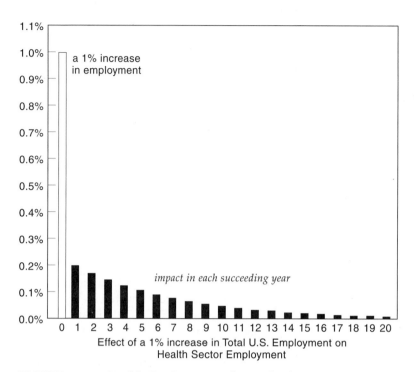

FIGURE 18.11   *Health Employment Adjusts Slowly*

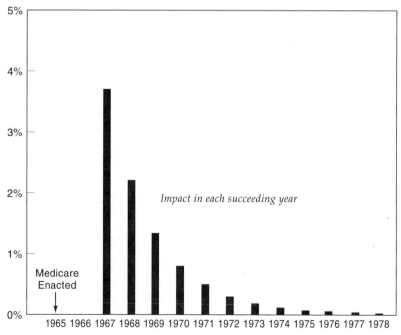

FIGURE 18.12   *Effect of Medicare on Health Employment in Subsequent Years*

and so consuming an ever-larger share of GDP. The labor portion of that 5 percent annual increase in expenditures can be decomposed into a 4 percent increase in employment and a 1 percent annual increase in real wages, so that increased intensity of medical services—more nurses and perfusionists and occupational therapists per patient day—is by far the more important cause of increased spending over this time span. However, since 1980 excessive compensation growth in the health sector relative to the rest of the economy has accounted for a significant proportion of spending increases. With both wages and employment increasing faster than in other occupations, it may well be that health care professionals are getting more than a fair share of the nation's economic growth, a concern that health economist Uwe Reinhardt of Princeton University has humorously identified as "feasting on healthcare, or the allocation of lifestyles to providers."

Although the power of licensed health professions to control entry and wages is a major cause of delayed adjustment, it is not the only one. The dominance of nonprofit firms and third-party financing is also an important factor in creating labor market rigidity. Health services in the United States are currently undergoing significant institutional changes. The pattern of slow and delayed adjustment over the last thirty years indicates that the ultimate outcome of these changes will not be revealed for a considerable period of time, and certainly will extend into the next century.

SUGGESTIONS FOR FURTHER READING _____

Katherine Levit, *et. al.*, "National Health Expenditures, 1994," *Health Care Financing Review* 17(3):205–242, Spring 1996.

Sally T. Burner and Daniel R. Waldo, "National Health Expenditure Projections, 1994–2005," *Health Care Financing Review* 16(4):221–242, Summer 1995.

Milton Friedman, *A Theory of the Consumption Function*, Princeton, N.J.: Princeton University Press, 1957 and with Simon Kuznets, *Income from Independent Professional Practice*, New York: National Bureau of Economic Research, 1945.

Thomas E. Getzen, "Macro Forecasting of National Health Expenditures" *Advances in Health Economics and Health Services Research*, Vol. 11, pp. 27–48, 1990.

Marian Osterweis, et. al, editors, *The U.S. Health Workforce: Power, Politics, and Policy*, Washington, D.C.: Association of Academic Health Centers, 1996.

Randall P. Ellis and Thomas G. McGuire, "Supply Side and Demand-Side Cost Sharing in Health Care," *Journal of Economic Perspectives* 7(4):135–51, Fall 1993.

SUMMARY _____

1. Consumption and savings decisions are based not on current income, but expected **permanent income** over the whole lifecycle.

2. Shared financing through government and insurance makes health care into a **quasi-public good** so that group or national income is the relevant budget constraint, not individual income.

3. The major determinants of total health spending are macroeconomic (inflation, population, GDP).

4. Professional licensure, nonprofit organization, third-party reimbursement, and other institutional features **make the health care sector slow in adjusting to changes** in macroeconomic conditions.

5. These delays in response create **pressures for regulatory change**.

6. Many of the "effects" associated with the passage of health care cost control regulations are actually **delayed effects** of inflation and recession.

7. A **major structural shift** took place around 1950 that increased the rate of growth in health spending. Another structural shift that will reduce the rate of growth is likely to occur "sometime" in the near future, but there is no sure way to know if that will be four or forty years.

8. **Spending increases are largely manpower increases.** Much of the growth shows up in the form of new occupations, and some shows up as higher wages and professional incomes.

PROBLEMS _____

1. {*dynamics, productivity*} How many nonphysicians are currently employed in the health sector for each M.D.? Is this ratio more or less than fifty years ago? Does the change in the ratio of physician to nonphysician labor imply that productivity has increased or decreased? Which adjusts more rapidly to changes in demand, ancillary employment or physician supply?

2. {*flow of funds*} Which factor has accounted for more of the increase in the cost of hospital care per patient: Increases in the number of physicians? Increases in the number of days of care? Increases in physician incomes? Increases in the wages of nonphysician employees? Increases in the number of nonphysician employees?

3. {*dynamics*} Do delays in adjustment cause deficits, surpluses, or both?

4. {*elasticity*} If the income elasticity of NHE spending is 1.4 and per capita income increases from $12,000 to $15,000, how much will health care spending increase? If income elasticity is 0.9?

5. {*elasticity, aggregation*} Since the amount of income spent on health for a group is just the sum of the amounts spent on each member, why would the income elasticity be different if the economist measured 1 person, groups of 10, or 100, or 1,000,000? Is individual income elasticity for health care spending larger or smaller than national income elasticity for health care spending? Why?

6. {*fallacy of composition*} What determines how much is spent on your health care, how sick you are, or how much money you earn? What determines how much is spent on average in the U.S., how sick people are, or how much money they earn?

7. {*price controls*} Suppose that you read Sunday's paper and find out that price

controls have been placed limiting the cost of health insurance to $2,500 per employee, significantly below the current average. What effects would you predict to occur?

8. {*inflation*} (A) Assume inflation is 4 percent for the years 19x0 to 19x4, jumps suddenly to 14 percent for the years 19x5 and 19x6, and then falls to 3 percent for 19x7 to 19x9. Calculate the price index using 19x0 as the base year. What is the price in each year of a good whose price changes matched the overall level of inflation and cost 27.42 in 19x2?

   (B) Suppose that service "L" has a price that adjusts with a lag, so that a third of the change in average prices shows up in L's price in each of the succeeding years. Calculate the annual percentage rates of price increase for L.

   (C) Suppose, there is a good A that anticipates future price increases, so that half of the change in next year's inflation rate will show up in its price in advance. Calculate the annual rate of price increase for A.

   (D) What prices in the health care system might be expected to show delayed adjustment, lagging behind changes in the general rate of inflation? What prices in the health care system might show anticipatory response, changing in advance of the general rate of inflation? What problems would this pattern of delay/advance present to administrators trying to work within a budget?

9. {*inflation*} Will changes in the rate of inflation affect health care spending? In your answer, distinguish between real and nominal expenditures, and between short- and long-run effects.

10. {*dynamics*} Are decisions regarding health care budgets and medical school enrollments based on the past or the future?

11. {*marginal consumption*} What is the difference between the Keynes and Friedman consumption functions? For which would the level of spending be higher at the mean? For which would the rate of increase (marginal propensity to consume) be higher? Which states that the marginal propensity to consume is above the average? Below the average? Equal to the average?

12. {*consumption*} What is the permanent income hypothesis? For which type of person would the permanent income hypothesis lead one to expect the greatest error from using tax returns to predict consumption?
    a. assistant manager at Macy's
    b. management intern at Macy's
    c. CEO at Macy's
    d. retired VP of Macy's
    e. college student
    f. medical student
    g. highschool teacher

13. {*dynamics*} Why might it take longer to adjust health expenditures downward than upward? Frame your answer in terms of the economic incentives facing those who would make the actual decisions.

14. {*equilibrium, segregation*} What determines the level of wages among health care occupations?

15. {*public good*} Why does insurance turn private medical care into a public good?

16. {*price controls, dynamics*} Did health care rise less rapidly after President Nixon introduced price controls in 1971? Why or why not?

17. {*dynamics, price controls*} What forces cause the public to want price controls?

18. {*price controls*} What was the effect of the Medicare Prospective Payment System (PPS), which paid a fixed price per diagnostically weighted hospital discharge (DRG) after 1983, on: Hospital length of stay? Outpatient surgery? Nursing home admissions? Total Medicare hospital expenditures? Total Medicare expenditures for all types of care?

19. {*voting*} If price controls and crazy tax proposals are the economic equivalent of voodoo, why do such proposal continue to gain support? (For that matter, why has voodoo continued to be profitable?)

20. {*dynamics*} How long is the "long run?" How much difference can the length of the periods chosen for measurement make on the estimates of price and income elasticity?

21. {*productivity*} Would it be possible to raise both employment and wages through the development of new technology that increased the productivity of medical care? Why or why not?

ENDNOTES

1. John Maynard Keynes, *The General Theory of Employment, Interest and Money*, London: Harcourt, Brace & Co., 1936.
2. Ernst Engel, "Die Productions und Consumtionsverhaltnisse des Konigreiches Sachsen," 1857, see commentary by George Stigler, "The Early History of Empirical Studies of Consumer Behavior," *Journal of Political Economy*, 62(2):95–113, 1954.
3. Simon Kuznets, "Proportion of Capital Formation to National Product," *American Economic Review: Papers and Proceedings*, 42:507–26, 1952.
4. Milton Friedman and Simon Kuznets, *Income from Independent Professional Practice*, New York: National Bureau of Economic Research, 1945.
5. Milton Friedman, *A Theory of the Consumption Function* (Princeton, N.J.: Princeton University Press, 1957).
6. Franco Modigliani, *The Collected Papers of Franco Modigliani: Vol. 2: The Life-Cycle Hypothesis of Saving*, Cambridge, Mass.: MIT Press, 1980.
7. Take-home advice: if you want to become rich, get in the habit of saving *now*, while you are still in school.
8. Thomas E. Getzen, "Macro Forecasting of National Health Expenditures," *Advances in Health Economics and Health Services Research*, Vol. 11, pp. 27–48, 1990.
9. Angus Deaton, "Involuntary Savings Through Inflation," *American Economic Review*, 67:899–910, 1977.
10. Thomas E. Getzen, "Macro Forecasting of National Health Expenditures," *Advances in Health Economics and Health Services Research*, Vol. 11, pp. 27–48, 1990.
11. David Dranove and Kenneth Cone,"Do State Rate Regulations Really Lower Hospital Expenses?" *Journal of Health Economics* 4(2):159–65, 1985; C. Eby and D. Cohodes, "What Do We Know About Rate Setting?" *Journal of Health Politics, Policy & Law* 10:299–327, 1985; Michael Morrisey, Douglas Conrad, Steven Shortell, and Karen Cook,

"Hospital Rate Review: A Theory and Empirical Review," *Journal of Health Economics*, 3(1):24–47, 1984.

12. Paul Ginsburg, "Impact of the Hospital Stabilization Program on Hospitals," pp. 293–323, in M. Zubkoff, I. E. Raskin and R. S. Hanft, eds., *Hospital Cost Containment—Selected Notes for Future Policy*, New York: PRODIST for Milbank Memorial Fund, 1978.

13. Congressional Budget Office, *Rising Health Care Costs: Causes, Implications and Strategies*, Washington, D.C.: U.S. Government Printing Office, 1991.

14. Karen Davis, Gerard Anderson, Diane Rowland, and Earl Steinberg, *Health Care Cost Containment*, Baltimore, Md.: Johns Hopkins University Press, 1990.

15. Prior to the efforts of the Committee on the Costs of Medical Care in the U.S. commencing in 1929, there are no surveys of national health expenditures as the term is now used. What is available are estimates of health expenditures of different types of workers, mostly factory workers. There exists an 1875 survey of 397 Massachusetts families carried out by Carroll Wright, who was later U.S. Commissioner of Labor and in 1889 conducted a massive and detailed representative survey of 6,000 workers for the whole U.S. and included comparable European Data (*Fifth and Sixth Annual Report of the Commissioner of Labor*, 1891). A "sick club" with contributions established by the Industrialist Matthew Boulton is reported in Ffrangcon Roberts, *The Cost of Health*, London: Turnstile Press, 1952. Budget surveys were carried out by David Davies in 1795 and Frederick Morton Eden in 1797. In Belgium, Eduard Ducepetiaux collected the data later analyzed by Ernst Engel in the 1840s. In France, the Frederic Le Play reports detailed budgetary expenditures, but only for a few families, in *Les Ouvriers Europeens*, 1855.

16. Michael Kendix and Thomas Getzen, "U.S. Health Services Employment: A Time Series Analysis," *Health Economics* 3(3):169–181, 1994.

CHAPTER 19

International Comparisons of Health and Health Expenditures

QUESTIONS

1. Which country provides the largest health care market?

2. Is health care trade more or less international than other goods and services?

3. Are the differences between countries larger in terms of doctor supply, hospital technology, or per capita spending?

4. Is it high income or high medical expenditures that make the wealthy countries more healthy?

5. Does the distribution of income within a country determine the distribution of health?

6. In which aspect of the health care system is there more trade between countries: goods, services, people, or ideas?

19.1 WIDE DIFFERENCES BETWEEN NATIONS _____

There were more than 5 billion people in the world in 1990, distributed across some 200 countries. Health care expenditures for those 5 billion people totaled $1,702 billion that year. The 260 million people living in the United States represented 5 percent of the worldwide total, but its healthcare expenditures of $690 billion accounted for more than 40 percent. Although China is the world's largest country, with 1.2 billion people, it accounted for less than 1 percent of global health spending, just $13 billion. Health expenditures per person in the United States were 10 times the worldwide average in 1990, and 250 times the average expenditure of $11 per person in China. The extra $500 billion purchased a lot more hospitals, physicians, drugs, and technologically sophisticated equipment for the use of U.S. citizens. But how many additional years of life, how much reduction in morbidity and mortality, did all of those extra medical inputs yield? Could the U.S. have done as well, or have become even more healthy, while spending less? Of course there are many factors other than hospitals and doctors responsible for differences in health between China, the U.S. and other countries, but $500 billion is sufficiently large that it could pay for changes in many other factors as well.

Any assessment of health economy across the world must deal with a tremendous diversity in population, economic growth, and health status. Mozambique, Tanzania, and Ethiopia are among the world's poorest countries. They are still dominantly rural and dependent upon subsistence agriculture, with limited government, little accumulation of savings or investment, per capita incomes of less than $200, and rapidly expanding populations that face repeated threats from starvation. In these countries, half of all the children who are born will die before reaching age 5, and life expectancy at birth is less than fifty years. At the other extreme sit Sweden and Switzerland, whose urbane citizens enjoy incomes of more than $30,000 per person, most deaths occur after age 75, and average life expectancy exceeds 78 years. Development economists categorize countries as low, middle, or high income. More than half of the world's population still falls into the low-income, rural agricultural category. Most countries in Africa are toward the bottom of the distribution. The two undeveloped giants are China and India, with 1,150 and 866 million people, respectively. This may change because China's recent development has been so rapid that it could, if maintained, transform the economy within twenty years. In the middle ($1,000 to $7,500 per capita) are 1.5 billion people—including much of Latin America, most of what used to be the socialist economies of Russia and Eastern Europe, South Africa, Saudi Arabia and other oil-rich states of the Middle East, and emerging Asian economies such as Korea. The high-income group (over $10,000) consists of 850 million people in Europe, the United States, Canada, Japan, Australia, and New Zealand.

A nation's health resources generally increase with income, while the extent of illness and need for medical care is reduced. The high-income group spent an average of $1,860 per capita on health care in 1990, and had 2.5 doctors and 8.3 hospital beds per 1,000 persons (see Table 19.1). The average life expectancy was 76 years, with more than half of all deaths occurring after that age. The perinatal mortality rate was 9 per 1,000 births, and the rate of tuberculosis (TB) infection

TABLE 19.1 Comparison of Health and Expenditures Across Nations, 1990

	Popu- lation	growth rate	% age <15	% age >65	% urban	female literacy	GNP/ capita	growth rate	Ag. %	food share	$ Health /capita	GNP Share	public share	doctors	hosp. /1,000 population	TB	infant mortality	median death	life expect.
World	5,267	1.7%	.33	.06	.51	.55	$4,010	1.2%	.05	**	$323	8.0	.61	1.34	3.6	1.4	5.3	55	65
Kenya	24	3.8%	.49	.02	.24	.58	$340	0.3%	.27	.38	$16	4.3	.63	0.14	1.7	1.4	6.7	15	59
Nigeria	96	3.0%	.47	.02	.36	.39	$340	-2.3%	.37	.48	$9	2.7	.44	0.15	1.4	2.2	8.5	7	49
India	850	2.1%	.36	.04	.27	.34	$330	3.2%	.31	.52	$21	6.0	.22	0.41	0.7	2.2	9.0	37	58
China	1,134	1.5%	.27	.06	.60	.62	$370	7.8%	.27	.61	$11	3.5	.60	1.37	2.6	1.7	3.8	64	69
Mexico	86	2.0%	.38	.02	.73	.85	$3,030	-0.5%	.09	.35	$132	3.2	.50	0.54	1.3	1.1	3.6	60	70
Turkey	56	2.3%	.35	.03	.63	.71	$1,780	2.9%	.18	.40	$76	4.0	.38	0.74	2.1	0.6	5.8	52	65
Japan	124	0.5%	.18	.12	.77	.99	$26,930	3.6%	.03	.17	$1,538	6.5	.74	1.64	15.9	0.4	0.5	78	79
Germany	79	0.1%	.16	.16	.85	.99	$23,650	2.2%	.02	.12	$1,511	8.0	.73	2.73	8.7	0.2	0.7	78	76
U.K.	57	0.2%	.19	.16	.89	.99	$16,550	2.6%	.02	.12	$1,039	6.1	.85	1.40	6.3	0.1	0.7	77	76
U.States	250	0.9%	.22	.13	.75	.99	$22,240	1.7%	.02	.10	$2,763	12.7	.44	2.38	5.3	0.1	0.9	76	76

Source: The World Bank, *World Department Report 1993: Investing in Health.*

was 0.2 per 1,000. In contrast, the low-income countries of sub-Saharan Africa could spend only $12 per person on health care and had just 0.1 doctors and 1.4 hospital beds per 1,000 persons. Life expectancy averaged 52 years in 1990, the perinatal mortality rate was 68 per 1,000 births, half of all deaths occurred to children under age 6, and the TB infection rate was 2.20 per 1,000.

Size of the Market

From the perspective of the marketing department of a profit-maximizing health care firm, the importance of a country is determined not by the number of people, illnesses treated, or unmet needs, but by the number of dollars spent there. In these terms, the United States is by far the largest market in the world, with a 41 percent share. In contrast, the world's most populous country, China, has only a 0.8 percent share. In dollar terms, China's market is roughly the same size as the state of Missouri. All of the low-income countries together, 3.2 billion people, account for less than 3 percent of world spending (about half as much as the state of California) (Figure 19.1).

The disparity in health resources is not quite as great as the disparity in health spending because wages are lower in low-income countries, so that 75 percent less health care spending usually translates into a somewhat less severe reduction in the number of doctors or nurses.[1] Still, it is clear after perusing Table 19.1 that the gap between high-income and low-income countries is substantial. Some goods, such as pharmaceuticals, are traded internationally, and have prices that are fairly constant across countries, so that any decline in spending causes an equivalent decline in usage. Such internationally traded items take a much larger portion of health budgets in low-income countries (25–50%) than in high-income countries (5–15%). The broad picture is one of vast disparities between rich and poor. Haves and have-nots face such different choices that they almost seem like inhabitants of different centuries, or different planets. What is common and readily accessible to most citizens of high-income countries becomes the favored privilege of a few government officials, industrialists, and celebrities in low-income countries.

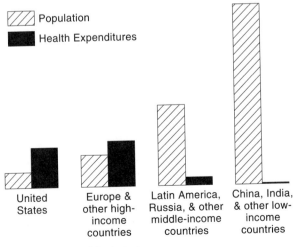

FIGURE 19.1 *Market size*

Medical care as practiced in the developed world is but a dream, as distant as Hollywood, for most of the world's population.

19.2 MICRO VERSUS MACRO ALLOCATION: HEALTH AS A NATIONAL LUXURY GOOD _____

Economists term entertainment, travel, and other expenditures "luxury goods," not by making any judgments regarding the necessity or importance of such items, but by observing changes in consumption spending as income increases. Items for which a 10 percent increase in income leads to a greater than 10 percent increase in spending (i.e., income elasticity > 1.0 are labeled luxury goods, whatever their use may be. The determination of income elasticity for services tends to be a bit more difficult than for goods due to the complication already noted: the same service usually costs more as per capita incomes rise because the wages of those providing the service also rise. In order to get around this difficulty, economists make use of the algebraic relationship between income elasticity and budget shares: if spending on an item rises by more than the increase in income, then its share of total consumption will increase. A country that spends 12 percent of GDP on health is using more of its resources for medical care than a country spending 8 percent, regardless of most differences in income-related wage rates.[2]

Nations spend more money on health care because they have the money to spend, not because they have greater medical needs. This conclusion is not very surprising when thinking about whether Bangladesh (GDP $200 per capita) will spend more or less than Canada (GDP $20,000 per capita), and is graphically obvious in Figure 19.2, yet the finding that health spending is unrelated or inverse to medical needs contradicts most personal experience, since an individual spends more on health care if they become sick. The choices made regarding how much is to be spent by or for a particular individual (micro) are very different from, and based on different factors than, national decisions made collectively through the political process about how much of the budget or GDP should be spent on health (macro). Health expenditures come mostly from pooled funds raised through taxes or employee benefit plans. Given that pooled set of funds, a decision will be made about how to spend it on a covered individual based on personal medical need. Insurance and government financing are ways of making sure that an individual's ability to pay does not limit the care that they can receive when they need it. Yet collectively, the ability of all to pay, their aggregate prior contributions in taxes or insurance premiums, puts an absolute limit on how much can be spent in total on all of the individuals treated. As the focus shifts from micro to macro allocation, the significant determinant of spending shifts from "medical need" to "available income" (Figure 19.3). For example, every country spends two to five times as much on elderly people as they do on young and middle-aged people. However, this does not mean that if a country's population is older it will spend more on health care (take it to the limit and suppose everyone were old and retired—who, then, would be working to pay for all of the extra nursing homes, hip replacements, and heart medications?)[3] As can be seen from Table 19.1, England has an older population than the United States, and a health service that is roughly equivalent on many measures (life expectancy

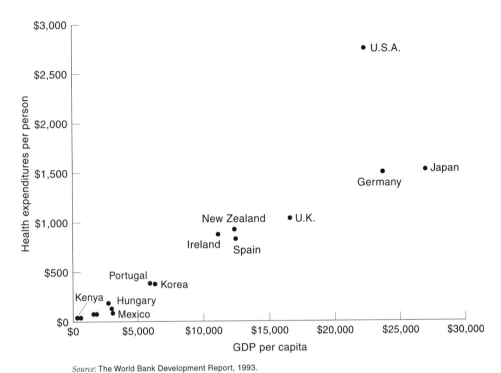

Source: The World Bank Development Report, 1993.

FIGURE 19.2   *Health expenditures versus income*

75 vs. 76, infant mortality 8 vs. 10) but spends significantly less on average ($1,039 vs. $2,763), largely because per capita income is lower ($16,550 vs. $22,240).[4]

19.3   CAUSALITY: DOES MORE SPENDING IMPROVE HEALTH? _____

Wealthier countries are healthier, and they spend more on medical care. Can one then conclude that more spending buys better health? Not necessarily. Many factors

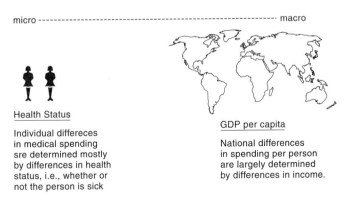

micro -- macro

Health Status

Individual differeces in medical spending sre determined mostly by differences in health status, i.e., whether or not the person is sick

GDP per capita

National differences in spending per person are largely determined by differences in income.

FIGURE 19.3   *Determinants of health spending*

associated with higher incomes such as education, nutrition, and sanitation are also known to improve health (see chapter 15). Furthermore, life expectancy has increased greatly in many poor countries over the last twenty years, even when the availability of doctors and GDP per capita declined. A full categorization of all the influences on health status and relative contribution of each factor is not possible, but a rough assessment of the relative importance of *economic growth,* advances in *public health and medical research,* and the *use of medical care services,* can be made. However, it must first be recognized that all of these influences interact with and modify one another. With no knowledge of what to do, money is worthless; and medical knowledge alone is helpless in the face of extreme poverty, which leads to death from starvation. Any categorical estimate of "how much" each factor contributes is to some extent artificial, and is also limited to what can readily be observed (i.e., differences noticeable within the range covered by statistics, such as those presented in Table 19.1). Perusal of data from many countries indicates that only large differences, increases of ten-fold or hundred-fold, consistently affect health outcomes. Income differences on the order of 50 percent or 100 percent are not reliably associated with increases or decreases in life expectancy, and appear to be within some range of indifference or minor variation or measurement error. Hence, they should either be treated with caution or ignored. It is the big picture that matters in this assessment of health.

Figure 19.4 graphically illustrates that there is a relationship between per capita

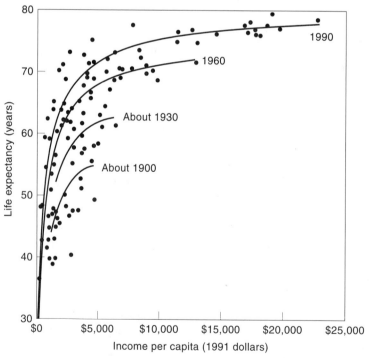

FIGURE 19.4 *Life expectancy and income per capita for selected countries and periods*

Source: World Bank Development Report, 1993, page 34.

income and average life expectancy, and that the relationship has changed over time. A plausible interpretation is that movements along the curve reflect the combined effects of more income and more medical care, while the shifting of the curve reflects the universal effect of increased knowledge, which is a public good. Between 1960 and 1990, life expectancy in Africa increased by about ten years, from 43 to 52, despite the lack of improvement in living standards or incomes. Another piece of evidence for the effect of knowledge on health is provided by studies of childhood mortality in the United States around 1900.[5] In that era, the children of well-to-do physicians were just as likely to die before age 5 as the children of poor laborers living in tenements, since both the wealthy and the poor used the same ineffectual health practices. As the importance of infection and nutrition were revealed, physicians' families were able to take advantage of their better education and resources, so that child mortality declined much more rapidly for this group than for low-income laborers. In poor countries today, sanitation, basic nutrition supplements for infants, and control of preventable disease are still of primary importance. In these situations, studies have indicated that maternal education and literacy is often more important than income in preventing childhood disease and death.

Separate assessment of the effects of living standards and utilization of medical care is difficult because both generally rise or fall together. Japan, for example, has achieved a phenomenal twenty-five-year increase in life expectancy since World War II, but there is no easy way to determine how much is due to the rapid economic growth, and how much to the deployment of modern medical care. The achievement of relatively high life expectancies in some low- or middle-income countries with relatively low use of sophisticated medical treatments (71 years in Malaysia, 72 years in Sri Lanka, 73 years in Chile) suggests that the incremental effect of medical care alone is probably modest. Analysis across many countries reveals that the absolute level of income may not be as important in many cases as **income distribution**.[6] Upon reflection, it is not surprising that where there is greater equality of income, the average level of health is higher. The relationship between income and health is nonlinear. A 20 percent drop means much less at the middle or top of the distribution than it does toward the bottom. High rates of illness are a function not of poverty, but of extreme deprivation. The greater the degree of inequality, the more likely it is that some families will be so lacking in food and amenities that deaths from infantile diarrhea, tuberculosis, and other preventable or treatable conditions occur.

19.4 LOW-INCOME COUNTRIES _____

Low-income countries face very different health care problems than wealthy, industrialized countries. Their populations are rural, with many children, and a heavy burden of infectious disease and stunting (abnormally low height and/or small body size) due to occasional malnutrition. However, the government officials living in the capital have incomes, tastes, and health care needs much more like those of developed countries. This can lead to a major misallocation of resources such as building a modern research hospital in the capital providing excellent tertiary care, while much of the country lacks access to a doctor or a nurse and children remain unvaccinated so that preventable epidemics remain common. It is not unusual for as much as half of the entire health budget of a low-income country to be spent in the capital city, with a large part going to equip and staff the leading hospital (in contrast, the Johns Hopkins University Hospital takes about 0.6 percent of the U.S. health budget). Convincing local medical leaders to change the allocation of resources to a more appropriate emphasis on low-technology primary care is difficult, since they do not wish to give up their expensive research hospital, which might bring the doctors and government officials prestige and international fame. The world may admire a European doctor trained at a leading university who spends years alone treating cases in an isolated river village, but a local physician who spends his days treating diarrhea and wound infections without any chance to practice in a modern surgical facility is simply considered to have minimal skills, and little of importance to outsiders. The incentives of the rulers and of the medical profession are not aligned with the health needs of the vast majority of the citizens. Both will naturally tend to favor maintaining a state of the art facility with modern technology and capability for research, even when doing so drains funds from the village clinics and nursing care that can do more to reduce infant mortality and raise life expectancy. Even in very-low-income countries, medical schools train too many specialists who want to perform technologically advanced procedures, rather than primary care generalists able to treat most common illnesses.

Studies by the World Bank have found that the status of women is a major determinant of health in low-income countries. Access to knowledge is one factor. In countries where most women are illiterate and have not been to school, there is no way for them to know about sterilization of water, proper nutrition, or care of childhood infections. Women are also more likely than men to make family health a priority. In subsistence economies where women have some control over spending (because of tradition, or because they have a job with wages), a larger fraction of the household budget gets spent on food, and less on alcohol and tobacco.

Starvation remains a problem in much of the lowest-income countries. In Nigeria, 43 percent of the children aged 2 to 6 are stunted (low height-for-age); in Kenya, 32 percent; and in India, 65 percent, compared to 22 percent in Mexico, 4 percent in Japan, and 2 percent in the United Kingdom and United States. It is not so much that food supply is insufficient, as that the supply is maldistributed. Organizational disarray, lack of transport, disruptions due to war and political upheaval, and poorly functioning markets mean that food does not get to where it is needed most. No simple solution presents itself, since the defects in economic organization that cause mismanagement of food are the same as those responsible for a lack of economic development in the first place. National governments that maintain order, handle their budget and money supply prudently, and support market-oriented policies are able to grow out of the low-income category.

Health Care in Kenya

The economy of Kenya is still dominated by agriculture. Its most significant exports are coffee, tea, cotton, and minerals. Its 24 million people had a per capita annual income of about $340 in 1990, although "income" is much more difficult to measure or define in a traditional agricultural economy, and so any figure should be considered very approximate. The population is still growing very rapidly (3.8% per year), with almost half still under the age of 15. Enrollment of children in primary school is 88 percent, and more than half of all adults are literate. About a quarter of the population lives in cities. The single-party KANU government is relatively stable for such a poor country, having been in power since 1963. Life expectancy at birth, 59 years, is among the highest in sub-Saharan Africa. Still, half of all deaths occur to children under the age of 15, and adults are about three times as likely to die in any given year as they are in the United States.

The health system is split almost equally between the public and private sector (see Table 19.2).[7] The ministry of health runs 80 hospitals, 41 District Health Centers in the provinces, 178 rural health centers, and about 1,200 sub-centers and dispensaries. District medical officers are always physicians, usually assisted by one or more nurses and a hospital secretary (administrator). Below the district level, most facilities are operated by para-professionals, and at the dispensary level, by community workers or untrained auxiliaries. Despite a stated emphasis on primary care and rural development, more than 35 percent of the entire national budget is spent on the showcase Kenya National Hospital in Nairobi. Some government agencies, such as the Ministry of Transport and the Coffee Board, run health services for their workers, as do the dozen or so corporations with more than 500 employees.

Religious missions are a very important part of the health care system, running 40 hospitals, 84 health centers, and 173 clinics. Although the origins and management of these facilities are religious, 60 percent of their funding comes from patient fees, about 25 percent from government subsidy, and only 15 percent from donations. Thus, they are correctly considered a part of the private sector. Overall, about 22 percent of Kenyan health expenditures are derived from foreign aid.

The government actively encourages private sector health care. Private hospi-

TABLE 19.2 Health Expenditures in Kenya, 1990 (*estimated*)

	$ millions	*percentage*
GOVERNMENT		
Ministry of Health	204	*42%*
Municipalities	27	*6%*
Other Government	6	*1%*
PRIVATE SOURCES		
Voluntary Agencies	6	*1%*
Religious Missions	28	*6%*
Corporate Clinics	2	*
Household Spending		
Hospitals	45	*9%*
Physicians & Healers	36	*7%*
Drugs	114	*24%*
Other	16	*3%*
Total	484	*approximately $20 per person*

Sources: The World Bank Development Report 1993, and Bloom *et al*, 1986.

tals, supported entirely by fees, are popularly viewed as being of higher quality and are growing rapidly. The government runs a National Hospital Insurance Fund for high-income workers through a mandatory 2 percent wage tax (there is no employer contribution) designed to reimburse stays in private and religious hospitals, or the private rooms of public hospitals. However, this plan covers just 12 percent of the population. The effectiveness of the plan may be further limited by its low payout rate: only 60 percent of the hospital insurance premiums collected were used to pay claims or administrative expenses, allowing 40 percent to be held by the central government.

Most physicians (70%) work full-time in private practice. The 30 percent that work for the government or missions also engage in private practice after clinic hours. There are, perhaps, 2,000 physicians actively in practice in Kenya, almost half of them in Nairobi (although it has only 7% of the nation's population). In contrast, there are about 19,000 traditional healers and herbalists practicing in Kenya, most of them in the countryside. A physician will earn roughly thirty times as much as a traditional healer from the practice of medicine. A small fraction of the population, the 2 or 3 percent that belong to upper-income families living in the major cities, accounts for more than half of all private expenditures for medical care. About one-third comes from the 10 percent that are middle-income city dwellers. All of the poor that have flocked to the cities account for less than 2 percent of private spending, and the vast bulk of the population still living in rural areas (about 75%) account for just 17 percent of private expenditures. The flow of medical resources clearly follows the flow of funds. The disparity between members of the elite who live in the capital and the vast rural population that subsists by farming is clearly visible in morbidity and mortality statistics, and remains the largest problem facing health care in Kenya.

19.5 MIDDLE-INCOME COUNTRIES _____

Turkey, Mexico, Thailand, and South Korea are all examples of countries that are in the process of industrialization. Subsistence agriculture and poverty is still the norm in the remote rural regions, but the bulk of the population has moved into cities and works for wages. The shift from rural agricultural labor to urban wage labor presents a major organizational problem: how to develop a comprehensive health insurance system able to fund a higher level of health care. Rapid economic growth allows some countries to expand government services, so a dominantly public system is created. In other cases, such as Korea, a strong tradition of industrial paternalism leads to private insurance based on employment benefits. Some countries have begun with a public system and switched to reliance on the private sector, while others are moving in the opposite direction. In almost every middle-income developing country the health insurance system is in transition. Even when coverage is universal by law, the reality is that access to medical care is still very uneven. The urban ghettos and impoverished rural villages still frequently lack sanitation. Restrictions and incompleteness in the health insurance system may prevent poor citizens from using medical facilities even when they are accessible geographically. Thus, the disadvantaged populations are disproportionately represented in the statistics for morbidity and mortality. At the same time, expanding incomes have brought the lifestyle illnesses of the wealthy countries, such as heart disease and lung cancer, to prominence. The growth markets for cigarettes in the twenty-first century are China, India, and Asia, not Europe and North America. Finally, the middle-income countries are still too likely to misallocate resources emulating the advanced health care systems of high-income nations: large research hospitals in the cities matched by a lack of village clinics in the countryside; training too many specialists and not enough primary care physicians or public health experts.

The Health Care System of Mexico

With a 1990 per capita GDP of $3,030, a population of 86 million with an average life expectancy of 70 years that is quite young (38% below age 15) and still growing rapidly (2% per year), Mexico is perhaps not dissimilar from many other transitional economies. The bulk of the people have moved off the farms into cities to find industrial and service jobs, but agriculture and export of raw commodities still make up a substantial part of the economy, and literacy is still a problem in the rural areas. The government is politically stable, although it has shown signs of strain in recent years as Mexico attempts to shift away from the eighty years of single-party rule to a more open, multi-party democracy.

The government enacted a comprehensive social security system, IMSS, in 1942, relatively early for a transitional economy, but it only covered industrial workers and their dependents.[8] A nationwide network of IMSS health centers, polyclinics, and hospitals was built. However, in order to accommodate all the beneficiaries, it was necessary for the system to contract with private doctors and hospitals as well. In 1960, a plan for government employees, ISSSTE, was established, and an even more modern and technologically sophisticated set of hospitals and clinics was built with generous funding to accommodate this favored group of employees. ISSSTE and IMSS provided the top two tiers of health insurance, and covered about half of the population. The agricultural workers, temporary workers, and the unemployed depended on private medical care, *curanderos* (native herb doctors), and public clinics. Public medical care has been repeatedly reorganized over the years into a social security system, SSA, so that most of the population receives coverage. Requirements that public facilities admit emergency cases regardless of insurance assure that everyone has some form of access to care (see Table 19.3).

Access to services is, however, rigidly segregated, and often of poorer quality and limited use to those most in need. There are IMSS and SSA hospitals virtually

TABLE 19.3 Health Insurance Coverage in Mexico

Mexican Institute of Social Security (IMSS)	39%
Institute for Governmental Workers (ISSSTE)	8%
Other federal agency health plans	2%
Secretariat of Health & Welfare (SSA)	21%
Marginal families program	13%
Private medical care	5%
Unprotected population	12%

Source: Milton Roemer, *National Health Systems of the World*, 1991.

across the street from each other, but the poor or marginally employed are only allowed to use the inferior SSA facilities. Much of the medical care in SSA clinics is provided by *pasantes,* young doctors just out of medical school fulfilling their one year of required government social service. Although the SSA facilities are free, they are not particularly attractive to patients. The doctors see an average of just eight patients a day, and although they could easily accommodate two or three times as many, the patients do not come. SSA hospitals are less than half full. It is clear that the reality of coverage for the poor falls far short of the promise. The private market provides services both at the bottom (where SSA is inadequate) and at the top (where wealthier people can buy state-of-the-art medical care), with the middle occupied by three separate tiers of public care. Most physicians in Mexico work in salaried positions for ISSSTE, IMSS, or SSA, and also have a private practice as well. Yet even though there are many fewer physicians per 100,000 population than in the United States (about one-fourth as many), there is a large pool of unemployed or under-employed physicians (15–25% of all physicians) who cannot find a government job or attract enough private patients to make a living from medicine. Relative to that in other transitional economies, the health care system in Mexico seems to work reasonably well. Yet despite (or because of) the active involvement of the government at many levels, and an emphasis on integration and coordination, the most glaring deficiencies appear to be organizational.

19.6 HIGH-INCOME COUNTRIES _____

Among the high-income countries, there is considerable variation in the use of medical care inputs (doctors/1,000 ranging from 1.4 to 4.3; hospital beds/1,000 from 3.9 to 16.1), organization of services, reliance on taxpayer financing, and total cost (from $383 to $2,763 per capita), but remarkably little variation in health outcomes. Life expectancy for the twenty-two high-income countries lies between 74 and 79 years, and infant mortality is between 5 and 9 per 1,000 births. There is much greater variation in health statistics between regions within any one of these countries, than across the twenty-two countries. Given the rather small differences in average health outcomes, it would be difficult to say that one country's system is better or worse. What is clear is that many health problems are concentrated in specific, underserved populations, usually ethnic minorities or areas of extreme poverty. Although tremendous resources are available for advanced experimental treatment, electronic scanning for diagnosis, and long-term rehabilitation, there is still a lack of primary care resources ensuring that every child is immunized, that all pregnant women receive adequate prenatal care and nutrition, that every person has a primary physician to contact when in need of advice or care. In many ways, the high-income countries face the same problems of maldistribution and misallocation in the delivery of medical care as the low-income countries, but at a different level (see Figure 19.5).

Costs and Cost Control

Rapidly rising health care costs created fiscal difficulties in all high-income countries during the 1970s. Although the attempts at control varied widely, there has

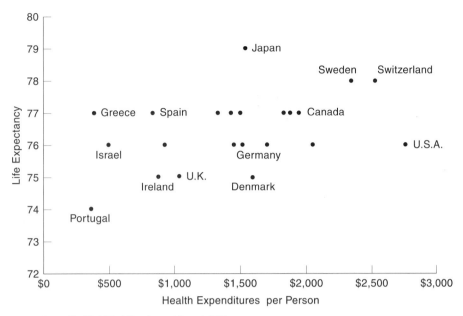

Source: The World Bank Development Report, 1993

FIGURE 19.5 *Health expenditures and life expectancy*

been a degree of convergence across nations so that most spend between 6 percent and 10 percent of GDP on health care, with the notable exception of the United States, which spent 14 percent in 1994. What is surprising is that the factors to which cost increases are usually attributed (increases in the number of services, of doctors, of hospitals, or increase in the extent of insurance coverage) appear to have no impact on the total cost of health care. For example, the United States spends by far the most on health care, yet ranks twenty-second out of twenty-three countries in number of patient bed days per 1,000 population (only Greece is lower), ninth out of fourteen in number of physician visits per person, and twelfth out of eighteen in number of prescriptions.[9] Controls at the micro level, reducing the number of services used, are not sufficient to control overall costs. Changes in the method of payment or system administration do not hold much promise, either. One comprehensive examination concluded "there appears to be no relationship between success in containing costs and ways of organizing services."[10]

How were Japan and Europe able to keep health care costs so much lower than the United States while maintaining equal or better health outcomes and patient satisfaction? Many of the attempts to control costs in the United States have been motivated at the individual level, using deductibles and copayments to moderate demand, yet the use of pooled financing that protects patients from risks also insulates them from costs. Consumer choice does not lead to lower expenditures when consumers are spending someone else's money. The European countries have operated largely on the supply side, constraining the provider system rather than individual demand. The number of health care workers, and their wages, have been limited, and are often subject to nationwide bargaining and controls.

TABLE 19.4   Medical Technology per Person in Three Countries, 1992–93

	Canada		Germany		United States	
	number	per million persons	number	per million persons	number	per million persons
Open-heart surgery	36	1.3	61	0.8	945	3.7
Cardiac catheterization	78	2.8	277	3.4	1,631	6.4
Organ transplant	34	1.2	39	0.5	612	2.4
Radiation therapy	132	4.8	373	4.6	2,637	10.3
Lithotripsy	13	0.5	117	1.4	480	1.9
MRI	30	1.1	296	3.7	2,900	11.2

Source: Dale A. Rublee, "Medical Technology in Canada, Germany and the United States: An Update," *Health Affairs,* 13(4):113–117, 1994.

Purchase of expensive new diagnostic and therapeutic technology has been re-stricted (See Table 19.4).[11] Open-ended entitlements that reimburse all bills have been avoided in favor of contracts for large groups of patients on a per-capita or fixed-budget basis. In analyzing the evolution of payment systems, it has been ar-gued that the flaws of bureaucratic governmental control (lack of innovation and consumer responsiveness) and of insurance markets (lack of cost control and gaps in coverage) are leading toward a convergence of public and private in a blended contractual model—what is known in the United States as managed care (chap-ters 10 and 11).[12] Government will be responsible for setting the rules and the overall limits on the amount to be spent, and making sure that everyone receives coverage, while market competition is used to maintain the quality and amenity of services, and provide local control.[13]

The Japanese Health Care System

Japan has the highest life expectancy in the world at 78 years, yet the level of health care spending is only half that of the United States, 7.3 percent of GDP, about $2000 per person in 1997. While the technology used in the Japanese health care system is quite similar to that in the U.S., the organization and flow of funds—and hence, the quantity and intensity of use—is quite different.[14]

In Japan, all citizens are covered by some form of insurance, and are able to choose any physician or hospital that they wish, with no bills other than modest copayments per visit or per day. Physicians are clearly split into two groups. Generalist physicians are private solo practitioners providing primary and sec-ondary care as small businesses, earning a substantial portion of their income from mark-ups on pharmaceuticals and laboratory tests. Specialist physicians work in hospitals on salary and generally earn much less. There is virtually no mi-gration or overlap between professional categories. Private practitioners cannot attend hospitalized patients, and hospital physicians are not allowed to have a private practice on the side.[15] Hospitals are also divided. Small facilities owned by a private practitioner provide less sophisticated treatments, and large public and university hospitals contain the medical schools and research facilities—but they may also have large outpatient departments providing primary care. For-profit investor-owned hospitals are prohibited in Japan.

Universal health insurance coverage is obtained through a myriad of funding bodies, all linked formally and informally by the Ministry of Health. It is possible to describe the system in broad outlines as follows (see Figure 19.6). The "society managed health insurers" (SMHI) cover the employees of the large corporations. Premiums for the SMHI are 6 to 10 percent of base salary, split equally between the employer and the employee. The large-company employees tend to have the best salaries and the best health, and these funds typically run a surplus. Some of the SMHI premiums are diverted to cover the elderly and other government subsidies. The small- and medium-sized corporations (less than 700 employees) and national government workers are covered by the government-managed Health Insurance (GMHI), and receive some subsidy from the Ministry of Health (about 14%). The self-employed, retirees, local government employees,

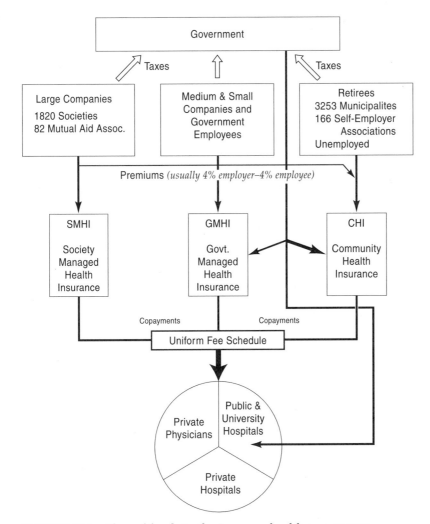

FIGURE 19.6   *Flow of funds in the Japanese health care system*

the unemployed, and others, are covered by community health insurance (CHI) using a combination of individual sliding-scale premiums and substantial government subsidy (about 50%). Hence, although the Japanese health care finance system superficially resembles a large number of independent insurance pools, the extent of transfers and cross-subsidies is such that these plans are linked through the Ministry of Health into what is, in effect, a form of social insurance that equalizes medical purchasing power across all types of persons.

With the exception of government subsidies for public and university hospitals, *all funding for providers comes through a single mechanism—the fee schedule*, which states what will be paid for each of thousands of different services and procedures. Hence, even though there are many different insurance plans on paper, they are all forced into uniformity by the fee schedule. No balance billing is allowed (i.e., the provider gets the specified insurance payment and copayment only. No extra charges to the patient or family are allowed, although the practice of giving gifts to the doctor, a form of tipping, is not infrequent). Fees have been set to generously compensate primary care services in physicians' offices, and under-compensate high-technology procedures. Thus, general physician office practice is highly profitable, while specialists such as neurosurgeons or radiologists all work on salary and earn only about half as much. Fees are set so low for most complex surgical and diagnostic procedures that only public university hospitals, which receive government subsidies, can afford to perform them. Since all funds pass through a single pipeline, it is possible for the government to exert rather rigid control over total expenditures, even in the absence of a global budget.[16] The egalitarianism of the Japanese health system, with all persons universally covered and treated by the same providers, reduces competitive pressures to fund expansion of the newest high-technology procedures.

The financial incentives regarding specialization and high technology are almost exactly opposite of those in the United States, where doctors doing high-technology procedures garner the most prestige *and* the most income. In Japan, a doctor who chooses to become a sub-specialist gets prestige, but must give up the lucrative office-based primary care practice. Academics compete for movement up the department ladder, not more income. General practitioners compete for income, not expertise.

The operation of the fee schedule system reverses the financial dynamics of health care. In a market, those services for which demand is increasing obtain higher prices, which, in turn, brings forth a larger supply. In Japan, if a procedure becomes popular, its fees are often cut to discourage provision. A notable effect of this shift in remuneration is that there are *two-thirds fewer* surgical operations in Japan than in the United States.

The fees in the Japanese system are negotiated provider payments, not "prices." Fees are adjusted in response to political agreements, not changes in demand.[17] There is an unstated principle that the relative shares of each constituency (e.g., surgeons vs. internists, hospitals vs. private practitioners, radiologists vs. psychologists) will stay relatively constant. Any group that reaps a windfall in one year is expected to give it up two years later in the next round. Across-the-board percentage adjustments are avoided for this reason. A detailed set of more than two thousand fees is agreed upon by a small group of participants meeting in a small room over the course of a few days. The Ministry of Health has its representatives on one side (and has agreed in advance to what is, in effect, an overall budget via its negotiations with the Ministry of Finance regarding how many trillion yen are available for health insurance subsidies during the next two years) and on the other side the Japanese Medical Association (JMA) speaks for all provider interests. The primary constituency of the JMA are the private practitioners delivering generalist care. The willingness of all other providers to defer to the JMA and so to perpetuate a division of funds that solidifies a political outcome from previous decades is intriguing from the perspective of an outsider not used to this form of decision making. This closed session of one-on-one bargaining works within an elaborate but unstated framework of rules. It is a way of reaching equilibrium through consensus vastly different from the sprawling mixture of regulated and competitive markets in the United States. Attention to the details of the system should not distract an economist from recognizing the direction of causality and the significance of the end result. In Japan, the health care financing mechanism flows from the medical (and political) culture. It binds and holds, both depending on and reinforcing a series of unstated understandings that have accumulated over the years.[18] Political and economic power is frozen into a structure in which most of the conflict is stylized or hidden. The contrast with the United States is obvious. Here the system is subject to market and scientific shocks that shift status and fortunes daily. Prices respond to demand and information more than precedent and tradition. Thus, financial incentives are somewhat more able to shape the medical culture instead of conforming to it. In the Japanese system of negotiated fee schedules, tradition and strong informal controls make it much easier to maintain the status quo.

19.7 INTERNATIONAL TRADE IN HEALTH CARE _____

Health care is among the world's largest industries, accounting for 8 percent of gross world product, but only a tiny fraction of world trade. Products (drugs, equipment) are much more likely to be bought and sold across national boundaries than services. Although in principle there is no reason why an X-ray performed in Seoul cannot be read in San Francisco, licensure and other regulations currently make such international service flows difficult or impossible. Trade in services is usually limited to a small amount of border crossing, as, for example, when a Canadian citizen disgruntled with a long wait for elective surgery crosses into the United States, or an uninsured Hispanic worker in Texas goes across to Mexico for cheaper hospital and physician care. The part of the health care system most subject to international movement does not appear in the world economic accounts: trade in people and skills.

Pharmaceuticals

The pharmaceutical trade is one of the world's truly global businesses (see chapter 13). Drugs made in England or France cross the counter as readily as drugs made in Des Moines, and research is as apt to be done in Genoa or Geneva as Georgia. Combinations such a Rhone–Poulenc Rhorer and Astra–Merck cross international boundaries and link the major markets. Protectionist legislation still gives local firms an advantage, but it is rare for any large pharmaceutical company to have less than 25 percent of its sales from countries outside its headquarters, and some, like Ciba–Geigy, are mostly international. There are three major markets: Japan, the United States, the European Union. The ability of Japanese doctors to profit from prescribing gives them the highest rate of drug use in the world, and because of this the Japanese market, with half as many consumers, is actually larger in dollar terms than the U.S. market ($51 billion vs. $48 billion in 1990). The European Union accounts for about $40 billion, and all of the developing low- and middle-income countries $44 billion.[19] Only the major market countries have the research infrastructure and a (protected) domestic market of sufficient size to cover the massive fixed costs of discovering and testing new drugs. Canada presents an interesting case. Since the nation lacked significant pharmaceutical development capacity, it decided to free-ride on the technology produced by the rest of the world. It refused to recognize the property rights created by patents, and mandated that foreign companies license their drugs for manufacture or use in Canada in return for set royalty payments. In this way they could obtain the benefits of research, but not pay the cost. Vigorous protests eventually led to this system being overturned, and now Canada recognizes international patent protection like other industrialized countries. However, free-riding is still the rule for many developing countries, either through mandatory licensing, or simple failure to enforce patents so that local companies can make copy-cat versions of brand-name drugs. Clinical tests of drugs constitutes a sizable portion of their costs, and provides an interesting opportunity for international trade. By carrying out trials in a foreign country, a firm may be able to significantly reduce the cost per patient, and may also face lower liability from any adverse reaction the experimental drug might produce.

Equipment

Medical equipment is less amenable to international trade because it cannot simply be packed in a box and shipped. Skilled technicians are required to maintain and use these sophisticated devices, and the ongoing labor costs are much larger than the manufacturing cost. Once a new technology is developed, it will usually be produced and supported by a local firm, or the local branch of a global firm, within a few years.

Services

Public health care is sharply demarcated at national boundaries. The U.S. Medicare program does not pay for operations in Mexico, nor will it cover Canadians who come to the U.S. Therefore the border-crossing trade in services that does occur is usually paid for privately. Private investment in the small fee-for-service or insured hospitals and clinics that exist alongside national health facilities in the United Kingdom, Sweden, and elsewhere is often international. The largest hospital in Singapore was owned by an American firm, National Medical Enterprises. Yet the true test of international trade in medical care looms in the proposals for full integration of service markets within the European union. There is no reason why a Belgian patient might not prefer heart surgery in one of the major Parisian hospitals, or a Swiss factory worker decide to seek psychiatric care in Germany. Conversely, a German hospital would find it cheaper to obtain nurses or doctors from Greece and pay travel expenses rather than hire them locally. To date, every country has jealously guarded its health care system, and such freedom of choice is available only to a few employees of international companies that provide special executive benefits.

People and Ideas

Standing in stark contrast to the lack of international trade in medical services is the substantial movement of medical people and ideas across national boundaries. Most of the specialists in developing countries receive some of their training in Europe or the United States, carrying back skills of immense value. The revolutionary increase in life expectancy that has swept over the world is perhaps one of the greatest benefits of international trade, made no less significant by the fact that, as public goods, information and scientific discoveries could not be owned or charged for by a particular firm or country. What is somewhat surprising is the extent of trade in the reverse direction, doctors and nurses who have come to work in the United States from low-income countries. At its peak, in 1978, more than half of all medical residents who were "in training" (and providing care) in urban teaching hospitals were foreign medical graduates. In the less remunerative and attractive specialties, like psychiatry, that is still the case today. More than 12 percent of all U.S. physicians are immigrant doctors. Similarly, a large number of licensed nurses were educated overseas. There are more Filipino nurses practicing in the United States and Canada than in the Philippines. The reason for this anomalous flow of highly trained labor from less-developed to more-developed countries has much to do with the economics of restrictions on labor supply, and with the incentive structure created by the size of the market. Limits on the numbers of physicians and nurses imposed through the U.S. educational system mean that there is room for those who have received training overseas and are willing to work for less. Also, a truly outstanding neurosurgeon is clearly able to earn more in the United States than in Mexico, and will be tempted to go where her skills command the highest reward, just as a movie actress or baseball player would. There is also a vacant niche at the bottom of the market that attracts foreign labor. Caring for the elderly in nursing homes is so demanding and underpaid that it is difficult to find competent staff willing to work for the minimum wage. These positions are attractive to immigrants who are able to obtain steady employment and benefits in jobs that require a lot in the way of patience, endurance, and strength, but not in language or education. The lack of dollar-denominated trade obscures the extent to which medicine and health care have become globalized in the twentieth century.

SUGGESTIONS FOR FURTHER READING _____

William Glaser, *Health Insurance In Practice: International Variations in Financing, Benefits and Problems*, San Francisco: Jossey-Bass, 1991.

Naoki Ikegami and John Campbell, Medical Care in Japan, *New England Journal of Medicine*, 333(19):1295-1299, 1995.

Alan Maynard and Karen Bloor, Introducing a Market to the United Kingdom's National Health Service, *New England Journal of Medicine* 334:604-608, 1996.

Milton I. Roemer, *National Health Systems of the World*, New York, Oxford University Press, 1991.

OECD, *The Reform of Health Care Systems: A Comparative Analysis of Seven OECD Countries*, 1992 and volume 2 :*A Review of Seventeen OECD Countries*, 1994, Paris: OECD.

The World Bank, *Better Health In Africa*, Washington, D.C.: The World Bank, 1994.

The World Bank, *World Development Report 1993: Investing in Health*, New York: Oxford University Press for the World Bank, 1993.

SUMMARY

1. **The U.S.A. is the world's largest health care market**, accounting for 40 percent of all health expenditures, even though it has just 5 percent of the world's population. U.S. health expenditures per person are 10 times the worldwide average, and 250 times the average per person in China. With more than 20 percent of world population, China accounts for less than 1 percent of the global health care market.

2. There is **a tremendous disparity in health** between rich and poor nations. The poor countries of sub-Saharan Africa have very little health care and low life expectancies. Half of all deaths there occur before a person reaches the age of 5 years. The wealthier countries of Europe, North America and Japan have many more health resources to be applied to much less need and enjoy a much longer life expectancy. Half of all deaths there occur after age 70.

3. Average **spending on health care is determined primarily by national income per capita, not the health needs of individuals**. Increased per capita income is also a major factor explaining increases in life expectancy.

4. More health expenditures usually means more health professionals and more use of technology, not more visits to physicians or days in the hospital. That is, it is the **intensity rather than the utilization of services** that increases as spending is increased.

5. Significantly **higher medical expenditures do not** appear to have made U.S. citizens significantly healthier. U.S. life expectancy ranks about in the middle of developed higher income countries.

6. The curve depicting the relationship between national income per capita and life expectancy has shifted upward over time. This illustrates the productive impact of **new knowledge**, as well as the **transmission of that knowledge across national boundaries**.

7. The **distribution of income** across people and social groups, as well as the average, is important in explaining differences in health and life expectancy.

8. **Lack of organization, maldistribution, and political instability** are perhaps even more important than low income in causing poor health among many low income countries. Even in mid- and high-income countries, many of the

worst health problems lie in the uneven distribution of health care and an inability to effectively target care to those most in need.

9. Most countries say that their health systems emphasize **primary care**, but their **funding favors specialty training and tertiary hospital care**.

10. **Cost control** in Europe, constraining supply and putting limits on the system as a whole, appears to have been more effective than in the United States. Japan's inexpensive health care system is much less technology-intensive than that of the United States, using only a third as much surgery, but more drugs.

11. There is very little **international trade** in health care services. Global trade in health care is dominated by pharmaceuticals. However, it is the "invisible" trade in knowledge and health professionals that has the largest effect on national health care systems.

PROBLEMS _____

1. {*flow of funds*} How many people are there in the world today? What fraction of them live in high-income developed economies? What fraction of total health expenditures are accounted for by high-income countries?

2. {*flow of funds*} How much is spent per person on health care in China? How much is spent per person on health care in the United States? In the United Kingdom? What are the primary factors accounting for these differences?

3. {*market size*} What is the largest global health care market?

4. {*correlation v. causality*} Is more spending on health care associated with more health?

5. {*incidence*} As an officer of the World Health Organization, what programs would you fund if you wished to make the largest impact on health, measured as the increase in life expectancy multiplied by the number of people affected, for a given budgetary allocation of $100 million?

6. {*nominal v. real*} Mexico spends less than a tenth as much per person on health care as the United States. Does it have more or less than a tenth as many hospital beds? physicians? Is the real amount of health care provided over- or under-estimated by dollar comparisons? Why?

7. {*international trade*} What types of health care labor are most likely to be traded between countries? Why?

8. {*international trade*} What types of health care goods are most likely to be traded between countries? Are there more or less barriers to trade in health care than in other sectors?

9. {*trade*} Which aspects of medical care are most international? The most parochial?

ENDNOTES _____

1. Victor Fuchs, "The Health Sector's Share of the Gross National Product," *Science* (2 February 1990):534–38.

2. Mark Pauly, "When Does Curbing Health Costs Really Help the Economy?" *Health Affairs*, 14(2):68–82, 1995.

3. Thomas Getzen, "Population Aging and the Growth of Health Expenditures," *Journal of Gerontology*, 47(3):S98–104, 1992.

4. Thomas E. Getzen, "An Income-Weighted International Average for Comparative Analysis of Health Expenditures." *International Journal of Health Planning and Management* 6:3–22, 1991.

5. Samuel H. Preston, *Fatal Years: Child Mortality in Late Nineteenth-Century America*, Princeton, NJ: Princeton University Press, 1991.

6. G. B. Rodgers, "Income and Inequality as Determinants of Mortality: An International Cross-Section Analysis," *Population Studies*, 33(2):343–51, 1979, also The World Bank, *Population Change and Economic Development*, New York: Oxford University Press, 1985.

7. Milton I. Roemer, *National Health Systems of the World*, New York: Oxford University Press, 1991, which includes information reproduced from G. M. Bloom, M. Segal and C. Thube, *Expenditure and Financing of the Health Sector in Kenya*, Nairobi: Ministry of Health, 1986. The World Bank Statistics, used for most of the tables in this chapter, estimate national health spending in Kenya at $375 million for 1990, of which 63 percent came from the public sector. Roemer argues that private sector spending is much less visible and usually under-reported since no regular statistics are kept. Bloom et al., through extensive surveys and several alternate methods, estimate that private sector spending actually slightly exceeded public sector spending, 51 percent to 49 percent, in 1986. Table 19.2 takes the World Bank estimate of public spending of 237 million dollars, derived from government budget reports, as correct. Private sector spending is then estimated to be 51 percent of the total, or $247 million, following Bloom et al. The percentages of total spending within each category in Bloom et al. for the year 1986 are then applied to the 484 million total to create breakdowns by category. The net effect of the adjustment for under-reported private expenditures is to raise the estimate of per capita health expenditures in Kenya from $16 per person to $20 per person.

8. Milton Roemer, *National Health Systems of the World*, New York: Oxford University Press, 1991, pp: 345–51.

9. *OECD Health Systems: Facts and Trends 1960–1991*, Paris:OECD, 1993.

10. Brian Abel-Smith, *The Reform of Health Care Systems: A Review of Seventeen OECD Countries*, Paris:OECD, 1994, p.49.

11. Dale A. Rublee, "Medical Technology in Canada, Germany and the United States: An Update," *Health Affairs*, 13(4):113–17, 1994.

12. Jeremy Hurst, *The Reform of Health Care: A Comparative Analysis of Seven OECD Countries*, Paris:OECD, 1992, p.140–51. See also, Alan Maynard and Karen Bloor, Introducing a Market to the United Kingdom's National Health Service, *New England Journal of Medicine* 334:604–608, 1996.

13. The fact that so many health policy experts in so many countries all agree on the essential elements of what the future of health care organization and financing will and should be is probably reassuring, although such a consensus has not always guaranteed either insight or good results in the past.

14. Much of the information presented here came from conversations with Naoki Ikegami, M.D., Professor of Health Administration at Keio University, and is well presented in Naoki Ikegami and John Campbell, "Medical Care in Japan," *New England Journal of Medicine*, 333(19):1295–99, 1995. See also Margaret Powell and Masahira Anesaki, *Health Care in Japan*, New York: Routledge, 1990; and Kyoichi Sonoda, *Health and Illness in Changing Japanese Society*, Tokyo: University of Tokyo Press, 1988.

15. Salaried hospital physicians are allowed to earn money on the side in private practice within many national health systems, such as, for example, those of England, Sweden, and Norway.

16. In contrast, Germany and the U.K. explicitly set budgets for part or all of their health care systems.

17. The adjustments to fees are primarily political and reflect budgetary considerations, not scientific ones. Changes are not based on cost–benefit analysis or new scientific information regarding efficacy or side-effects, as might be the case with pharmaceutical prices. See the comments by Ikegami, and William E. Steslicke, *Doctors in Politics: The Political Life of the Japan Medical Association*, New York: Praeger, 1973.

18. Can you imagine a group of U.S. executives or lawyers suspecting heart failure being willing to wait patiently for hours in a public clinic to be served alongside the unemployed, or accepting a situation in which two out of three who currently would be receiving a bypass graft or new pacemaker are sent home with pills instead? Then, when adversity strikes, can you further imagine that they would not sue? The sources of such a disparity go beyond language, currency, and government. Although cultural studies lie a bit beyond the scope of this book, it is clear that culture profoundly affects the health systems of the two countries just by looking at the differences in physician salaries, relative differences in the uses of drugs vs. invasive therapy, and ownership of facilities and equipment.

19. The World Bank, *World Development Report 1993: Investing in Health*, New York: Oxford University Press for the World Bank, 1993, p.145.

CHAPTER 20

Value for Money in the Future of Medical Care

QUESTIONS

1. *What, how, and for whom is medical care produced?*
2. *Is Medicare likely to go broke, or continue to grow?*
3. *Will investors put more money into biotechnology or nursing homes?*
4. *How will economists affect the allocation of health care? Of health care incomes?*
5. *Are people willing to spend more and get less health?*
6. *Why is it so hard to reach a consensus if everyone knows what the problem is?*

20.1 FORCING THE QUESTION: WHO GETS HEALTHY AND WHO GETS PAID?_____

The most important contribution economists can make to the operation of the health care system is to be relentless in pointing out that every choice involves a trade-off; that certain difficult questions regarding who gets what, and who must give up what, are inevitable, and must be faced even when politicians, the public, and patients would rather avoid them. In the words of Paul Samuelson, "every economy must answer a triad of questions: *what, how* and *for whom*".[1] With regard to cancer for example, one could ask what symptoms or diagnoses are to be treated, whether inpatient or outpatient by generalists or specialists, and who is to receive first priority for treatment (those who are most ill, most likely to recover, best insured, or those who plan ahead and show up first). Although these questions can be stated independently, the answer to any one influences all of the others:"for whom" affects "what" and "how," and vice versa. Any answer also determines who pays, who gets paid, and how much; that is, it determines the distribution of income as well as the distribution of health care.

It is the job of economists to give advice, not patient care. They estimate, evaluate, and elucidate the decisions to be made; they do not make the decisions or carry them out. The analysis of decision making can be divided into three levels:

WHAT ARE THE QUESTIONS?

WHO IS GOING TO DECIDE?

WHAT ARE THE ANSWERS?

For most economists it is necessary to work backward, starting with the data collection required to make comparisons among different treatments (i.e., cost–benefit analysis); then considering how different systems for making medical care decisions can affect efficiency (e.g., indemnity insurance v. managed care, networks v. solo providers), and only then approaching the top level—framing the questions. Tracing the flow of money over the last nineteen chapters reveals that while data can be used for clarification, the questions are fundamentally *economic*: about values rather than numbers. Are some lives worth more than others? What does it mean to be human? How much should a surgeon be paid for a one-hour operation if it saves a life? Which product of the health care system is more important, social justice or cancer mortality?

The pragmatic and detailed collection of data in order to compare the costs and outcomes of different drugs, different surgical procedures, and different treatment settings has grown rapidly over the last decade. Doing such work requires a tremendous amount of clinical knowledge, and an understanding of basic economic principles: equilibrium at the margin, production functions, comparative advantage, opportunity cost, and so on. Increasingly, such work is being carried out by clinicians who have been trained so that they are literate in economic concepts, while economists concentrate on developing theory and new measurement techniques.

Upon this mass of detailed data collection and analysis rests the second layer of issues regrading how to design a better health care system. At this level, the question is not whether radiation is better than chemotherapy, but whether capitation or fee-for-service leads to better decisions, or whether group practice is more efficient than solo practice. The focus shifts from the particular decision being made to the issue of who is making the decision—physicians, patients or payers?

As economists trace how the flow of money follows the path of decision making, the assumptions embedded in the current medical care system become more evident. Analysis at the third level becomes reflective. What does "better" mean? According to what value system? Better for whom? Analysis transcends the current system as it is by asking, "What are the questions?" Reaching beyond the veil of money and grasping that every dollar spent on health care is a dollar earned by a health care provider starts to make plain how the distribution of income and health are connected, and suggests some fruitful directions for assessing the health implications of changes in economic organization.

20.2 SPENDING MONEY OR PRODUCING HEALTH? _____

The distribution of health is very unequal, and has a profound impact on economic well-being. Some people work productively for years, and contentedly die with wealth and happiness in old age, while others struggle for a few months or decades in agony as they are drawn remorselessly down into premature mortality. The question is not whether the distribution of health is fair, or whether it determines or is determined by income, but whether it is amenable to change. More precisely, the questions are: How, and how much, change can be brought about by spending more on medical care? What is that change worth? The marginal productivity of medical care spending declines as more is spent. Increasing spending from $4,000 to $5,000 per person increases average life expectancy, but not by as much as increasing spending from $2,000 to $3,000, which, in turn, would not have as large an effect as going from $0 to $1,000. As more and more is spent, fewer and fewer gains are achieved in life expectancy as one reaches the "flat of the curve" where marginal productivity, although still positive, is barely above zero.

Reaching a consensus about how much to spend becomes more complicated when there are two (or more) types of people who are to receive care. Suppose one group is relatively healthy, and would have a high level of health even if no money were spent on them, while another group begins at a disadvantage, and even with maximal effort would still remain less healthy. If the same amount is spent per person on each group, then the total and marginal impact of medical care will be very low in the healthy group, which seems wasteful, while the sicker group would still be forced to do without a lot of potentially beneficial care. In order to jointly maximize the average healthiness of all the groups for a given health care budget, it would be necessary to equalize the marginal productivity of medical care (increase in health per additional dollar spent) across both groups, spending much more per person on the sicker people. Such an allocation of medical care resources might seem both fair and efficient, but it also might not. Suppose the healthy group were all of the working people who paid insurance premiums while the sicker group were intravenous drug users. Most voters would not be willing to cut funding for those who take care of themselves and go to work every day in order to provide more to those who live on the streets and stick needles in their arms. Further complications are posed by groups like infants born with genetic defects who are likely to die young even with the best of medical care. Should they be denied any treatment on the grounds that it would not do them much good anyway?

Although describing the goal of medical care as "maximizing health" seems superficially accurate and appropriate, a little reflection (or reading the last nineteen chapters) shows how inaccurate and irrelevant such a measure often is. If taken literally, maximizing health would mean that most of the hospitals in the United States would close so that more food, clothes, books, and medicine could be consumed in China, India, Mozambique, and other undeveloped countries. It would also force most surgeons to give up their operating rooms in favor of sewage treatment, and force psychiatrists to give up therapy and the prescription of psychoactive drugs in favor of immunization campaigns and early childhood education. Stating that the goal of medical care is "maximizing health for all" is not only inaccurate, but profoundly misleading. It confuses a measure of social welfare with the incentives of the groups that make up society to maximize their own welfare. Doctors, nurses, hospital supply company executives, NBA basketball players, healthy industrial workers, college students, and other definable groups have multiple objectives, including the health of their families and their own incomes, many of which are more important to them that the advancement of global health averages.

It is relatively easy to understand why most Americans do not want all of their hospitals to close, and why most of the doctors who work in them are not anxious to practice in Mozambique, even if they are quite certain that the number of additional life-years produced would be higher. It is less obvious why Americans keep spending more and more on medical care if technological advances are making medicine more productive and efficient. Given that the baseline life expectancy at birth, even in the absence of medical care, is now much higher than it was a century ago, each year of life expectancy added becomes more difficult and more expensive to obtain. It is almost certain that if the nation was to spend the same amount per person on medical care in 1999 as it did in 1959, then the marginal productivity (gain in life expectancy per additional dollar spent) would be lower. If society was optimizing by choosing the point at which the value of health matched the price of health, and the value of health were the same, then less money would be spent as technology improved.[2] In fact, we now spend more per person implying that the incremental increase in health per additional dollar is even smaller. Extrapolating from the comparisons with Japan, Germany, and England in chapter 19, it appears that it would be possible to cut spending by a third or more, with only a minor decrease in health, leaving average life expectancy in the United States almost unchanged at 78 years.

The declining marginal productivity of health care is offset, to some extent, by the increasing aggregate wealth of society, which raises the dollar value of each additional year of health gained. The increased medical buying power of specific groups of persons who are likely to be high utilizers of care (the elderly, the disabled) is perhaps more important as a factor in augmenting demand. Yet even so, the vastness of the increase in medical spending cannot be explained purely in terms of productivity and relative prices. It must be recognized that medical care has become largely a consumption good. Economists do not seek to explain increased spending on clothes in terms of warmth or durability, nor should they try to explain all of the increase in medical expenditures in terms of analogous quality dimensions. Although it may seem inappropriate to compare arthroscopic surgery to the cut of a jacket, or the organ transplant to the installation of a quadraphonic stereo system in a car, it is impossible to avoid the conclusion that medical care has a significant consumption component that is not well explained by production theory. Medicine is coming more and more to resemble the service industries studied by marketing researchers.

If surgery is being sold like automobiles, and mental health like entertainment,[3] what role is there for the dismal science of economics with its insistent "on the other hand . . . ?" Perhaps economists relate to the public and politicians a bit like the way personal athletic trainers relate to their affluent and often overweight clients: someone whose expertise is required in order to establish authority and make compliance with an unpleasant regime easier even though all of the exercises and advice are pretty simple and mostly well known in advance. It may be that economists, like politicians, are being paid to talk about the old-fashioned values of thrift and efficiency that everyone is anxious to hear about, if not always to follow.

20.3 ALLOCATION, ALLOCATION, ALLOCATION _____

When asked what three factors are most important in determining value, real estate appraisers reply, "location, location, and location." In a similar vein, health economists asked to determine the value of the money spent on health care must focus primarily on allocation: the distribution of resources, the distribution of health, the distribution of medical care, and the distribution of provider incomes. Although a high value is often placed on the quality of nursing care, the skill of the physician, or the use of new medical technology, none of these matters much if the care is provided to the wrong person, or at the wrong time. The health economist is asked to assess economic efficiency, how well the health care system has used the resources available to achieve its stated (and unstated) goals. The following short list contains a few of the questions that must be answered in this regard:

- Which diseases are to be treated?
- Which people are to be treated?
- How much care should be given?
- Who is to pay?
- If the money is to come from taxes, who should be taxed most—those who benefit most, or those who can afford to pay the most?
- Should more money be spent on prevention or cure?
- How much are the healers to be paid?
- Is treatment to be carried out by specialists or primary care providers?
- How is the power to make decisions to be allocated?

Allocation is the subject of economics. Why, then, haven't economists been more successful in reforming health care? First of all, it must be recognized that the study of health economics has indeed improved efficiency to some degree. It has made the system better, although it is still far from perfect. Cost–benefit analysis has lead to a reduction in the over-investment in hospitals, to the support and improvement of immunization programs, and to the more rapid and objective evaluation of new drugs. Assessment of incentives and risk-bearing has led to the creation of new forms of insurance, and to the refinement of managed care contracting. The application of microeconomics to decisions regarding individual allocation has only limited potential, however, because the most crucial issues in health are likely to involve public goods, macro allocation, and the contentious questions of how the costs and benefits are to be distributed between different groups of producers and consumers.

It is quite possible to spend less on health care and simultaneously improve the average level of health by changing the allocation of resources. Yet just as U.S. citizens are unlikely to vote for a program that cuts Medicare in half and sends 75 percent of the remaining funds overseas for clinics in poor countries so that the overall global average level of health can be raised to offset the declines in the United States, almost any reallocation that improves efficiency makes some concerned group with decision-making power worse off, and is therefore likely to be opposed even if overall efficiency is clearly improved. The difficulty for health economists is that the question of "how to improve efficiency" is far less relevant to the reform of health care systems than the question of "how to make a deal" so that the various interests can agree to make a change that, at the cost of harming some identifiable groups, yields an increase in average benefits.

20.4 DYNAMIC EFFICIENCY _____

Deals are hard to make, even when clearly beneficial overall, because the groups that are to be harmed find it difficult to be sure that their concerns are adequately weighed, and that the harm done them is somehow offset by benefits gained from other programs and policies. Assurances of fair treatment are harder to believe the more distant in time and uncertain the compensating benefits are. Thus, while a group of elderly persons might be willing to accept less technologically advanced treatment for a reduction in their premiums and out-of-pocket costs, they might not be willing to make such a sacrifice in order to fund research that might bring results in the future. Although this reluctance may be short-sighted, it is perfectly reasonable.

The problems of allocation are often formalized by economists in terms of technical productivity (maximizing the output from any given set of resource inputs), cost minimization (choosing the least expensive set of inputs), and current economic efficiency (balancing marginal costs and marginal benefits). More sophisticated analyses may also consider how systems are structured to deal with transactions costs and public goods. In medicine, the most important allocation may be that between current consumption and future productivity. The difference between adequate and outstanding current practice is far smaller than the gap between what was possible twenty years ago and what is expected within the next decade (gene therapy, real-time imaging, robotic laser surgery, in-vitro diagnoses). The challenge is to structure a health care system for *dynamic efficiency,* creating technological and organizational change to improve health and productivity. Some current allocative efficiency must be sacrificed for scientists to spend time tinkering to make new discoveries, and to give managers the slack to come up with ideas for new products and service delivery systems. A purely cost-minimizing organization is not creative enough to be economically efficient in the long run.

20.5 THE FUTURE

What can be said with some confidence about the future of health and medical care over the next fifty years? Table 20.1 lists expected trends. It is relatively certain that there will be continued increases in longevity, greater technological capability to treat disease, and continuous increases in expenditure. There will be more spending overall, and the sources and uses of funding will change rather markedly. An older and healthier population implies more long-term care, with greater emphasis on caring and rehabilitation. Thus, the fraction of medical spending accounted for by acute illnesses of the tax-paying population will fall. The tension between public and private financing is likely to remain unresolved, with managed care organizations operating under a mixture of market incentives and regulatory structures to provide a kind of middle ground. Treatment and production will become less and less important relative to the provision of caring and information. The best prototypes for studying health economics in the next century are probably biotechnology and hospice. Physicians will become technical team leaders operating within a corporate organization, rather than independent medical practitioners. Cost-shifting in the form of marked-up prices and open-ended reimbursement will continue to wither away, and be replaced by new forms, such as mandated benefits pools. The use of economic information and cost accounting for comparative decision making will continue to increase. Greater

TABLE 20.1 Future Trends

- Greater longevity, better health
- More long-term and chronic care, less acute illness
- More spending overall, but a smaller fraction spent on the working population
- Less ability to shift costs by overcharging for treatment
- Managed care as a middle ground, mixing public and private
- Less dependence on trust and tradition, more assessment of costs and outcomes
- Physicians lead technical teams within corporate organizations, not independent solo medical practices
- Successful organizations based on information (e.g., biotechnology) and caring (e.g., hospice)
- Special characteristics previously found primarily in medical care become typical of many service organizations in a post-industrial service economy

knowledge about actual costs and the actual effectiveness of clinical practice will force greater clarity in the questions raised about the trade-off between dollars and health. Some fields (mental health and substance abuse, rearing disabled children, dietary modification) are increasingly being spun off, and are less likely to be counted as an integral part of medicine. Others, such as information systems and genetic engineering, are becoming more integrated, and will tend to blur the traditional boundaries between what is medicine and what is information or environmental modification.

The special institutional features that set medicine and health apart from the rest of the economy will become less and less distinctively special over the coming years. In part, this is because medicine is becoming more organized and more corporate, more subject to a bottom-line assessment of cost and benefits. Yet the extent to which medicine is becoming like the rest of the economy is probably of far less importance that the extent to which the rest of the economy is becoming like medicine: where information, service, and public goods matter more than commodities. Previously, health economists have taken models from the study of industrial production and applied them to health and medical care. Ideas may increasingly flow in the other direction as the issues of special interest to health economists—uncertainty, agency, trust, service delivery and quality—become central to the economy as a whole in a post-industrial era. Models developed for the study of medical care may in the future be applied to banking, entertainment, automation, fashion, and other industries.

SUGGESTIONS FOR FURTHER READING _____

Victor Fuchs, "Economics, Values and Health Care Reform," *American Economic Review,* 86(1):1-24, 1996.
William Kissick, *Medicine's Dilemmas,* New Haven, Conn: Yale University Press, 1994.

SUMMARY _____

1. A primary role of health economists is to **force consideration of the trade-offs** implicit in every choice made regarding health and medical care. They should help the public and politicians to ask: who gets helped, who gets hurt, and who makes money?

2. Health economics can be viewed as dealing with questions in levels of ascending generality. At the base, **which treatments are better,** and **how much do they cost?** At an intermediate level, **who is going to have the power to make decisions?** And finally, **what are the questions to be asked** in order to shape and judge the health care system?

3. The purpose of the health care system is to **satisfy the interests of the groups that participate** in it. Maximizing health is but one of many objectives. The average health of the population may often matter much less than *who* in particular gets healthy.

4. The increase in health and life expectancy that can be obtained from any given set of medical resources depends largely upon the **allocation** of treatment to those most likely to benefit. Often, this is not the group that is most able or willing to pay.

5. Major **difficulties in economic appraisal** of health care policies arise because the most important issues frequently involve **public goods** and the **distribution of benefits and incomes** to different groups, as well as technical questions regarding productive efficiency.

6. Differences in the quality of care at any point in time are usually dwarfed by changes in the effectiveness of care over time. Hence, a health care system must provide resources and slack to achieve **dynamic efficiency**, fostering technological and organizational change.

7. **Values** ultimately mean more in health economics than the efficacy of medical technology or the estimation of costs. Analysis will increasingly be focused on **the economics of caring and information**, not production.

PROBLEMS _____

1. {*allocation*} Will health care be more or less efficient in 2020? Will people spend more or less money on health care?

2. {*budget*} Will Medicare go broke by 2007, as some analysts predict? Why or why not? What historical evidence could you give to support your answer?

3. {*distribution*} Which matters more, how healthy we are on average or *who* gets healthy?

4. {*values*} Economists debate the future of Medicare by arguing about which set of numbers best represents reality. Do these numbers represent objective or subjective values?

5. {*economic organization, distribution*} Who will make the decisions regarding medical care in the year 2010? Which of these groups will have more or less power in 2010?
   physicians
   nurses
   biotechnology investors
   U.S. Senators
   AARP (American Association of Retired Persons)
   disability advocates
   children
   economists

6. {*productivity*} As medical technology continues to develop, will the marginal productivity per dollar spent increase or decrease?

7. {*economic organization, distribution*} Are health care funds spent to maximize health or to maximize the welfare of those who get to make the decisions?

ENDNOTES ————————————————————————————

1. Paul Samuelson and William Nordhaus, *Economics*, 14th ed., New York: McGraw-Hill, 1992 p.19.
2. It is possible to construct a production function that moves up and yet is steeper, with greater average productivity and yet lower marginal productivity for a given set of inputs, but it requires some contortion to do so, and such quirks are unlikely to explain the large and persistent rise in health care spending that has accompanied the twentieth-century advance of health care technology. Some other explanation must be found if the attempt is to remain plausible.
3. In the words of Dr. John R. Ball, president of the nation's oldest hospital, "Health care used to be something perceived as mystical. Now it's something closer to marketing a product or a service," as quoted in Eric Hollreiser, "Nation's Oldest Hospital Coping With New Age," *Philadelphia Business Journal,* March 22, 1996, p.25.

Glossary

Activities of Daily Living (ADLs) A checklist measure of the extent of disability and functional status.

Actuarially Fair Premium A premium equal to the expected value of the loss, although in practice all premiums must be set higher in order to cover overhead costs.

Actuary Accredited insurance mathematician who calculates premium rates and company reserve requirements using statistical studies.

Administered Prices Prices which are specified by an administrative agency, rather than being set in the market.

Administered Service Only (ASO) A self-insured health plan in which the employer bears all the risk of losses, but hires an administrator to process claims.

Administratively Necessary Days (ANDs) Payment for days when a patient's medical status is such that they should have been discharged from the hospital but were not because no nursing home beds were available.

Adverse Selection A disproportionate share of bad risks. When given a choice, the people who choose to purchase insurance are likely to be a group with higher than average losses.

Agency The process of having one party (the agent) make decisions on behalf of another (the principal).

Aggregation The process of clumping together; the creation of summary measures for a population as a whole; study at the system or group level.

Allocative Efficiency Allowing those who value a good more to consume more. Total consumption value is maximized by allowing the process to continue toward an equilibrium where for each individual, marginal benefit = marginal cost. Also, targeting medical care to those most in need so as to maximize average life expectancy.

American Medical Association (AMA) The professional organization which represents the interest of MD physicians in the United States and lobbies government agencies on their behalf.

Anti-trust Legal restrictions relating to collusion between firms and market domination.

Assignment An agreement by a physician to take payment directly from Medicare, and to accept the amount as payment in full (i.e., with no balance billing).

Average Cost The total cost divided by the number of units.

Balance Billing Making the patient pay for the balance of any charges in excess of the amount allowed by the insurance company.

Branded Drugs Drugs whose production and sale are protected by a patent. Also, the brand-name drug produced by the initial firm even after its patent expires and other firms begin to sell competing generic versions.

Cap A limit on the amount that an insurance company will pay. The cap may be an overall maximum, such as a lifetime maximum of $250,000, or may apply to specific services, such as a $500 per year cap on outpatient mental health counselling.

Capitation Paying a fixed amount per enrolled person per month for a defined set of services which does not vary with **utilization**.

Case-Mix Reimbursement Adjustment of reimbursement to account for differences in patient diagnoses, and sometimes for the severity of illness as well.

Certificate of Need (CON) A legal requirement that approval from a state agency to certify need (CON) must be obtained before a health care facility is built or remodeled.

Ceteris Paribus All other factors being held constant.

Charges The amount appearing on the patient's bill.

Chiropractic An alternative form of medical practice which emphasizes spinal manipulation in the treatment of disease, often to the exclusion of drugs and surgery. Although chiropractors are found in most communities, they are often not accepted by the organized medical profession.

Circular Flow of Funds The circulation of money facilitates exchange; it is not used up or consumed. Each dollar spent by a consumer goes to a producer, who in turn gives it to an owner, worker or supplier, who as consumers send those dollars on to another producer, and so on in an unending circular flow.

Clinical Pathways A protocol, or defined standard set of tests and procedures to be used in diagnosing or treating a particular symptom or disease.

Clinical Trials Testing of new drugs or medical technology on humans.

Coase Theorem The assertion that the type of economic organization (profit or non-profit, one firm or many, capitalist or socialist) and which party holds ownership rights (e.g., chemical firms or fishermen, homeowners or airport operators) would not matter if there were no transaction costs.

Coinsurance The amount of the bill not paid by insurance, but by the patient. A plan with 15% coinsurance means that the insurance company pays 85% and the person pays 15%.

Community Rating Setting the same premium rate for every person in the community regardless of age, sex or previous illness.

Comparative Statics The study of a system by comparing how the state of equilibrium differs when some set of parameters (incomes, prices, fertility) differs; in contrast to **dynamics** in which the process of change is the focus of study.

Compounding Adding to; the accumulation of growth over time; how a small percentage increase eventually leads, with interest on the interest, to doubling, quadrupling and manyfold increasing.

Concurrent Review Daily checks by an HMO on the status of a patient to monitor, and if necessary, modify or terminate, the provision of services.

Consumption Function The relationship between consumption and income as income changes; the fraction of total income saved as the level or composition of aggregate income changes.

Continuing Care Retirement Communities (CCRCs) Living quarters for elderly persons with provisions for meals, transportation, therapy and other assistance, usually constructed with an adjacent nursing home. Financial risks to the individual are often reduced through prepayment. Also known as lifecare communities.

Copayment A copayment is a specified amount that the patient must pay with each service received, such as the $2 for each prescription that many drug plans make the pharmacist collect, $10 for each day in the hospital under Medicare, $5 for each visit to the doctor under some HMO plans, etc. One of the purposes of copayments is to discourage overutilization. Thus while deductibles and coinsurance may sometimes be covered under a spouse's plan or other insurance, the insured must usually pay the copayment out of pocket.

Cost Reimbursement Retrospective payment for services based upon audited cost reports, often including complex limits and rules for allocation.

Cost Shifting The process of using excess revenues from one set of services or patients to subsidize other services or patient groups.

Cost-Benefit Analysis (CBA) A set of techniques for assisting in the making of decisions, which translates all relevant concerns into market (dollar) terms.

Cost-Effectiveness Analysis (CEA) Comparison of the costs of different ways of achieving an objective (cases prevented, years of life saved). Similar to CBA, except that CEA does not require benefits to be expressed in dollar terms.

Cream Skimming Choosing to provide only the most profitable services, or to insure only the healthiest patients, so as to avoid subsidizing public goods (education, research, indigent care) and thus obtaining extra profits.

Cross-Sectional Analysis Statistics constructed using observations across different individuals or groups at one point in time, as opposed to **longitudinal** or **time-series** analysis.

Deductible An amount that must be paid by the individual before the insurance company begins to pay. For example, many policies have a $100 per year deductible. This means that if total insured medical bills were $730, the insurance would apply only after the person had paid the first $100, that is, to $630.

Demand A schedule of the amount that will be consumed in the market at varying prices.

Demographic Transition The period of rapidly increasing population which usually occurs during economic development as a poor society with high mortality and high birth rates transitions to a wealthy society with low mortality and low birth rates.

Demographics Age, sex, and other characteristics of populations.

Derived Demand The demand for an input due to the demand for output; demand for a good due to its use, rather than in itself (e.g., the demand for x-ray film is derived from the demand for medical diagnoses, which in turn are derived from a consumer's demand for health).

Detailing Marketing of pharmaceuticals to physicians by drug company representatives (detailers); offers of free samples and advice in order to increase the number of times a drug is prescribed.

Diagnostically Related Grouping (DRG) A system of reimbursement which compensates by the case (rather than per day or per charged item) based on the diagnosis of the patient.

Discounted FFS Contracts with providers to pay a specified percentage of usual charges.

Discounting Adjustment of valuation for the passage of time, reflecting the fact that the present value of a future good is smaller. Also, adjustments to reflect risk, reductions in the quality of life, and other factors.

Diseconomies of Scale The average cost per unit rises as the quantity produced increases.

Dynamic Efficiency Use of inputs so as to maximize long-run value over time, taking account of the need for tinkering to bring about technological and organizational advances.

Dynamic Shortage A temporary deficit in supply caused by a sudden increase in demand, or sudden drop in supply.

Dynamics The process of change; the study of how change occurs over time, including the order, timing and strength of interacting forces.

Economies of Scale The average cost per unit decreases as output increases.

Efficacy The ability to actually cure a disease; how well a treatment works in practice.

Elasticity The percentage change in one variable when another variable changes by one percent.

Enrollee A person covered by a health benefits plan.

Entitlements Social insurance payments to which beneficiaries are entitled by law with little regard to actual contributions or premiums, or income qualifications (e.g., Medicare, Social Security).

Entrepreneur The person who undertakes the effort to create an organization and the network of contracts necessary for its success.

ERISA The "Employee Retirement And Income Security Act of 1974" and subsequent amendments which govern most health insurance contracts, and in particular, exempt self-insured plans from most state regulation.

Expected Value The value of an outcome multiplied by its probability of occurring. Also, the probability-weighted average of all possible outcomes.

Experience Rating Setting a group premium based on the actual losses experienced by that group during the prior year or years.

Externalities The effects of a transaction between parties on outsiders; the uncompensated effects of an action (e.g., pollution); side-effects.

Fallacy of Composition The logical error of assuming that what holds true for the individuals within a group must also hold true for the group collectively, or vice-versa.

Fee Schedule A list of approved fees for each service promulgated by an insurance company, government agency, or professional society.

Fee-For-Service (FFS) Payment for health care based on the charges for each service or item used.

Flexible Budget A budget that is adjusted for changes in the volume of service.

Flexner Report The critique written in 1910 which led to the reform of medical education and established the MD degree as a qualification for licensure.

Flow The amount over a period of time (i.e., income, annual mortality rate).

Food and Drug Administration (FDA) The federal agency with jurisdiction over labelling, manufacture, and sale of food and drugs for human consumption.

Formulary A list of approved drugs for reimbursement with all non-approved drugs paid at a lesser rate or not at all.

Free Rider A person who allows others to produce a public good, and then uses it without paying. For example, most poor country prevention programs are free-riders, dependent upon the research of rich countries to do the research and produce the vaccines needed to control infectious diseases.

Full Time Equivalents (FTE) A measure of the quantity of labor used.

Fundamental Theorem of Exchange Any voluntary exchange between persons must make both of them better off since they willingly agreed to trade.

Gatekeeper A primary physician who manages and approves all services for the patient who enrolls in his practice.

Generic Drugs Drugs which are identical in chemical composition to a brand name pharmaceutical preparation, but produced by competitors after the firm's patent expires.

Global Budget A fixed total budget for all health services.

Grandfathering Approving those who are already in practice to continue even if they do not meet the new standards.

Gross Domestic Product (GDP) The total market value of all production in a nation.

Group Insurance Contract for insurance made with an employer or other entity, called the policyholder, that covers a group of persons as a single unit.

Health Maintenance Organization (HMO) An organization that contracts to provide comprehensive medical services (not reimbursement) for a specified fee each month. The term health maintenance organization arose because doctors under this arrangement have a financial incentive to keep their patients healthy, since they are not paid more for providing more services.

Health Care Financing Administration (HCFA) The federal agency responsible for administering Medicare and Medicaid.

Homeopathy An alternative form of health practice emphasizing natural remedies used in extremely dilute solutions.

Hospital Privileges The rights of those doctors who have been voted acceptance on the hospital's medical staff to admit patients and perform surgery.

Human Capital Analysis of investments of time, effort, and money in education or health that improve productivity as analogous to investments of financial capital.

Income Distribution The fraction of all income earned by the top 10 percent of the population, the second 10 percent, and so on; the degree of disparity in incomes between the rich and the poor.

Income Elasticity The percentage change in expenditures due to a one percent change in income. Income elasticities below 1.0 mean that although spending on a good rises with income, it rises less than proportionately so that the fraction of total income spent on that good is reduced. With income elasticities greater than 1.0 (luxury goods), spending rises more than proportionately so that the share of total income spent on the good increases as income increases.

Indemnity Benefit A specified dollar amount reimbursed for a particular injury or type of care, such as $15 for each x-ray or $475 for gall bladder removal, is an indemnity benefit. Life insurance, which provides a specified dollar amount in case of death, has an indemnity benefit.

Independent Practice Association (IPA-HMO) An HMO formed by non-exclusive contracts with many providers who operate independently, as opposed to closed group staff HMO where physicians work exclusively for the HMO and are often on salary.

Inflation A measure of the reduction in the real purchasing power of currency over time.

Information Asymmetry The disparity in information between a buyer and a seller in a transaction.

Inpatient Services or goods provided within a hospital or nursing home.

Intensity (of services) The amount of inputs used to provide each unit of service. For example, an urban university hospital will typically provide complex services of high intensity, while a primary care doctor on an emergency call in an isolated rural area will use far fewer resources to treat the same injury.

Investigational New Drug (IND) A designation of FDA approval to begin the testing of a drug.

Kickbacks Surreptitious payments made in order to obtain business.

Licensure The establishment of legal restrictions specifying which individuals or firms have the rights to provide services or goods.

Life-cycle Hypothesis Assertion that individual spending at any point in time is based on their long-run expected income over the life-cycle rather than just current income at that point in time; a common form of the **permanent income** hypothesis.

Loading factor (or load) The percentage of total premiums used for administrative costs, profits, and all items other than medical benefits.

Long-Term Care (LTC) Nursing homes, visiting nurses, home I.V. and other services provided to chronically ill or disabled persons.

Longitudinal Analysis Study of a set of individuals or groups tracking how they change over time.

Major Medical In order to compete with the Blue Cross service benefits, commercial insurance companies came up with plans with deductibles and coinsurance that could be sold for much less. Often today, major medical is used as a supplement, while some basic services, such as hospital and doctor visits, are covered in full.

Malpractice The legal framework for failure to meet professional standards.

Malthusian Hypothesis The expectation that any increase in food supply would eventually lead to a matching increase in the number of people living at a subsistence level, so that on average, living conditions would be no better off than before.

Managed Behavioral Health Mental health and substance abuse services managed by an MCO.

Managed Care The use of a manager to control utilization of medical services and control costs. Often associated with HMOs, other forms of managed care include peer review panels, pre-approval procedures for surgery, case management for the chronically ill, formularies limiting pharmacy reimbursement to an approved list, and other contractual provisions.

Managed Care Organization (MCO) An HMO, PPO, or other organization that accepts financial risk and manages care.

Managed Competition A policy of increased reliance on competing HMO's and a fixed limit to tax subsidies so that employees would bear the full marginal cost of their health benefit plans.

Mandated Benefits Specific services (e.g., pregnancy, alcoholism detoxification) for which a state requires all health plans to provide coverage.

Marginal Propensity to Consume The fraction of an additional dollar that would be spent on consumption, and thus not invested as savings.

Marginal Productivity The incremental output obtained with one more unit of input.

Marginal Cost The increase in total costs caused by the production of one more unit of output.

Market Failure The inability of the market to arrive at a reasonably efficient equilibrium under certain conditions, notably the existence of public goods and externalities, lack of clear property rights, inability of some consumers to act in their own best interest, natural monopoly due to constantly declining average costs of production, and excessive transaction costs or information asymmetry.

Means Testing Setting a standard of low income in order to qualify for a government benefit, e.g., Medicaid.

Medicaid Combined state/federal program to insure people whose incomes are insufficient to pay for health care; primarily those on welfare or older people in nursing homes.

Medical Savings Account (MSA) A proposal to replace regular health insurance and HMOs by allowing people to place money in a tax-free savings account to be used for medical expenses, in conjunction with the purchase of a catastrophic stop-loss health insurance plan covering expenses in excess of $3,000.

Medicare A Federal government insurance program that provides hospital benefits (part A) and medical benefits (part B) to persons over age 65 and some qualified widows and disabled.

Medigap A policy designed to pay coinsurance, deductibles, drugs, and other expenses not fully covered by Medicare.

Monopoly Rents Profits in excess of competitive market returns due to a monopolist's ability to unilaterally increase prices.

Moral Hazard Any change in individual behavior due to insurance which increases expected losses, such as the higher utilization of covered services.

Morbidity Illness or disability, especially when expressed as a rate (e.g.; sick days per year per 1,000 employees).

Mortality Death, usually expressed as a rate per one hundred, thousand, or hundred-thousand.

Need A professional determination of the quantity that should be supplied (as distinct from market demand).

Normative Shortage When too little is supplied according to professional opinion, although not necessarily according to market behavior (e.g., there is a shortage of raw vegetables in the diet of teenagers).

Occupancy Rate The percentage of a hospital's beds filled at a specific time.

Opportunity Cost What must be given up in order to do or obtain something; the highest-valued alternative which must be foregone. For example, the opportunity cost of taking the final exam may be missing out on a trip to Bermuda.

Option Demand Willingness to pay for access to a good which may or may not be used, e.g., emergency services.

Osteopathy An alternative form of medical practice which emphasizes spinal adjustment as well as surgery and drugs in the treatment of disease. Originally quite distinct from mainstream allopathic medicine, osteopathy is now almost identical so that MDs and DOs usually practice together, although DOs are more likely to be generalists focusing on primary care.

Out-of-Pocket Payments made by individuals or their family, rather than an insurance company, HMO, government, or other third party, for medical care.

Outpatient Services provided in a physicians' office, clinic, or other ambulatory setting.

Patents A legal monopoly for a specified period of years given to a firm which makes a discovery.

Per Diem Per day payment for services.

Per Member Per Month (PMPM) The standard form of HMO payment, also known as **capitation.**

Permanent Income Expected long-run average income, as opposed to the transitory income which a person (or group) may have during the current month or year.

Pharmacoeconomics Cost-benefit analysis of drugs; assessment of the market for a drug.

Point of Service Plan (POS) An HMO which offers partial reimbursement for services which a patient chooses to obtain outside of the HMO network.

Population Medicine Analysis and assessment of health care on the basis of the community or group rather than the individual; design of a system with services targeted to those of greatest need; making trade-offs to optimize average health, rather than doing the best possible for one specific individual under treatment.

Practice Variation Differences in the number of medical services provided not explainable by any differences in the population served. Also known as small area variation.

Pre-authorization A requirement that the doctor or the patient obtain approval from the HMO before the service is provided.

Pre-existing Condition An insurance contract may specify that it will not pay for medical problems already diagnosed or under treatment before the policy is purchased, known as pre-existing conditions. A person with AIDS who bought a policy with such a clause would find that it paid for his broken leg, and maybe even to have his tooth drilled, but not for anything related to AIDS. Often the pre-existing condition exclusion will only apply to the first 6 months or year of coverage. This, and other exclusionary clauses, are a major way of reducing adverse selection when medical insurance is marketed to individuals.

Preferred Provider Organization (PPO) A health insurance plan which offers enrollees a discount for using hospitals and physicians within an approved network of contracted providers.

Premiums Payments made in advance to provide medical services or reimbursement in the future.

Price Discrimination Charging different people different prices for the same good.

Price Index A measure of the purchasing power of money, usually set arbitrarily equal to 100 at one specific point in time (or space). The average change in prices weighted by the expenditure on each item.

Primary Care The basic medical attention provided by a physician to a patient seeking care, as distinct from referral services obtained from specialists, or tertiary care provided in technologically sophisticated hospitals.

Property Rights The right to use, sell, or to derive income from a good.

Prospective Payment Payments set in advance, especially in contrast to retrospective **cost reimbursement**.

Provider Network The set of physicians, hospitals and others with which an MCO has signed a contract to provide care for enrollees.

Public Goods Goods that are consumed or financed collectively (e.g., clean air, national defense, discovery of penicillin) either because it is impossible to include/exclude any consumer who does not pay (see **free rider**), or because once produced, there is no additional cost for additional consumers.

QALYs (Quality Adjusted Life-Years) A way of measuring the value of a medical intervention by the increase in life expectancy, adjusted for difference in disability and timing.

RBRVS The "resource-based relative value system" developed for Medicare to reimburse ambulatory services based on the estimated time, effort, skill, equipment, and other resources needed to provide each service.

RCCAC The "ratio of costs-to-charges applied to charges" methodology used to apportion cost reimbursements.

Redistribution Policies that have the effect of changing the pattern of consumption by different income classes; allowing the poor to consume a larger share of GDP.

Regulatory Balloon The observation that any regulation pushing costs down on one side is apt to exert pressure pushing costs up in some other direction.

Regulatory Capture The subtle takeover of a regulatory agency by the industry it was meant to regulate, so that it tends to represent the interests of the industry, rather than the public.

Reimbursement The process of paying for the costs incurred, especially through a third party.

Reinsurance Acceptance by a second insurer (the reinsurer) of all or part of the risk undertaken by the first insurer; usually used to cover very large losses and protect against bankruptcy. For example, a reinsurer may agree that if total losses exceed the $5 million in expected claims by more than $1 million, they will, for a price, pick up 90% of the extra losses.

Relative Value Scales A list of point scores for each service to be used in setting reimbursement.

Rents Profits in excess of those necessary in order to call forth the requisite supply of inputs in the market. Compensation above competitive amounts obtained by professionals who are able to control supply.

Retention Ratio Agreement A contract specifying an allowed ratio of premiums to medical expenses with some fraction of any excess underwriting gains to be returned to the firm or used to reduce premiums in the following year.

Retrospective Review Monitoring records after discharge and disallowing (refusing to pay for) any services that do not meet specified standards of medical necessity and timeliness.

Revolving Door Term used to describe staff that leave a regulatory agency to work within the industry which is supposed to be regulated, and vice-versa. Such changes in employment may compromise the agency's objectivity.

Risk The chance or probability that an event will occur.

Risk Aversion The extent to which an individual is willing to pay to reduce variation in losses or income due to random events.

Risk Pooling Forming a group so that individual risks can be shared among many people.

Risk Selection Enrollment of healthier-than-average persons into an insured group.

Sanitary Revolution The 19th-century campaign to clean up the environment and change personal behavior to conform to Victorian notions: "cleanliness is next to godliness."

Selection Bias A disproportionate share of above- or below-average persons in the group.

Self-Insurance A health plan funded and controlled by the firm itself, so that no risk is transferred to an insurance company, although benefits may be administered by an outside party. Self-insurance often enables a firm to avoid regulations governing purchased health insurance.

Service Benefits If the insurance company contracts directly with the doctor or hospital to provide the service rather than setting up some form of financial reimbursement, this is a service benefit. Blue Cross provides service benefits through its contracts with hospitals. An advantage of a service benefit to the insurance company is that they usually get a discount off the price that the patient would have to pay directly for the services rendered.

Shared-Income Hypothesis Income becomes more and more important as a determinant of health-care spending as the unit of observation increases in size from the individual to the nation.

Social Insurance Pooling funded through taxes for protection against risks provided by the government for all (or almost all) of the citizens in a society. Social Security in the United States and the National Health Service in England are examples of social insurance plans.

Spend-down The process of spending or giving away assets by elderly persons so as to qualify for Medicaid reimbursement of long-term care expenses.

Stock The amount at a point in time (i.e., total assets, population).

Stop-Loss A limit on the maximum amount a person would ever have to pay is known as a stop-loss. If a family has a $1,000 stop-loss, then the insurance company will pay everything after the family's out-of-pocket expenses reach $1,000.

Sub-capitation Carving out a specialized service (physical therapy, mental health) and paying the specialized provider on a per-member per-month basis.

Subsistence Having barely enough food and other resources to sustain life.

Third-Party Administrator An organization that processes claims for a self-insured firm, but bears no financial risk for losses.

Third-Party Transaction An exchange which is indirect and often pools the funds of many individuals with money collected and disbursed by a third party such as an insurance company, voluntary non-profit organization, or government agency.

Time-Series Analysis Statistics using multiple observations of an individual or group over time; statistical analysis of the dynamics of change.

Transaction Costs All costs, monetary and non-monetary, whether counted or not, of carrying on trade.

Triple-Option A complete array of plans consisting of an HMO, a PPO, and an indemnity plan, offered by an insurer as a package. The package as a whole is experience rated, so that any one option may be significantly over- or under-priced to create cross-subsidies between plans.

Two-Party Transaction An exchange between a buyer and seller, usually trading money for goods or services.

Underwriting gains (losses) The amount by which premiums received exceed (fall short of) benefits paid out.

Universal Health Insurance A national plan providing health insurance or services to all citizens, or to all residents.

Usual, Customary, and Reasonable (UCR) A method for setting the maximum allowed fee for each service based on usual charges by other physicians in the area, the customary charge by this particular doctor over the preceding year, and "reasonable" adjustments for severity or special conditions.

Utilization The number of services used, often expressed per 1,000 persons per month or year.

Utilization Review (UR) Monitoring of medical records to determine if services are appropriate and should be paid for.

Variability The extent of random changes over time or between persons.

Voluntary Organization A nonprofit organization, such as a hospital or social service agency, governed by a board of concerned citizens rather than owners or elected officials.

Welfare Loss The decline in social welfare (total value of consumption/production) due to monopoly supply restrictions, price controls, rationing, taxes, or other interventions that cause misallocation of resources. Also known as deadweight losses.

Welfare Triangle The reduction in consumer's surplus caused by a reduction in quantity sold due to monopoly supply restrictions, price controls, or other distortion.

Willingness to pay (WTP) How much a person is willing to give up in order to obtain some specified improvement in quality of life.

Withhold A pool of money for providers which is held back and distributed by the HMO only if total expenses for the year end up being at or below acceptable levels.

Workers Compensation A mandatory insurance program covering the costs of medical treatment and disability due to work-related accidents and illness.

Wrap-Around An insurance policy designed to create a more comprehensive set of coverages sold with an underlying base policy.

Index

Page references followed by lowercase Roman f indicate illustrations, while page references followed by lowercase Roman t indicate material in tables. Page references followed by lowercase italic n indicate footnotes in the body of the text; if a number follows the italic n a back-of-chapter note is indicated.